Sectional Anatomy

for Imaging Professionals

Sectional Anatomy
for Imaging Professionals

Lorrie L. Kelley, MS, RT(R)(MR)(CT)
Associate Professor, CT/MRI Program Director,
Boise State University,
Boise, Idaho

Connie M. Petersen, MS, RT(R)(CT)
Instructor, Radiologic Sciences Program,
Boise State University,
Boise, Idaho

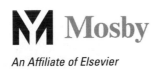 Mosby

An Affiliate of Elsevier

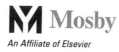

Copyright © 1997 by Mosby, Inc.

Printed in the United States of America

Mosby, Inc.
11830 Westline Industrial Drive
St. Louis, Missouri 63146

Library of Congress Cataloging-in-Publication Data
Kelley, Lorrie L.
    Sectional anatomy for imaging professionals/ Lorrie L. Kelley,
Connie M. Petersen.
        p.   cm.
    Includes index.
    ISBN 0-8151-8665-7 -- ISBN 0-8151-8665-7
    1. Human anatomy--Atlases.   2. Tomography--Atlases.   3. Magnetic
resonance   imaging--Atlases.   I. Petersen, Connie M.   II. Title.
    [DNLM: 1. Anatomy.   2. Diagnostic Imaging.   QS 4 K29s 1997]
QM25.K45   1997
611' .022'2--dc20
DNLM/DLC
                                                            96-41242

04 05 06 07 08 / 14 13 12 11 10

Reviewers

Steven J. Bollin, Sr., MPA, RT(R)
Special Procedures Technologist
Department of Radiation Oncology
Arthur G. James Cancer Hospital
Ohio State University Medical Center
Columbus, Ohio

Robert Entel, MD, MPH
Staff Radiologist
Department of Radiology
Mease Hospital

Clinical Assistant Professor of Radiology
University of South Florida College of Medicine
Safety Harbor, Florida

John Fries, MD
Clinical Professor of Radiology
School of Radiologic Technology
St. Louis University School of Medicine
St. Louis, Missouri

Ginger S. Griffin, RT(R)
Education Coordinator and Program Director
School of Radiologic Technology
Baptist Medical Center
Jacksonville, Florida

Kenneth K. Helfrick, BA, RT(R)
Program Director
School of Radiologic Technology
West Park Hospital
Cody, Wyoming

Kathleen O. Kienstra, BS, RT(T)
Program Director
School of Radiation Therapy Technology
Barnes-Jewish Hospital
St. Louis, Missouri

Michael Kleinhoffer, BS, RT(R)
Clinical Research Scientist
Highland, Illinois

Eric J. Lantz, MD
Medical Director and Staff Radiologist
Department of Radiologic Technology
School of Health Related Sciences
Mayo Foundation
Rochester, Minnesota

Sherry Ann Masotto, BS, RT(R)
Clinical Coordinator
School of Radiologic Technology
Gannon University
Erie, Pennsylvania

Tina Phillips, BS, RT(R)
Clinical Instructor
School of Radiologic Technology
Brandywine Hospital
Coatesville, Pennsylvania

Keith Steeves, RT(R)
Chief CT Technologist
CT Scan Department
William W. Backus Hospital
Norwich, Connecticut

To James,
min beste venn og evig ledsager,

and to Kristina, Jennifer, Michael, and Angela,
my greatest treasures,
for enriching my life with your gifts of laughter and love.

To my mother
Darhl Buchanan
for inspiring the best,
and my father
Keith Botkin,
for showing continuous support.

LLK

To my husband, Grant, and son, Brady,
for so generously giving me the gifts
of never-ending love, support, and adventure.

To my parents
Carl and Ellen Collins
for giving me a life filled
with endless encouragement and love.

CMP

Preface

This text was written to address the needs of today's practicing health professional. As technology in diagnostic imaging advances, so does the need to competently recognize and identify cross-sectional anatomy. Our goal was to create a clear, concise text that would demonstrate in an easy-to-use yet comprehensive format the anatomy the health professional is required to understand to optimize patient care. Included are over 600 high-quality MR and CT images for every feasible plane of anatomy most commonly imaged. The text was purposely designed to be used both as a clinical reference manual and as an instructional text, either in a formal classroom scene or as a self-instructional volume. When used as the latter, the text allows individuals the freedom to learn sectional anatomy in a variety of settings (at home, work, or school) and at their own pace.

CONTENT AND ORGANIZATION

The images include identification of vital anatomic structures to assist the health professional in locating and identifying the desired anatomy during actual clinical exams. The narrative accompanying these images clearly and concisely describes the location and function of the anatomy in a format easily understood by health professionals. The text is divided into nine chapters, each covering a separate portion of the anatomy.

Each chapter of the text contains an outline, which provides an overview of the chapter's contents; a CT or MR image in each chapter opener, which is intended to interest and quiz the reader on an element of the anatomy discussed within the chapter; text boxes throughout the chapter, which provide brief examples of pathology for the anatomy being discussed; tables designed to organize and summarize the anatomy contained in the chapter; and reference illustrations, which provide the reader with the correct orientation for scanning the anatomy of interest.

Several of the CT and MR images in the book also have a corresponding reference illustration in the chapter opener. The legends with these figures contain a number that is cross-referenced to a drawing at the beginning of the chapter. A reader can easily use that reference number to match the CT scan or MR image to its appropriate reference illustration. The angle and level at which the scan was taken can be visually confirmed, which should enable the health professional to duplicate each individual scan and to identify the anatomy in the images.

ANCILLARIES

A Study Guide, Pocket Guide, and an Instructor's Manual complement the text. When used together, these additional tools create a virtual learning system/reference resource.

Study Guide: The purpose of the Study Guide is to provide practice opportunities for the user to identify specific anatomy. The study guide includes learning objectives that focus on the key elements of each chapter, a variety of practice items to test the reader's knowledge of key concepts, labeling exercises to test the reader's knowledge of the anatomy, post test questions, and answers to practice items and post test questions.

Pocket Guide: The Pocket Guide is an easy-to-use, ready reference for the practicing health professional. It includes essential anatomic images from the text with accompanying descriptions and organizational tables and charts.

Instructor's Manual: The Instructor's Manual may be used in a formal academic setting as desired. The primary elements of the Instructor's Manual are Key Terms and Glossary, Lecture Outlines, Diagnostic Tests specific to chapter content, Supplemental Readings and Resources, and in-depth discussion of key concepts.

Lorrie Kelley
Connie Petersen

Acknowledgments

This project is the product of the efforts of numerous people. The authors would like to express their gratitude to the following individuals who have contributed immeasurably to the quality of this project.

- James M. Prochaska, MD, for not only encouraging this project but for also providing invaluable advice regarding the organization and scope of the neuroanatomy content.
- Paul D. Traughber, MD, Tim Hall, MD, and Ronald J. O'Reilly, MD, for graciously taking time out of their busy schedules to answer our last minute questions and ensure the accuracy of many of the images.
- Debbie Pope, Chris Hayden, Art Rinehart, Glen Lopez, Dennis Swaer, and Laura Smith for spending countless hours reviewing cases, generating images, and helping with the many network and archive disasters.
- Craig Schonhardt and Barbara Kirk for their wonderful illustrations produced in record time.
- Saint Alphonsus Regional Medical Center and employees of the CT department for providing the majority of the CT images.
- The MRI Center of Idaho and employees for providing the majority of the MR images.
- Our colleagues in the Radiologic Sciences Department at Boise State University for their patience and understanding.
- Turn-Key Medical Systems for providing the network setup to transfer the images digitally.
- Jeanne Rowland, Carole Glauser, and Jeanne Genz from Mosby for their encouragement of the project and for pulling it all together.
- The many reviewers who examined the text and images for accuracy and provided valuable advice and comments regarding the format of the text.

Contents

1 Cranium and Facial Bones, 1

Cranium, 3
Facial Bones, 12
Temporomandibular Joint, 18
Paranasal Sinuses, 22
Petrous Portion of the Temporal Bone, 27
Orbit, 30

2 Brain, 36

Meninges, 38
Ventricular System, 40
Cerebrum, 45
Brain Stem, 55
Cerebellum, 60
Cerebral Vascular System, 63
Cranial Nerves, 72

3 Spine, 82

Vertebral Column, 85
Ligaments of the Spine, 93
Muscles of the Spine, 97
Spinal Cord, 100
Plexuses, 105
Vasculature of the Spine, 107

4 Neck, 110

Organs, 112
Muscles, 123
Vascular Structures, 130

5 Thorax, 136

Bony Thorax, 138
Lungs, 140
Pleural Cavities, 143
Bronchi, 143
Mediastinum, 144
Azygos Venous System, 159
Muscles of the Thorax, 160
Breast, 163

6 Abdomen, 164

Abdominal Cavity, 166
Liver, 173
Gallbladder and Biliary System, 178
Pancreas, 178
Spleen, 181
Adrenal Glands, 182
Urinary System, 184
Stomach, 187
Intestines, 188
Abdominal Aorta and Branches, 190
Inferior Vena Cava and Tributaries, 196
Abdominal Muscles, 199

7 Pelvis, 202

Bony Pelvis, 204
Muscles of the Pelvic Region, 209
Pelvic Viscera, 217
Pelvic Vasculature, 231
Lymph Nodes, 234

8 Upper Extremity Joints, 236

Shoulder, 238
Elbow, 247
Wrist, 257

9 Lower Extremity Joints, 262

Hip, 265
Knee, 274
Ankle, 280

Appendix, 288

Chapter 1

Cranium and Facial Bones

Gentlemen, damn the sphenoid bone!

Oliver Wendell Holmes (1809-1894)
Opening of anatomy lectures at Harvard Medical School

In Figure 1.1, which facial bones have been fractured as a result of trauma? (Answer on p. 35)

If you can identify the fractured bones in Figure 1.1, you have a good understanding of facial bone anatomy. If you are unable to identify the abnormal facial bones, read this chapter, and then try to answer this question again.

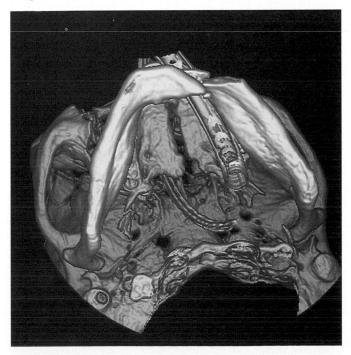

Figure 1.1 3D CT scan of traumatized face.

The complex anatomy of the cranium and facial bones can be intimidating. However, with three-dimensional (3D) and multiple imaging planes, the task of learning these structures can be simplified. It is important to understand normal sectional anatomy of the cranium and facial bones to identify pathologic disorders and injuries that may occur within this area. This chapter demonstrates the sectional anatomy of the following structures:

Cranium
occipital bone
temporal bone
sphenoid bone
ethmoid bone
frontal bone
parietal bone
sutures

Facial Bones
nasal bone
lacrimal bone
maxilla
palatine bone
zygoma
inferior nasal conchae
vomer
mandible

Temporomandibular Joint
bony anatomy
articular disk and ligaments
muscles

Paranasal Sinuses
ethmoid sinuses
maxillary sinuses
sphenoid sinuses
frontal sinuses
osteomeatal complex

Petrous Portion of the Temporal Bone

Orbit
bony orbit
eye

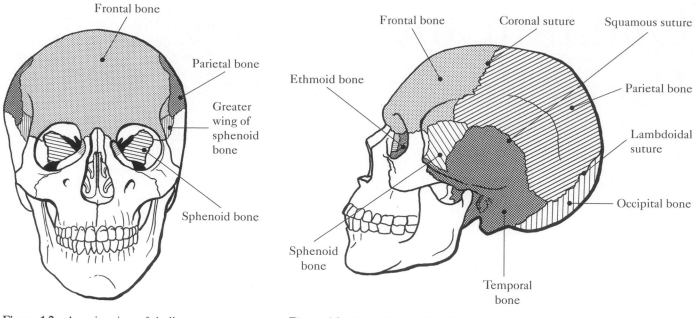

Figure 1.2   Anterior view of skull.

Figure 1.3   Lateral view of skull.

Key.   **E** ethmoid bone; **F** frontal bone; **O** occipital bone; **P** parietal bone; **T** temporal bone; **ve** vertex.

Figure 1.4   3D CT scan of anterior skull.

Figure 1.5   3D CT scan of lateral skull.

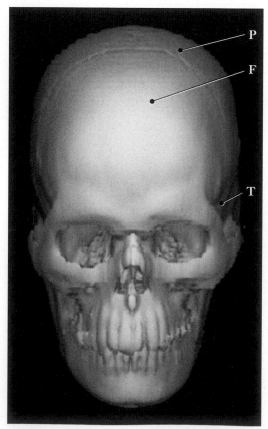

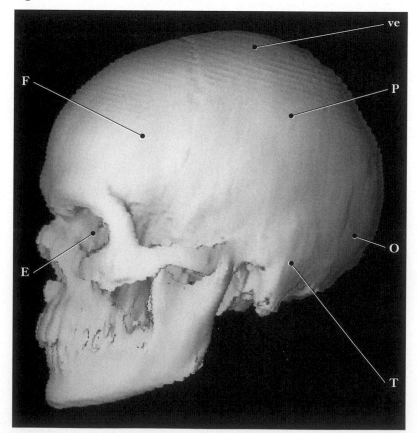

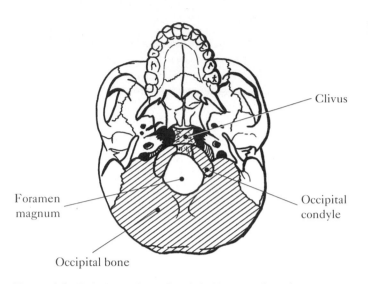

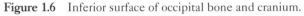

Figure 1.6   Inferior surface of occipital bone and cranium.

CRANIUM

The cranium is composed of eight bones that surround and protect the brain. These bones include the **occipital** (1), **temporal** (2), **sphenoid** (1), **ethmoid** (1), **parietal** (2), and **frontal** (1). Each bone is structurally unique, which can make identification of the physical components very challenging (Figures 1.2 through 1.5).

OCCIPITAL BONE

The occipital bone forms the inferoposterior portion of the cranium and the **posterior cranial fossa** (Figure 1.6). On the inferior portion of the occipital bone is a large oval aperture called the **foramen magnum**. This opening allows the brain stem to continue as the spinal cord. The occipital bone can be divided into four portions: lateral **condyles** (2), **basilar portion** (1), and **squamous portion** (1). The lateral condyles project inferiorly to articulate with the first cervical vertebra (atlas) at the atlanto-occipital joint (Figure 1.7). Located obliquely at the base of the condyles are the **hypoglossal canals** through which the hypoglossal nerve (CN XII) courses. The basilar portion forms the **clivus,** which curves anterosuperiorly to articulate with the sphenoid bone (Figures 1.8 and 1.9). Fat contained within the clivus causes it to appear bright on MR images (Figure 1.10). The squamous portion curves posterosuperiorly from the foramen magnum to articulate with the parietal and temporal bones.

Key.   FM foramen magnum; **Oco** occipital condyle.

Figure 1.7   Axial CT scan of occipital bone at level of foramen magnum and lateral condyles.

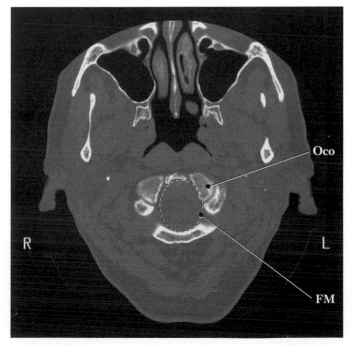

Key.   Cl clivus; **FM** foramen magnum; **HyC** hypoglossal canal.

Figure 1.8   Axial CT scan of occipital bone at level of clivus.

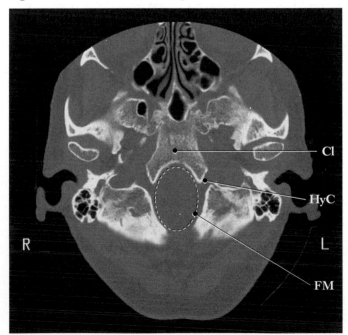

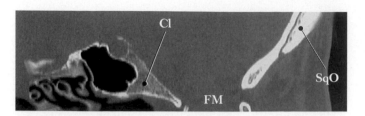

Figure 1.9   Sagittal CT reformat of occipital bone.

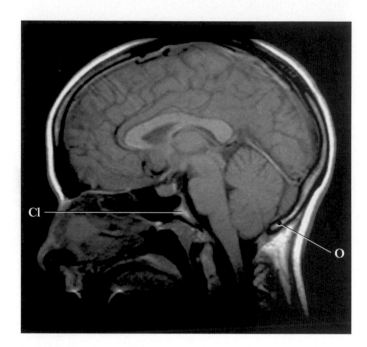

Figure 1.10   Sagittal MR scan of occipital bone.

Key. **Cl** clivus; **FM** foramen magnum; **O** occipital bone; **SqO** squamous portion of occipital bone.

Figure 1.11   Inferior surface of temporal bone and cranium.

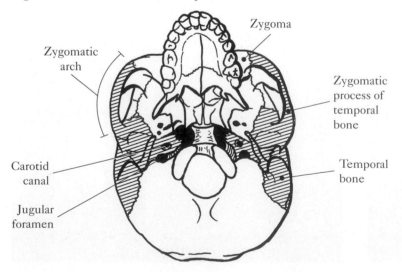

TEMPORAL BONE

The two temporal bones contain many complex and important structures. They form part of the sides and base of the cranium and, together with the sphenoid bone, create the **middle cranial fossa** (Figures 1.11 and 1.12). The temporal bone can be divided into four portions: **squamous, tympanic, mastoid,** and **petrous.** The thin squamous portion projects upward to form part of the side walls of the cranium. Extending from the squamous portion is the **zygomatic process,** which projects anteriorly to the zygoma of the face to form the **zygomatic arch.** The tympanic portion forms the walls of the **external auditory meatus** and the posterior section of the **mandibular fossa.** The mandibular fossa is the depression that articulates with the mandible. The mastoid portion encloses the **mastoid air cells** and forms part of the base of the skull (Figures 1.13 and 1.14). The petrous portion is pyramidal in shape and is situated at an angle between the sphenoid and occipital bones. This petrous portion is the thickest and densest area of the cranium. This attribute is important because the petrous portion serves to protect and house the delicate middle and inner ear structures. In addition to the four portions of the temporal bone, it is advantageous to identify the three major foramina associated with the temporal bone. These paired openings—**jugular foramina, carotid canals,** and **foramen lacerum**—serve as pathways for nerves and vessels through the petrous bone (Figure 1.15).

Key. **ACF** anterior cranial fossa; **Cl** clivus; **FM** foramen magnum; **MCF** middle cranial fossa; **PCF** posterior cranial fossa.

Figure 1.12   3D CT scan of cranial fossa.

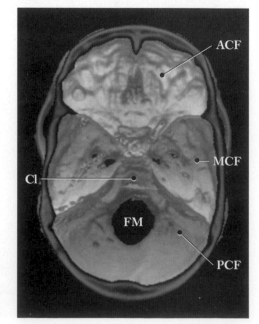

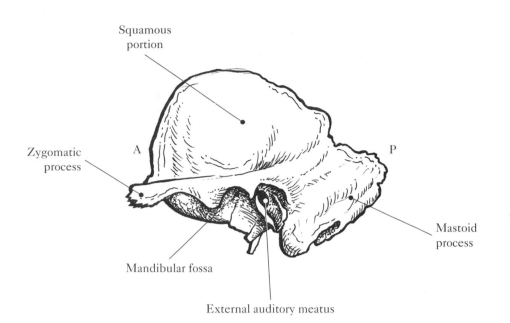

Squamous portion

Zygomatic process

A

P

Mandibular fossa

Mastoid process

External auditory meatus

Figure 1.13   Lateral view of temporal bone.

Key. ArE articular eminence;   **CC** carotid canal;   **EAM** external auditory meatus; **FL** foramen lacerum; **JF** jugular fossa; **Mac** mastoid air cells; **MC** mandibular condyle; **MF** mandibular fossa; **ZyP** zygomatic process.

Figure 1.14   Sagittal CT reformat of temporal bone.

Figure 1.15   Axial CT scan of temporal bone with foramen lacerum.

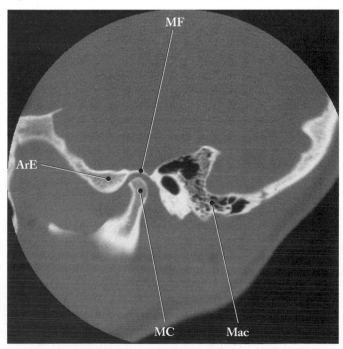

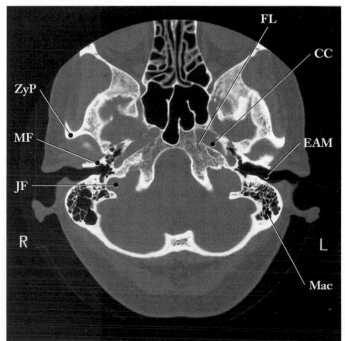

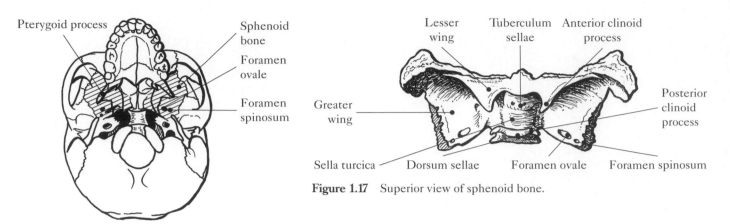

Pterygoid process

Sphenoid bone

Foramen ovale

Foramen spinosum

Lesser wing   Tuberculum sellae   Anterior clinoid process

Greater wing

Posterior clinoid process

Sella turcica   Dorsum sellae   Foramen ovale   Foramen spinosum

Figure 1.17 Superior view of sphenoid bone.

Figure 1.16 Inferior surface of sphenoid bone and cranium.

Figure 1.18 Sagittal CT reformat of sella turcica.

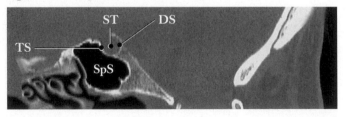

ST   DS

TS

SpS

Figure 1.19 Axial CT scan of sphenoid bone with foramen ovale and spinosum.

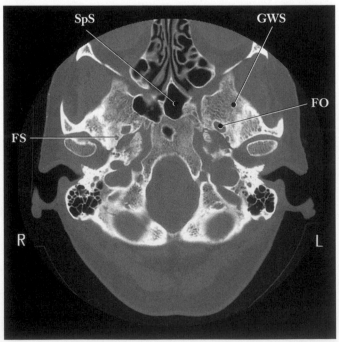

SpS   GWS

FS   FO

R   L

Key. **DS** dorsum sella; **FO** foramen ovale; **FS** foramen spinosum; **GWS** greater wing of sphenoid bone; **SpS** sphenoid sinus; **ST** sella turcica; **TS** tuberculum sella.

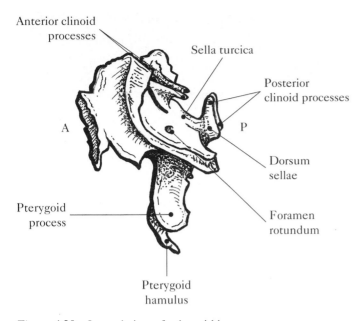

Anterior clinoid processes

Sella turcica

Posterior clinoid processes

A   P

Dorsum sellae

Pterygoid process

Foramen rotundum

Pterygoid hamulus

Figure 1.20   Lateral view of sphenoid bone.

Key.   aCl anterior clinoid processes; **FR** foramen rotundum; **GWS** greater wing of sphenoid bone; **PHS** pterygoid hamulus of sphenoid bone; **PPS** pterygoid process of sphenoid bone; **SpS** sphenoid sinus.

Figure 1.21   Coronal CT scan of sphenoid bone.

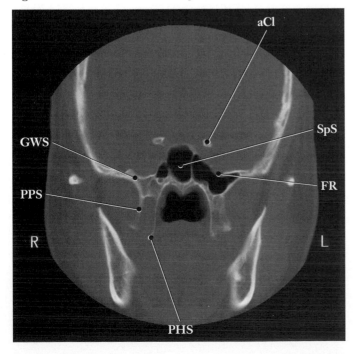

SPHENOID BONE

The butterfly-shaped sphenoid bone extends completely across the floor of the middle cranial fossa. This bone forms the majority of the base of the skull and articulates with the occipital, temporal, parietal, frontal, and ethmoid bones (Figure 1.16). The main parts of the sphenoid bone are the **body, lesser wings** (2), and **greater wings** (2) (Figure 1.17). Located within the body of the sphenoid bone is a deep depression called the **sella turcica,** which houses the **hypophysis (pituitary gland).** Directly below the sella turcica are two air-filled cavities termed **sphenoid sinuses** (Figure 1.18). The anterior portion of the sella turcica is formed by the **tuberculum sellae** and the posterior portion by the **dorsum sellae.** The dorsum sellae gives rise to the **posterior clinoid processes.** The triangular-shaped lesser wings attach to the superior aspect of the body and form two sharp points called **anterior clinoid processes.** The greater wings extend laterally from the sides of the body and contain three paired foramina—**rotundum, ovale,** and **spinosum**—through which nerves and blood vessels course (Figure 1.19). Extending from the inferior surface of each greater wing is a **pterygoid process,** which is divided into medial and lateral sections. The medial section is longer and has a hook-shaped projection on its inferior end termed the **pterygoid hamulus** (Figures 1.20 and 1.21). The pterygoid processes articulate with the palatine bones and vomer to form part of the nasal cavity.

ETHMOID BONE

The ethmoid bone is the smallest of the cranial bones and is situated in the **anterior cranial fossa.** This cube-shaped bone can be divided into four parts: horizontal portion, vertical portion, and two lateral masses (labyrinths). The horizontal portion, called the **cribriform plate,** articulates with the frontal bone. This plate contains many foramina for the passage of olfactory nerves. The **crista galli,** a bony projection stemming from the midline of the cribriform plate, projects superiorly to act as an attachment for the connective tissue that anchors the brain to the anterior cranial fossa. The vertical portion of the ethmoid bone, called the **perpendicular plate,** projects inferiorly from the cribriform plate to form a portion of the bony nasal septum (Figures 1.22 through 1.24). The **lateral masses** are thin-walled processes that contain many **ethmoid air cells.** Projecting from the lateral masses are two scroll-shaped processes called the **middle** and **superior nasal conchae (turbinates)** (Figure 1.25).

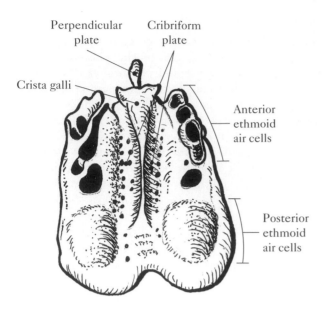

Figure 1.22   Superior view of ethmoid bone.

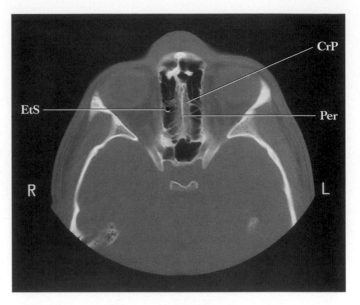

Figure 1.23   Axial CT scan of ethmoid bone.

Key. CrP cribriform plate; **EtS** ethmoid sinus; **Per** perpendicular plate of ethmoid bone.

Key.   CG crista galli; **CrP** cribriform plate; **eac** ethmoid air cell; **lm** lateral mass; **Per** perpendicular plate.

Figure 1.25   Coronal CT scan of ethmoid bone with crista galli.

Figure 1.24   Anterior view of ethmoid bone.

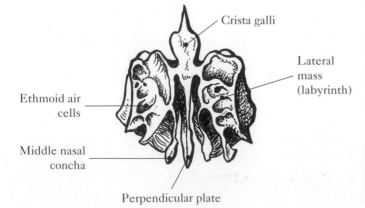

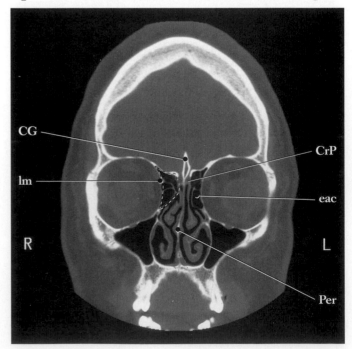

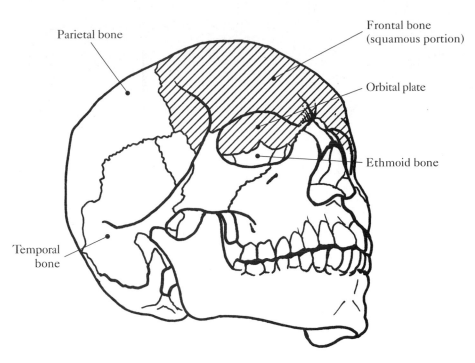

Figure 1.26   Oblique view of frontal bone and cranium.

FRONTAL BONE

The frontal bone consists of a vertical and a horizontal portion. The vertical or squamous portion forms the forehead and anterior vault of the cranium (Figure 1.26). The vertical portion contains the **frontal sinuses,** which lie on either side of the midsagittal plane (Figure 1.27). The horizontal portion forms the roof over each orbit termed the **orbital plate** (Figure 1.28).

Key. **FrS** frontal sinus; **OrP** orbital plate of frontal bone; **SqF** squamous portion of frontal bone.

Figure 1.28   Axial CT scan of orbital plates.

Figure 1.27   Coronal CT scan of frontal bone.

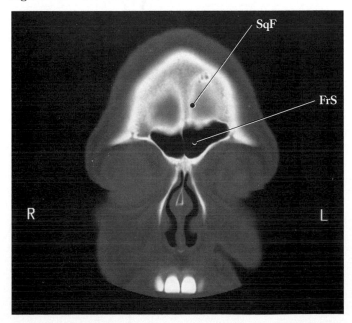

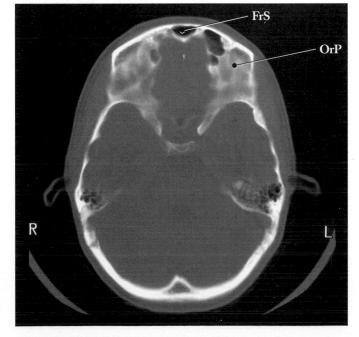

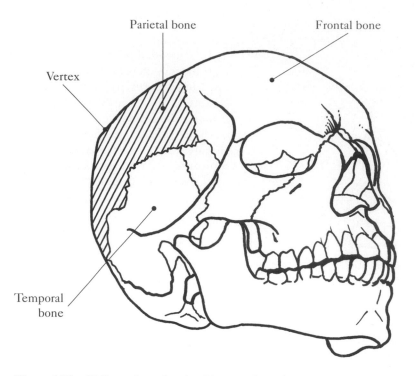

Figure 1.29   Oblique view of parietal bone and cranium.

Table 1.1   Foramina of the cranium

Foramen	Corresponding bone
Hypoglossal canal	Occipital
Foramen magnum	Occipital
Jugular foramen	Temporal, occipital
Carotid canals	Temporal
Internal and external auditory meatus	Temporal
Foramen lacerum	Temporal, sphenoid, occipital
Foramen rotundum	Sphenoid
Foramen ovale	Sphenoid
Foramen spinosum	Sphenoid
Superior orbital fissure	Orbit (between sphenoid wings)
Inferior orbital fissure	Orbit (sphenoid, zygoma, maxillae)
Optic canal	Apex of orbit
Olfactory foramina	Ethmoid

Key.   P parietal bone.

Figure 1.30   Axial CT scan of parietal bone.

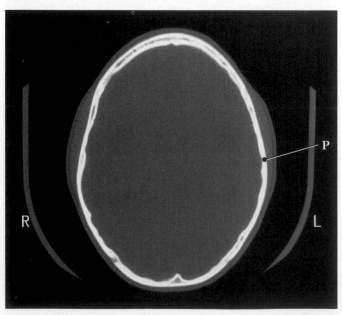

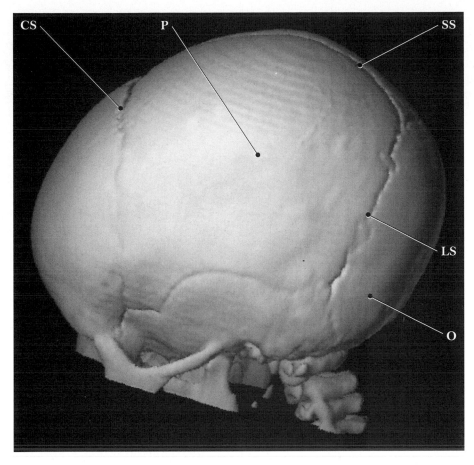

Figure 1.31   3D CT scan of lateral surface of pediatric cranium.

Key. CS coronal suture; **LS** lambdoidal suture; **O** occipital bone;
P parietal bone; **SS** sagittal suture.

Figure 1.32   Axial CT scan of lambdoidal suture.

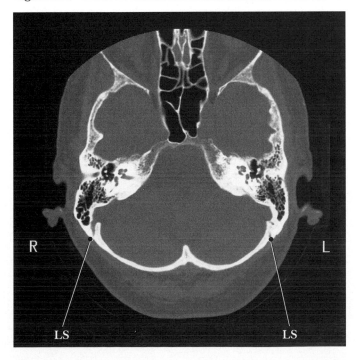

PARIETAL BONE

The two parietal bones form a large portion of the sides of the cranium. The parietal bones articulate with the frontal, occipital, temporal, and sphenoid bones. The superior point between the parietal bones is the **vertex,** which is the highest point of the cranium (Figures 1.29 and 1.30).

SUTURES

The cranial bones are joined together by four main articulations termed **sutures.** The **squamous suture,** which is located on the side of the cranium, joins the squamous portion of the temporal bone to the parietal bone (see Figure 1.3). The **coronal suture** runs transversely across the top of the cranium and is the articulation between the frontal and parietal bones. The **sagittal suture** provides the articulation between the parietal bones along the midsagittal plane. The **lambdoidal suture** is located posterior in the cranium and joins the occipital and parietal bones (See Figures 1.2, 1.31 and 1.32).

The sutures in neonates are not fully closed, allowing for growth of the head after birth. Craniosynostosis is the result of the premature ossification of one or more of the cranial sutures, which causes abnormal growth of the cranium.

FACIAL BONES

The face is made up of fourteen facial bones. The facial bones can be difficult to differentiate because of their relatively small size and irregular shape. They consist of **nasal** (2), **lacrimal** (2), **maxilla** (2), **zygoma** (2), **palatine** (2), **inferior nasal conchae** (2), **vomer** (1), and **mandible** (1) (Figures 1.33 and 1.34).

NASAL BONE, LACRIMAL BONE, MAXILLA, PALATINE BONE, AND ZYGOMA

The two nasal bones form the bony bridge of the nose. Posterior to the nasal bones are the lacrimal bones, which are situated on the median wall of each orbit (Figures 1.35 and 1.36). The junction of the lacrimal bones to the maxillae form the **lacrimal canals,** which act as passages for the drainage of excess lacrimal fluid (tears). The largest of the immovable facial bones is the maxilla. Fused at the midline, the maxillae extend to the frontal and zygoma bones. The inferior border of the maxilla has several depressions that form the **alveolar process,** which accepts the roots of the teeth. The **palatine process** of the maxilla extends posteriorly to form three fourths of the **hard palate.** The posterior one fourth of the hard palate is created by the horizontal portion of the palatine bones (Figures 1.37 through 1.39). The palatine bones also extend vertically to form part of the nasal cavity (Figure 1.40). The zygoma (malar bone) creates the prominence of the cheek and contributes to the lateral portion of the bony orbit (Figures 1.41 and 1.42).

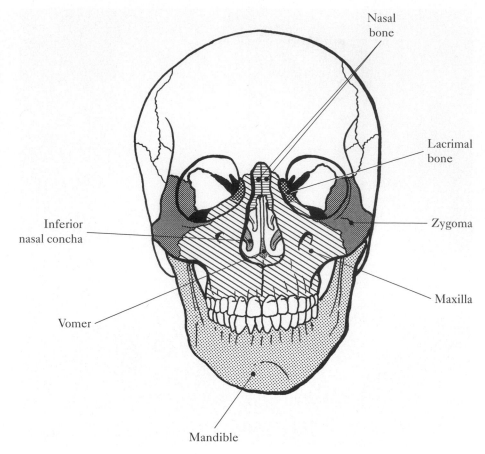

Figure 1.33   Anterior view of facial bones.

Figure 1.34   Lateral view of facial bones.

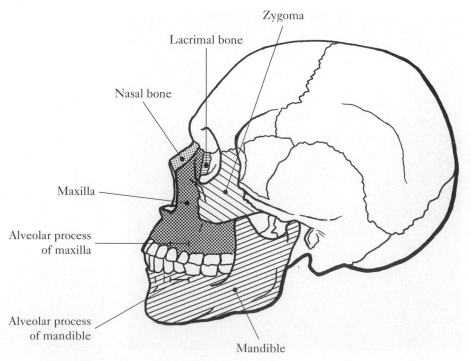

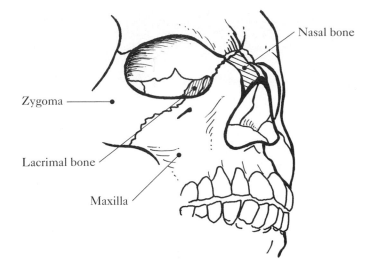

Figure 1.35   Oblique view of nasal and lacrimal bones.

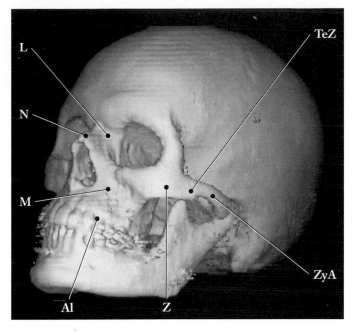

Figure 1.36   3D CT scan of oblique aspect of facial bones.

Key.   **Al** alveolar process of maxilla; **L** lacrimal bone; **M** maxilla; **N** nasal bone; **TeZ** temporal process of zygoma; **Z** zygoma; **ZyA** zygomatic arch.

Key.   **Hor** horizontal portion of palatine bone; **Pal** palatine process of maxilla; **PPS** pterygoid process of sphenoid bone.

Figure 1.38   Axial CT scan of hard palate.

Figure 1.37   Inferior view of facial bones and cranium.

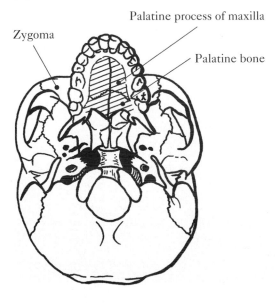

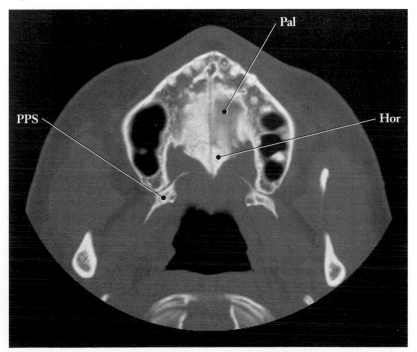

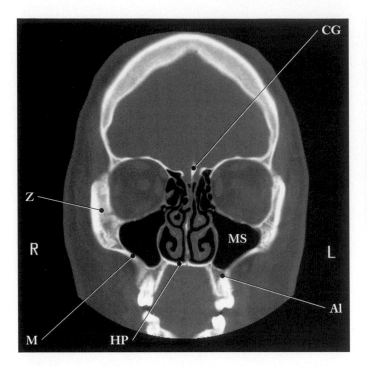

Figure 1.39 Coronal CT scan of maxilla and zygoma.

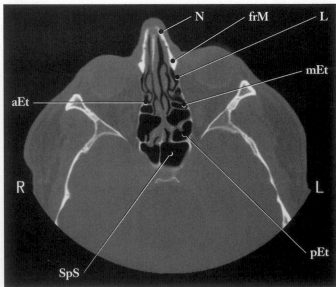

Figure 1.40 Coronal CT scan of nasal bones.

Key. **aEt** anterior ethmoids; **Al** alveolar process of maxilla; **CG** crista galli; **frM** frontal process of maxilla; **HP** hard palate (horizontal plate of palatine bone); **iNC** inferior nasal conchae; **L** lacrimal bone; **M** maxilla; **mEt** middle ethmoids; **MS** maxillary sinus; **N** nasal bone; **NaS** nasal septum; **pEt** posterior ethmoids; **SpS** sphenoid sinus; **Z** zygoma.

Figure 1.41 Axial CT scan of facial bones.

Figure 1.42 Axial CT scan of facial bones and ethmoid sinuses.

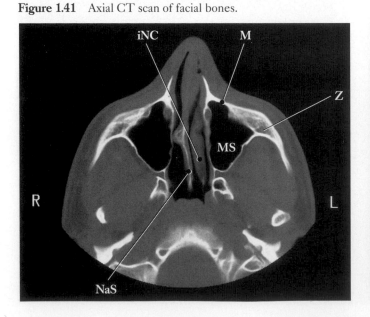

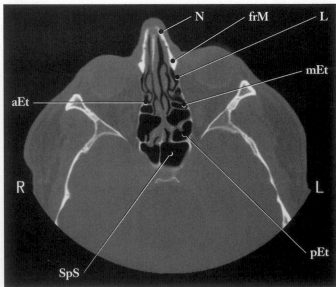

INFERIOR NASAL CONCHAE AND VOMER

The **inferior nasal conchae** project medially and inferiorly along the nasal cavity. They can be identified by their scroll-like appearance. These conchae, in conjunction with the superior and middle nasal conchae of the ethmoid bone, divide the nasal cavity into **superior, middle,** and **inferior meatus** (Figures 1.43 through 1.45). The **vomer** projects superiorly from the base of the nasal cavity to form the inferior portion of the **bony nasal septum** (Figure 1.46).

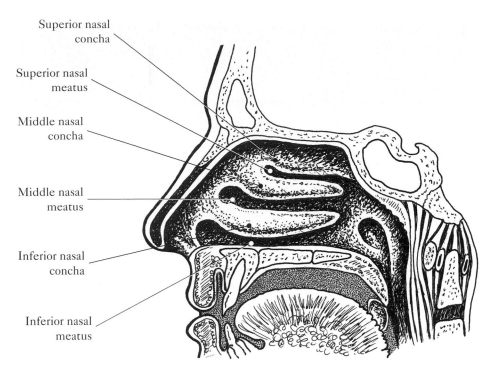

Superior nasal concha
Superior nasal meatus
Middle nasal concha
Middle nasal meatus
Inferior nasal concha
Inferior nasal meatus

Figure 1.43   Sagittal view of nasal meatus.

Key.   EtS ethmoid sinus; **FrS** frontal sinus; **iME** inferior meatus; **iNC** inferior nasal conchae; **mME** middle meatus; **mNC** middle nasal conchae; **SER** sphenoethmoidal recess; **sME** superior meatus; **sNC** superior nasal conchae; **SpS** sphenoid sinus.

Figure 1.44   Sagittal CT reformat of nasal meatus.

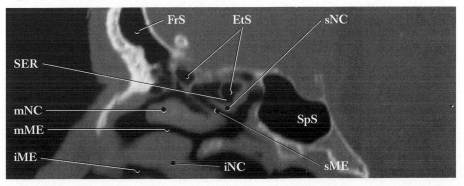

FrS   EtS   sNC
SER
mNC
mME
iME   iNC   sME   SpS

Figure 1.45   Axial CT scan of inferior nasal conchae.

Key. **iNC** inferior nasal conchae; **M** maxilla; **MS** maxillary sinus; **NaS** nasal septum; **Z** zygoma.

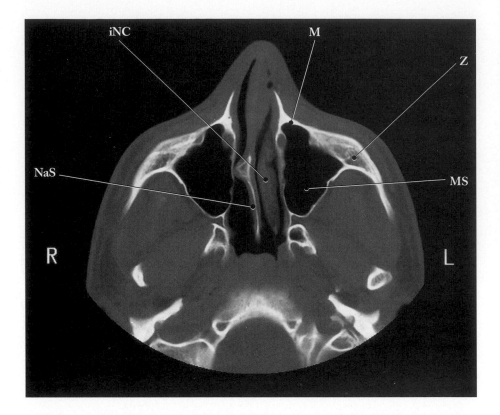

Figure 1.46   Coronal CT scan of nasal conchae and vomer.

Key. **iME** inferior meatus; **iNC** inferior nasal conchae; **mME** middle meatus; **mNC** middle nasal conchae; **NaS** nasal septum; **V** vomer.

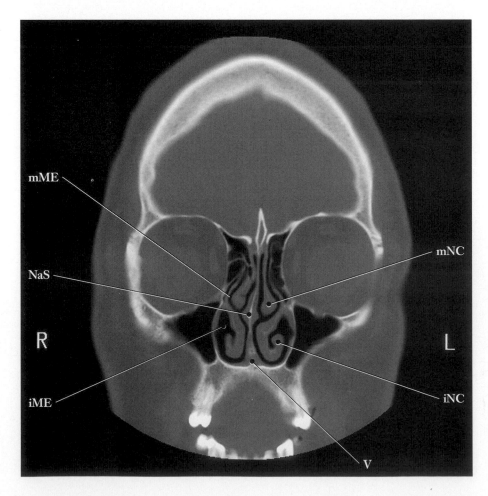

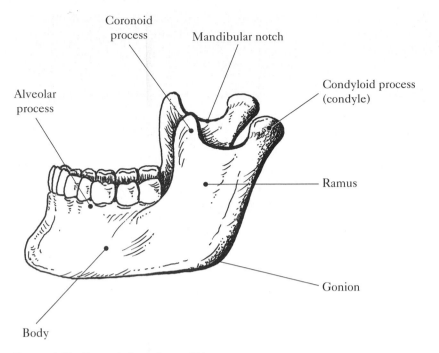

Coronoid process

Mandibular notch

Alveolar process

Condyloid process (condyle)

Ramus

Gonion

Body

Figure 1.47   Lateral view of mandible.

MANDIBLE

The largest facial bone is the **mandible.** This bone is composed primarily of horizontal and vertical portions. The angle created by the junction of these two portions is termed the **gonion.** The curved horizontal portion, called the **body,** contains an **alveolar process** that receives the roots of the bottom teeth. The vertical portion of the mandible is called the **ramus.** Each ramus has two processes at its superior portion: anterior **coronoid process** and posterior **condyloid process** (Figures 1.47 and 1.48). They are separated by a concave surface called the **mandibular notch.** The condyloid process articulates with the **mandibular fossa** to form the **temporomandibular joint** (Figure 1.49).

Key.   **Al** alveolar process of mandible; **Con** condyloid process of mandible; **Cor** coronoid process of mandible; **Mb** body of mandible; **Mn** mandibular notch; **Mr** ramus of mandible.

Figure 1.48   3D CT scan of lateral aspect of mandible.

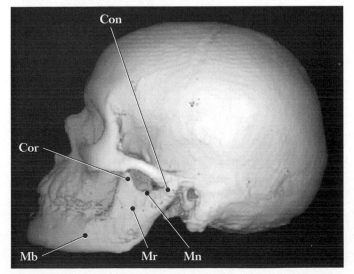

Con

Cor

Mb   Mr   Mn

Figure 1.49   Sagittal oblique CT reformat of mandible.

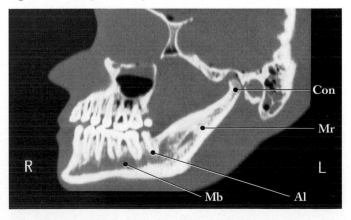

Con

Mr

R   L

Mb   Al

Temporomandibular Joint

The temporomandibular joint (TMJ) is a modified hinge joint that permits the necessary motions of mastication.

Bony anatomy

The **mandibular fossa** and **articular eminence** of the temporal bone form the superior articulating surface for the mandibular condyle. The articular eminence creates the anterior boundary of the joint, preventing the forward displacement of the mandibular condyle (Figures 1.50 through 1.52).

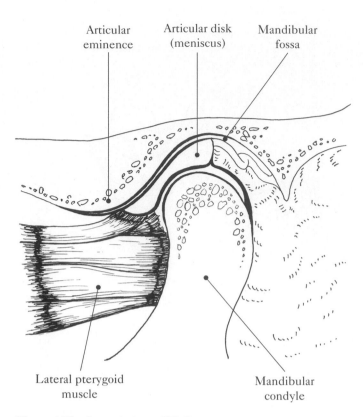

Figure 1.50 Lateral view of TMJ.

Key. **ArE** articular eminence; **Con** condyloid process of mandible; **EAM** external auditory meatus; **Mac** mastoid air cells; **MC** mandibular condyle; **MF** mandibular fossa; **ZyP** zygomatic process.

Figure 1.51 Sagittal CT reformat of TMJ.

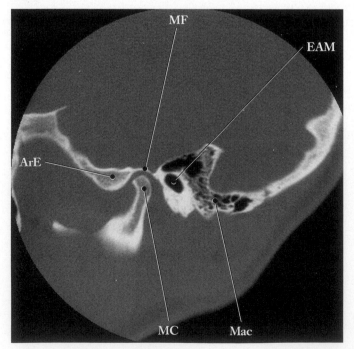

Figure 1.52 Coronal CT scan of TMJ.

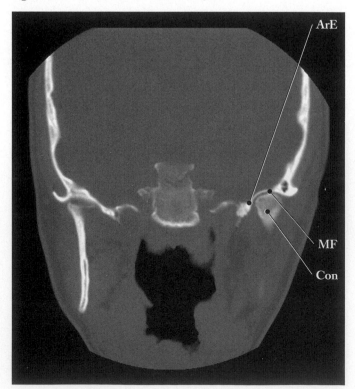

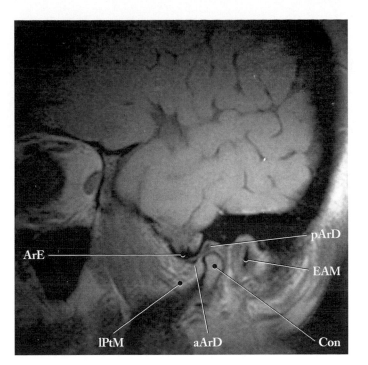

Figure 1.53   Sagittal MR scan of TMJ and articular disk.

Key.   aArD anterior band of articular disk; **ArE** articular eminence; **Con** condyloid process of mandible; **EAM** external auditory meatus; **lPtM** lateral pterygoid muscle; **pArD** posterior band of articular disk.

ARTICULAR DISK AND LIGAMENTS

The **articular disk,** frequently called the meniscus, is shaped like a bow tie because it is interposed between the condyle and fossa (Figures 1.50 and 1.53). The anterior surface attaches to the **lateral pterygoid muscle** and is secured posteriorly with fibrous connections to both the temporal bone and the posterior aspect of the condyle (Figure 1.54). The articular disk is not tightly bound to the fossa but moves anteriorly with the condyle. Several ligaments help to maintain the position of the articular disk. The articular disk is attached to the medial and lateral surfaces of the condyle by the **collateral ligaments** (Figures 1.55 and 1.56). Lateral stability is provided by the TMJ ligament (lateral ligament), which extends from the articular eminence and zygomatic process to the posterior aspect of the articular disk and the condylar head and neck (Figure 1.57). In addition, this ligament restricts the posterior movement of the condyle and articular disk.

Key.   Con condyloid process of mandible; **lPtM** lateral pterygoid muscle; **MaM** masseter muscle; **mPtM** medial pterygoid muscle.

Figure 1.54   Axial MR scan of TMJ.

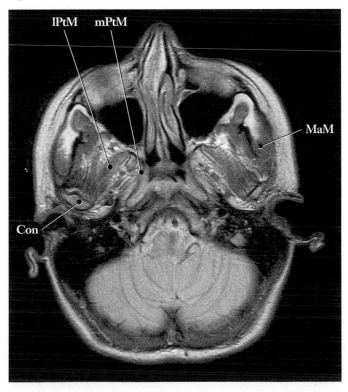

MUSCLES

The cooperative action of the muscles of mastication provides the movement of the mandible (Figure 1.58). The **temporalis muscle** originates on the temporal bone, inserts on the mandible, and elevates the mandible. The **masseter muscle,** located on the lateral ramus of the mandible, acts to elevate the mandible as well (Figure 1.59). The pterygoid muscles (medial and lateral) originate from the pterygoid processes of the sphenoid bone and insert on the mandible. The **medial pterygoid muscle** closes the jaw, whereas the **lateral pterygoid muscle** opens the jaw and protrudes and moves the mandible from side to side (Figures 1.60 and 1.61).

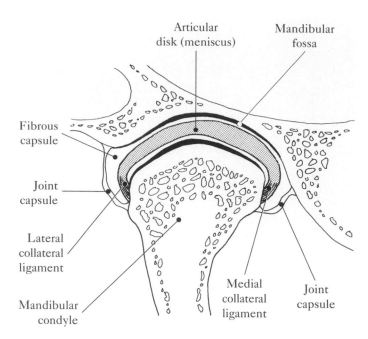

Figure 1.55   Coronal view of TMJ and collateral ligaments.

Key.   ArD articular disk; **Con** condyloid process of mandible; **LCoL** lateral collateral ligament.

Figure 1.56   Coronal MR scan of TMJ and collateral ligaments.

Figure 1.57   Lateral view of TMJ and lateral ligament.

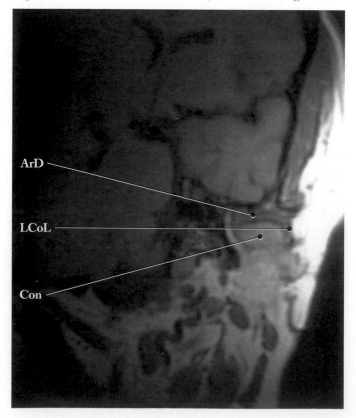

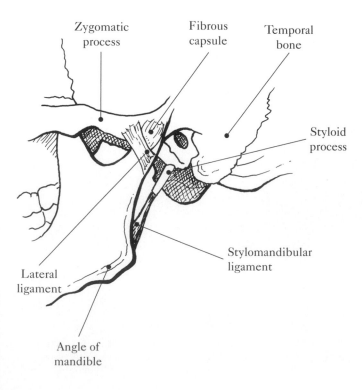

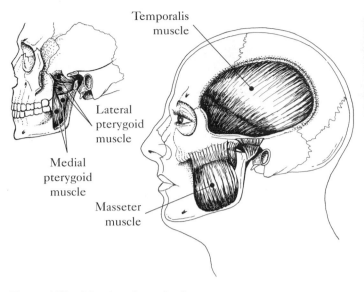

Temporalis muscle

Lateral pterygoid muscle

Medial pterygoid muscle

Masseter muscle

Figure 1.58 Muscles of mastication.

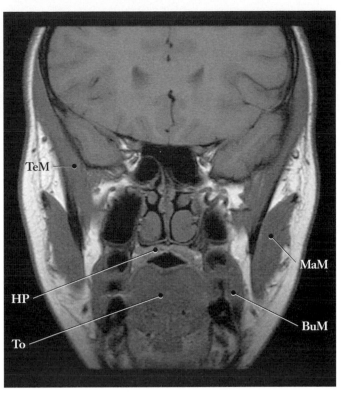

Figure 1.59 Coronal MR scan of muscles of mastication.

Key. BuM buccinator muscle; **Con** condyloid process of mandible; **HP** hard palate; **lPtM** lateral pterygoid muscle; **MaM** masseter muscle; **mPtM** medial pterygoid muscle; **PPS** pterygoid process of sphenoid bone; **TeM** temporalis muscle; **To** tongue.

Figure 1.60 Axial MR scan of TMJ and muscles of mastication.

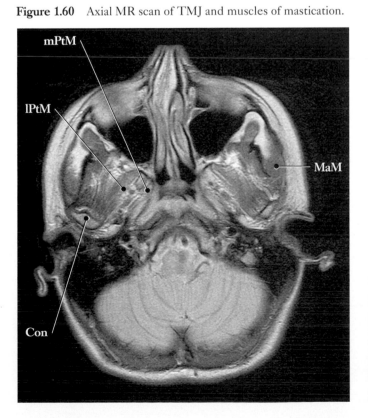

Figure 1.61 Axial CT scan of TMJ and muscles of mastication.

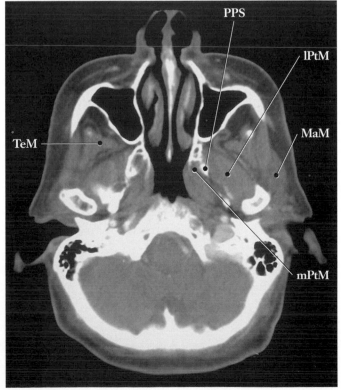

PARANASAL SINUSES

The **paranasal sinuses** are air-containing cavities within the facial bones and skull that communicate with the nasal fossa. The sinuses are named after the bones in which they originate: **ethmoid, maxillary, sphenoid,** and **frontal.** There is great variance in the size, shape, and development of these sinuses in each individual (Figures 1.62 and 1.63).

ETHMOID SINUSES

The **ethmoid sinuses** are contained within the lateral masses (labyrinths) of the ethmoid bone. They are composed of a varying number of air cells and can be divided into three groups: **anterior, middle,** and **posterior.** The anterior and middle groups drain into the **middle nasal meatus,** and the posterior group drains into the **superior nasal meatus** (Figures 1.64 through 1.67; see Figure 1.44).

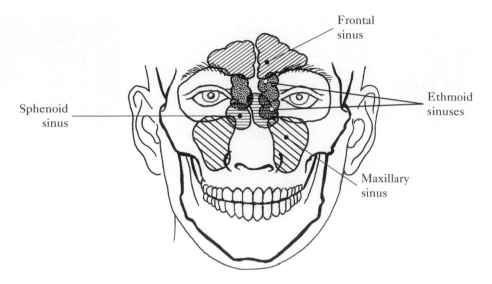

Figure 1.62   Anterior view of paranasal sinuses within cranium.

Figure 1.63   Lateral view of paranasal sinuses within cranium.

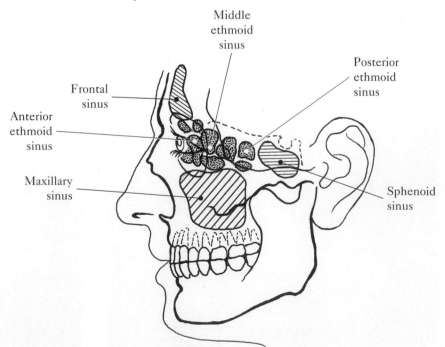

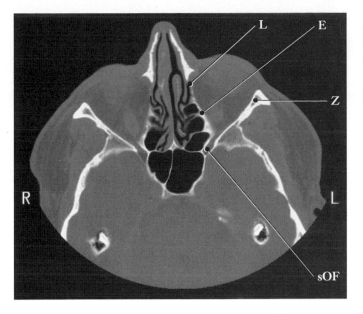

Figure 1.64   Axial CT scan of sphenoid and ethmoid sinuses.

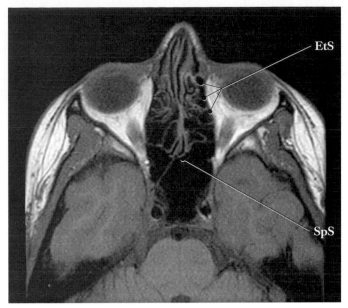

Figure 1.65   Axial MR scan of ethmoid and sphenoid sinuses.

Key.   E ethmoid bone; **EtS** ethmoid sinus; **iME** inferior meatus; **iNC** inferior nasal conchae; **L** lacrimal bone; **mME** middle meatus; **mNC** middle nasal conchae; **MS** maxillary sinus; **SER** sphenoethmoidal recess; **sME** superior meatus; **sNC** superior nasal conchae; **sOF** superior orbital fissure; **SpS** sphenoid sinus; **Z** zygoma.

Figure 1.66   Sagittal MR scan of sphenoid sinus.

Figure 1.67   Coronal CT scan of ethmoid and maxillary sinuses.

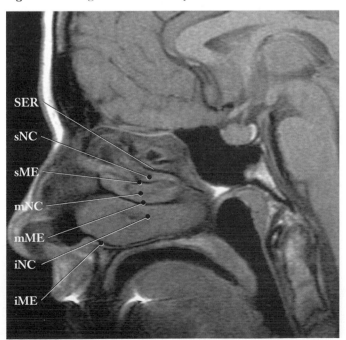

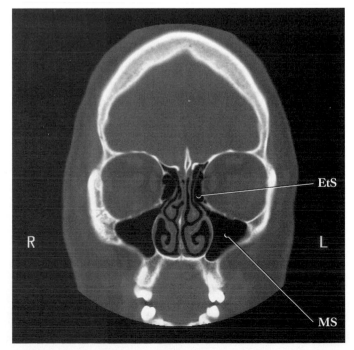

MAXILLARY SINUSES

The paired **maxillary sinuses (antrum of Highmore)** are located within the body of the maxilla. They are the largest sinuses and are triangular in shape. The maxillary sinuses and the roots of the teeth are separated by a very thin layer of bone. Often it is difficult to differentiate between the symptoms of sinusitis and infection of the teeth. The maxillary sinuses drain into the middle nasal meatus (Figures 1.67 and 1.68).

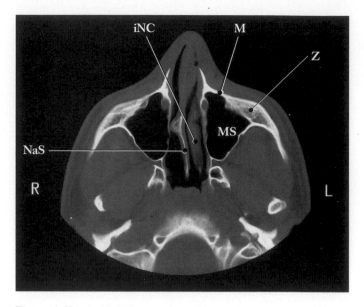

Figure 1.68   Axial CT scan of maxillary sinuses.

Key.   **iNC** inferior nasal conchae; **M** maxilla; **MS** maxillary sinus; **NaS** nasal septum; **Z** zygoma.

Key.   **aCl** anterior clinoid process; **FR** foramen rotundum; **ICA** internal carotid artery; **mNC** middle nasal conchae; **Och** optic chiasm; **Pit** pituitary gland; **sOF** superior orbital fissure; **SpS** sphenoid sinus.

Figure 1.69   Coronal MR scan of sphenoid sinuses.   **Figure 1.70**   Coronal CT scan of sphenoid sinuses.

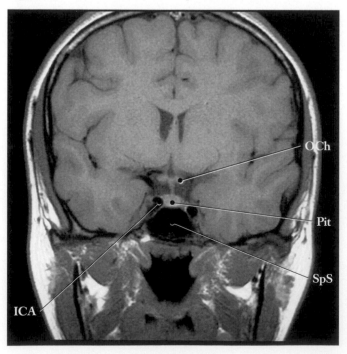

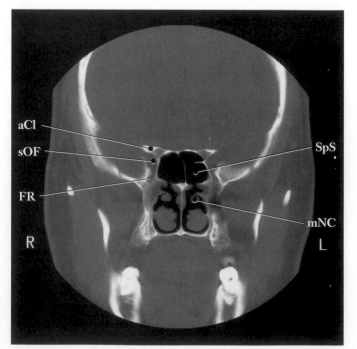

SPHENOID SINUSES

The **sphenoid sinuses** are typically paired and occupy the body of the sphenoid bone just below the **sella turcica.** Each sphenoid sinus opens into the **sphenoethmoidal recess** directly above the **superior nasal concha** (Figures 1.65 through 1.70).

FRONTAL SINUSES

The **frontal sinuses** are located within the **vertical portion** of the frontal bone. These sinuses are typically paired and are separated along the midsagittal plane by a **septum.** The frontal sinuses are rarely symmetric, vary in size, and can contain numerous septa. The frontal sinuses drain into the middle nasal meatus (Figures 1.66 and 1.71).

Table 1.2   Paranasal sinus drainage location

SINUS	DRAINAGE LOCATION
Ethmoid: anterior and middle	Middle nasal meatus
Ethmoid: posterior	Superior nasal meatus
Maxillary	Middle nasal meatus
Sphenoid	Sphenoethmoidal recess
Frontal	Middle nasal meatus

Key.   **FrS** frontal sinus; **N** nasal bone; **Per** perpendicular plate of ethmoid bone; **s** septum.

Figure 1.71   Coronal CT scan of frontal sinuses.

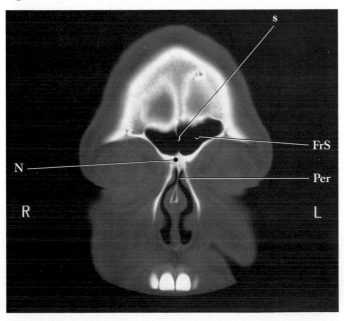

OSTEOMEATAL COMPLEX

The **osteomeatal complex** is made up of several structures that create the drainage pathways of the frontal, maxillary, and anterior and middle ethmoid sinuses. This complex is located in the area of the superomedial maxillary sinus. The key structures to identify are the **infundibulum, middle nasal meatus, uncinate process,** and **ethmoid bulla.** The infundibulum is the main drainage pathway of the maxillary sinus into the middle nasal meatus. The medial wall of the infundibulum is created by the uncinate process. Also draining into the middle nasal meatus is the ethmoid bulla, located superoposterior to the infundibulum, which receives drainage from the anterior and middle ethmoid air cells (Figures 1.72 and 1.73). CT imaging in a direct coronal plane with a bony algorithm will provide the best demonstration of these structures.

> Obstruction of the middle meatus can lead to maxillary, ethmoid, and frontal sinusitis.

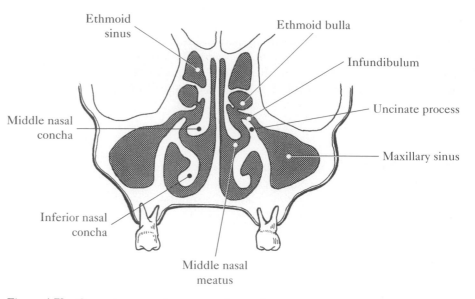

Figure 1.72   Coronal aspect of osteomeatal complex.

Key. EtB ethmoid bulla; **Inf** infundibulum; **mME** middle meatus; **Unc** uncinate process of ethmoid bone.

Figure 1.73   Coronal CT scan of osteomeatal complex.

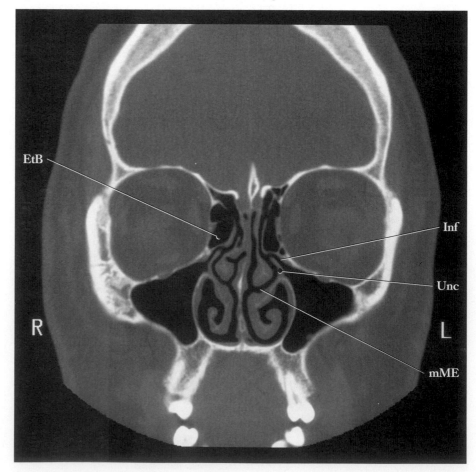

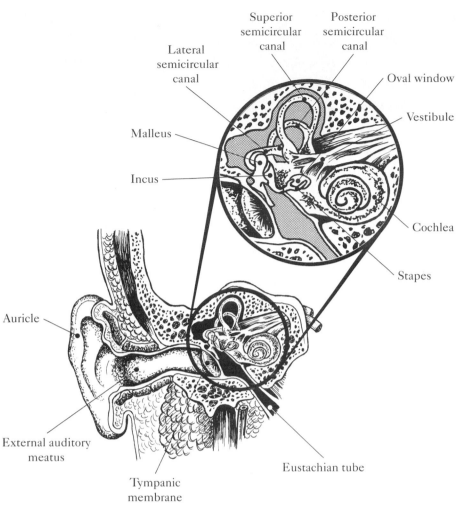

Superior semicircular canal

Posterior semicircular canal

Lateral semicircular canal

Oval window

Malleus

Vestibule

Incus

Cochlea

Auricle

Stapes

External auditory meatus

Eustachian tube

Tympanic membrane

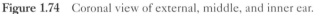

Figure 1.74   Coronal view of external, middle, and inner ear.

PETROUS PORTION OF THE TEMPORAL BONE

The **petrous portion of the temporal bone** contains all the structures of the middle and inner ear. This wedge-shaped bone forms a portion of the skull base between the occipital and sphenoid bones.

The structures of the ear can be divided into three main portions: **external, middle,** and **inner.** The external ear consists of the **auricle** and the **external auditory meatus.** The external auditory meatus is a sound-conducting canal that terminates at the tympanic membrane of the middle ear. The air-containing middle ear (tympanic cavity) consists of the **tympanic membrane** and three **auditory ossicles (malleus, incus,** and **stapes)** (Figure 1.74). The tympanic membrane transmits sound vibrations to the auditory ossicles (Figures 1.75 and 1.76).

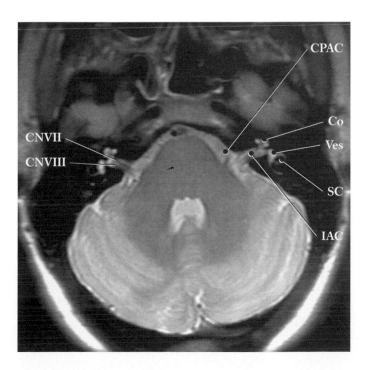

CPAC

CNVII

CNVIII

Co

Ves

SC

IAC

Figure 1.75   Axial MR scan of inner ear.

Key. **Co** cochlea; **CNVII** facial nerve; **CNVIII** vestibulocochlear nerve; **CPAC** cerebellopontine angle cistern; **IAC** internal auditory canal; **SC** semicircular canal; **Ves** vestibule.

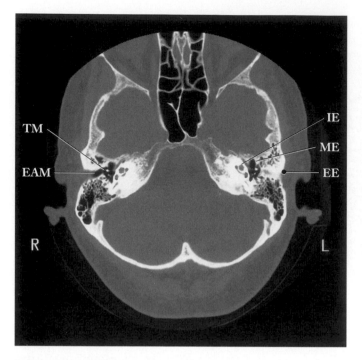

Figure 1.76 Axial CT scan of petrous portion at level of external auditory meatus.

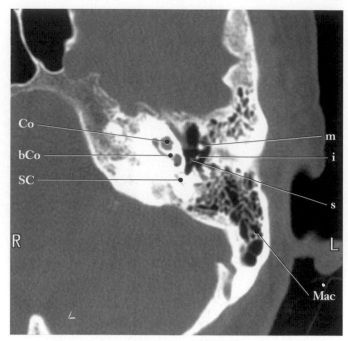

Figure 1.77 Axial CT scan of unilateral petrous portion at level of external auditory meatus.

Key. **bCo** basilar turn of cochlea; **Co** cochlea; **EAM** external auditory meatus; **EE** external ear; **i** incus; **IAC** internal auditory canal; **IE** inner ear; **m** malleus; **Mac** mastoid air cells; **ME** middle ear; **s** stapes, **SC** semicircular canal; **TM** tympanic membrane; **Ves** vestibule.

Figure 1.78 Axial CT scan of petrous portion at level of internal auditory canal.

Figure 1.79 Axial CT scan of unilateral petrous portion at level of internal auditory canal.

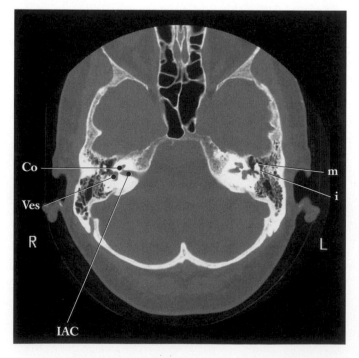

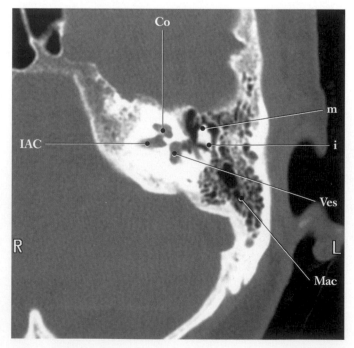

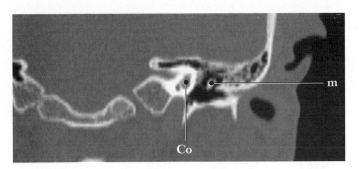

Figure 1.80   Coronal CT reformat of unilateral petrous portion with ossicles and cochlea.

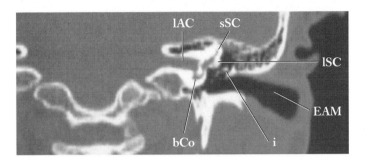

Figure 1.81   Coronal CT reformat of unilateral petrous portion with internal auditory canal, external auditory meatus, and semicircular canals.

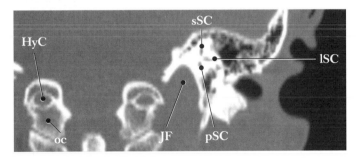

Figure 1.82   Coronal CT reformat of unilateral petrous portion with semicircular canals.

Key. **bCO** basilar turn of cochlea; **Co** cochlea; **EAM** external auditory meatus; **HyC** hypoglossal canal; **i** incus; **IAC** internal auditory canal; **iSC** inferior semicircular canal; **JF** jugular fossa; **lSC** lateral semicircular canal; **m** malleus; **oc** occipital condyle; **pSC** posterior semicircular canal; **sSC** superior semicircular canal.

The auditory ossicles, which are suspended in the middle ear, conduct sound vibrations from the tympanic membrane to the oval window of the inner ear. The inner ear is fluid filled and contains the **vestibule** and **semicircular canals,** which control equilibrium and balance, and the **cochlea,** which is responsible for hearing (Figures 1.77 through 1.80). The vestibule is a small compartment located between the semicircular canals and snail-shaped cochlea that communicates with the middle ear at the **oval window.** The semicircular canals are easily identified because of their three separate passages that are at right angles to each other. Located within the basilar turn of the cochlea is the **round window,** which allows the fluid of the inner ear to move slightly for propagation of sound waves (Figures 1.81 and 1.82).

Table 1.3   Sections of the ear

SECTION	STRUCTURES
External	Auricle, external auditory meatus
Middle	Tympanic membrane, auditory ossicles (malleus, incus, stapes)
Inner	Vestibule, semicircular canals, cochlea

ORBIT

BONY ORBIT

The bony **orbit** is a cone-shaped structure that serves to surround and protect the eyeball and associated structures. The orbit is created by the junction of the frontal, sphenoid, and ethmoid bones of the cranium and the lacrimal, palatine, maxillary, and zygomatic bones of the face (Figures 1.83 and 1.84).

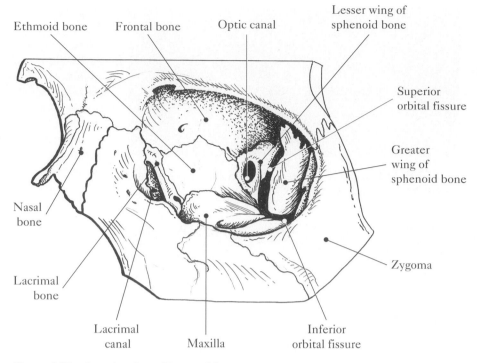

Figure 1.83   Anterior view of bony orbit.

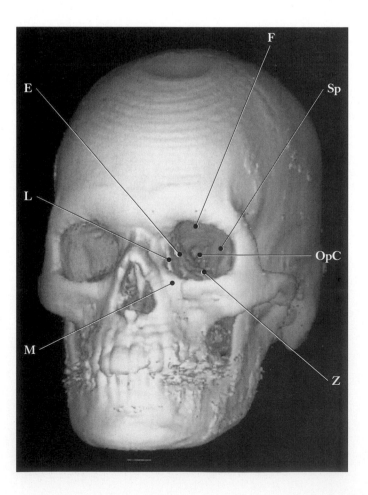

Figure 1.84   Oblique 3D CT scan of bony orbit and optic canal.

Key. E ethmoid bone; **F** frontal bone; **L** lacrimal bone; **M** maxilla; **OpC** optic canal; **Sp** sphenoid bone; **Z** zygoma.

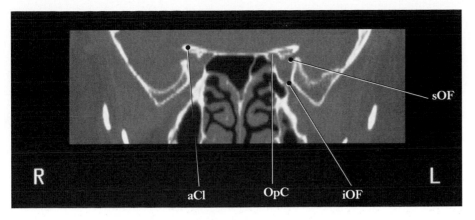

Figure 1.85   Coronal CT reformat of orbital fissures and optic canal.

Key.   **aCl** anterior clinoid process; **iOF** inferior orbital fissure; **OpC** optic canal; **sOF** superior orbital fissure.

Three openings in the orbit serve as passageways for nerves and vessels: **superior orbital fissure, inferior orbital fissure,** and **optic canal (foramen)** (Figure 1.85). The superior orbital fissure is a triangular opening located between the greater and lesser wings of the sphenoid bone. The inferior orbital fissure is located in the lower outer aspect of the orbit. Located in the posterior part of the orbit is the optic canal, through which the ophthalmic artery and optic nerve course (Figures 1.86 and 1.87).

Structures That Form Bony Orbit
Cranial bones   Frontal, sphenoid, ethmoid
Facial bones   Lacrimal, palatine, maxilla, zygoma

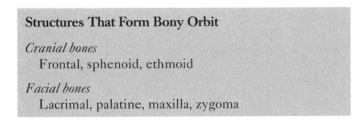

Key.   **aCl** anterior clinoid process; **DS** dorsum sella; **E** ethmoid bone; **L** lacrimal bone; **OpC** optic canal; **sOF** superior orbital fissure; **Z** zygoma.

Figure 1.86   Axial CT scan of inferior orbital fissure.

Figure 1.87   Axial CT scan of optic canal.

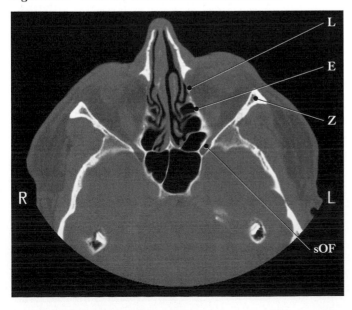

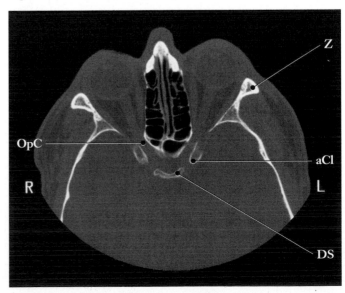

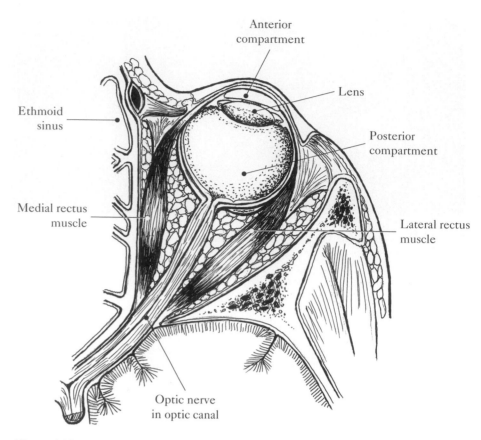

Figure 1.88 Axial view of orbit.

Key. **aCh** anterior chamber of globe; **l** lens; **lRm** lateral rectus muscle; **mRm** medial rectus muscle; **ON** optic nerve; **pCh** posterior chamber of globe.

Figure 1.89 Axial MR scan of orbit at midglobe.

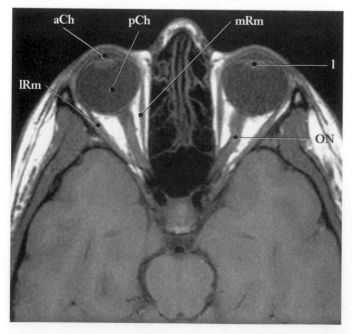

Figure 1.90 Axial CT scan of orbit at midglobe.

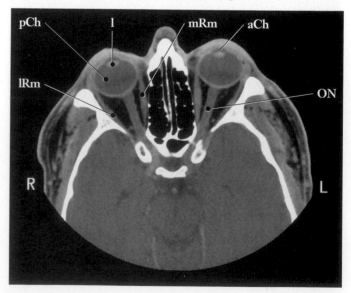

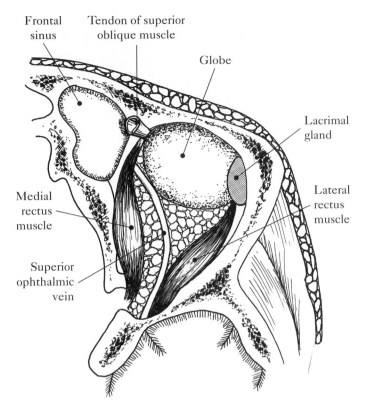

Figure 1.91   Axial view of orbit at lacrimal gland.

EYE

GLOBE.   The globe of the eye dominates the structures of the anterior orbit. The **globe** is divided into **anterior** and **posterior compartments.** The anterior compartment is a small cavity located anterior to the **lens.** It contains the **cornea** and **iris** and is filled with **aqueous humor,** which helps to maintain intraorbital pressure. Located behind the lens, the larger posterior compartment is surrounded by the **retina.** It contains a jellylike substance called the **vitreous humor,** which helps to maintain the shape of the eyeball (Figures 1.88 through 1.90). Located in the superolateral portion of the orbit is the **lacrimal gland** that produces tears (Figures 1.91 through 1.93).

Key.   G globe; **LG** lacrimal gland; **of** orbital fat; **SOV** superior ophthalmic vein.

Figure 1.92   Axial MR scan of orbit with lacrimal gland and ophthalmic vein.

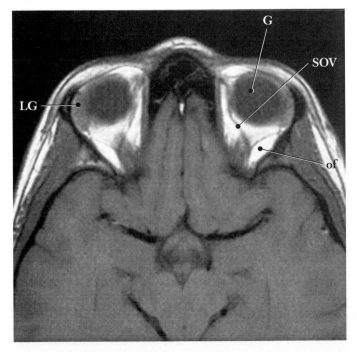

Figure 1.93   Axial CT scan of orbit with lacrimal gland and ophthalmic vein.

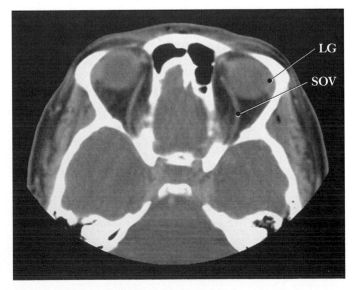

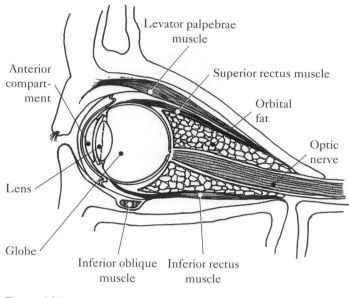

Figure 1.94   Sagittal view of orbit.

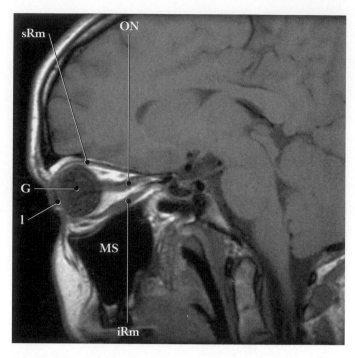

Figure 1.95   Sagittal oblique MR scan of orbit and optic nerve.

Key.   **G** globe; **iRm** inferior rectus muscle; **l** lens; **MS** maxillary sinus; **ON** optic nerve; **sRm** superior rectus muscle.

Figure 1.96   Coronal view of orbit through optic nerve.

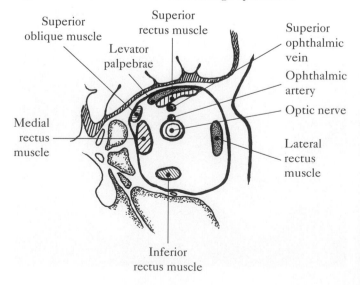

Key.   **iRm** inferior rectus muscle; **lRm** lateral rectus muscle; **mRm** medial rectus muscle; **ON** optic nerve; **OpA** ophthalmic artery; **SOV** superior ophthalmic vein; **sRm** superior rectus muscle.

Figure 1.97   Coronal CT scan of orbit through optic nerve and vessels.

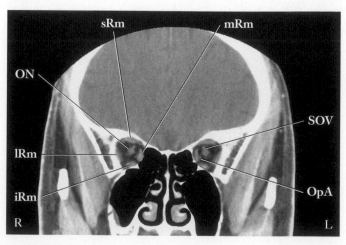

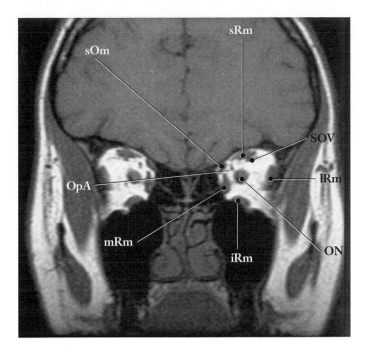

Figure 1.98   Coronal MR scan of orbit with rectus muscle group.

MUSCLES.   Six major muscles work together to control the movement of the eye. The **rectus muscle group** consists of four muscles named for their location in reference to the globe. The **superior, inferior, medial,** and **lateral rectus muscles** abduct and adduct the eyeball. Two **oblique muscles, superior** and **inferior,** abduct and rotate the eyeball (Figures 1.88, 1.94, and 1.95). The superior oblique muscle extends obliquely to the superior rectus muscle, whereas the inferior oblique muscle lies below the inferior rectus muscle (Figures 1.96 through 1.99).

OPTIC NERVE.   The **optic nerve** is the nerve of sight. It originates at the posterior surface of the globe and courses posteromedially to exit the orbit through the optic canal (Figures 1.88 through 1.90, 1.94 through 1.96, and 1.98). The **ophthalmic artery** runs inferior to the optic nerve initially, but then crosses over the nerve to supply the globe. It also exits the orbit through the optic canal. The **superior ophthalmic vein** is easily recognized because it originates from the medial orbit and courses below the superior rectus muscle (Figures 1.91 through 1.93, and 1.97). **Retroorbital fat** surrounds the muscular and vascular structures within the orbit, which allows for optimal visualization of these structures in cross-sectional imaging.

Table 1.5   Muscles of the orbit

GROUP	INDIVIDUAL NAMES	FUNCTION
Rectus	Superior, inferior, medial, lateral	Abduct and adduct eyeball
Oblique	Superior, inferior	Abduct and rotate eyeball

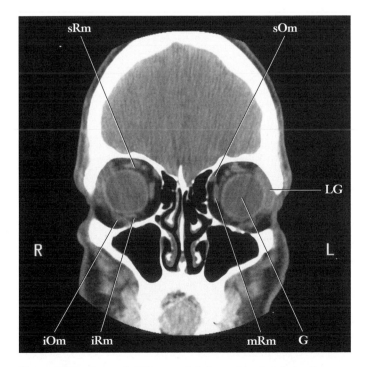

Figure 1.99   Coronal CT scan of globe and lacrimal gland.

Key.   **G** globe; **iOm** inferior oblique muscle; **iRm** inferior rectus muscle; **LG** lacrimal gland; **lRm** lateral rectus muscle; **mRm** medial rectus muscle; **ON** optic nerve; **sOm** superior oblique muscle; **SOV** superior ophthalmic vein; **sRm** superior rectus muscle.

ANSWER TO FIGURE 1.1

Several facial bones are fractured. The palatine process of the maxilla, the horizontal process of the palatine bones, and the body of the mandible are fractured. In addition, the zygoma is fractured (which is evident by the separation of the zygoma from the zygomatic process of the maxilla).

Chapter 2

1

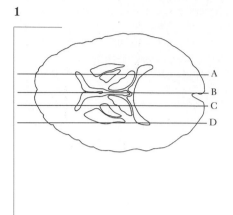

2

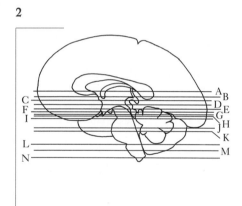

3

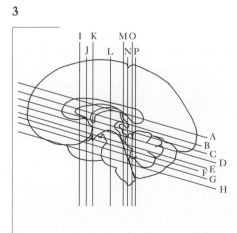

Reference illustrations

Brain

From the brain, and from the brain only, arise our pleasures, joys, laughter and jests, as well as our sorrows, pains, griefs, and tears.

Hippocrates (460?-377? B.C.)
The Sacred Disease

In Figure 2.1, Which portions of the ventricular system are being compressed by the mass? (Answer on p. 81.)

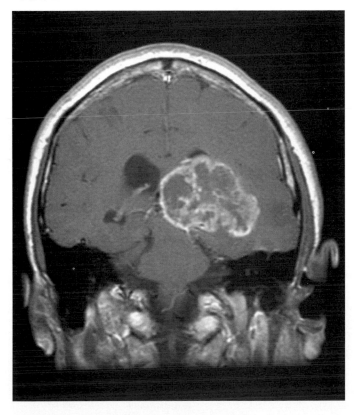

Figure 2.1   Coronal MR scan of abnormal brain.

The brain regulates and coordinates many critical functions from thought processes to bodily movements. For this reason, it is important to identify the anatomy of the brain.

Meninges

Ventricular System
ventricles
cisterns

Cerebrum
cerebral cortex
cerebral lobes
limbic system
basal ganglia
hypothalamus

Brain Stem
midbrain
pons
medulla oblongata

Cerebellum

Cerebral Vascular System
arterial supply
 internal carotid arteries
 vertebral arteries
 circle of Willis
dural sinuses
superficial cortical and deep veins

Cranial Nerves
olfactory nerve (CN I)
optic nerve (CN II)
oculomotor nerve (CN III)
trochlear nerve (CN IV)
trigeminal nerve (CN V)
abducens nerve (CN VI)
facial nerve (CN VII)
vestibulocochlear nerve (CN VIII)
glossopharyngeal nerve (CN IX)
vagus nerve (CN X)
accessory nerve (CN XI)
hypoglossal nerve (CN XII)

MENINGES

The brain is a delicate organ that is surrounded and protected by three membranes called the **meninges** (Figure 2.2). The outermost membrane, the **dura mater** (tough mother), is the toughest. This double-layered membrane is continuous with the periosteum of the cranium. Between the layers of dura mater are the meningeal arteries and the **dural sinuses.** The dural sinuses provide venous drainage from the brain. Folds of dura mater help to separate the structures of the brain and provide additional cushioning (Figure 2.3). Two dural folds are the **falx cerebri,** which separates the cerebral hemispheres, and the **tentorium cerebelli,** which rises up like a tent and forms a partition between the cerebrum and cerebellum (Figures 2.4 through 2.6).

Figure 2.2 Coronal cross section of meninges and subarachnoid space.

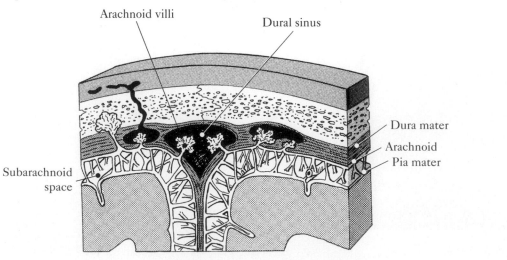

Figure 2.3 Sagittal view of falx cerebri and tentorium cerebelli.

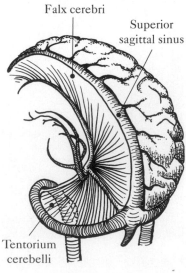

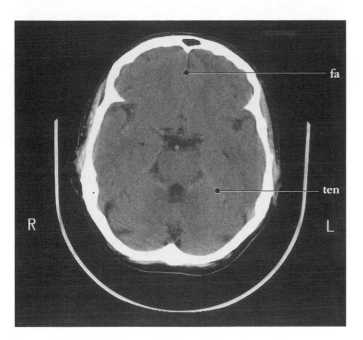

Figure 2.4   Axial CT scan of falx cerebri and tentorium cerebelli.   (R2.F)

Another dural fold, the **falx cerebelli,** separates the two cerebellar hemispheres. The middle membrane, known as the **arachnoid** (spiderlike), is a delicate, transparent membrane that is separated from the dura mater by a potential space called the **subdural space.** The arachnoid membrane follows the contour of the dura mater. The inner layer, or **pia mater** (delicate, tender mother), is a highly vascular layer that adheres closely to the contours of the brain. The **subarachnoid space** separates the pia mater from the arachnoid mater. This space contains cerebrospinal fluid, which circulates around the brain and spinal cord and provides further protection to the central nervous system (CNS).

Skull fractures with rupture of the meningeal arteries can cause a life-threatening condition known as an epidural hematoma.

Figure 2.5   Coronal MR scan of falx cerebri and tentorium cerebelli.   (R3.O)

Key.   du dura mater; **fa** falx cerebri; **ten** tentorium cerebelli.

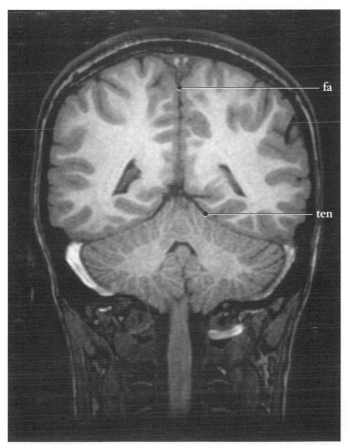

Figure 2.6   Sagittal MR scan of tentorium cerebelli.   (R1.B)

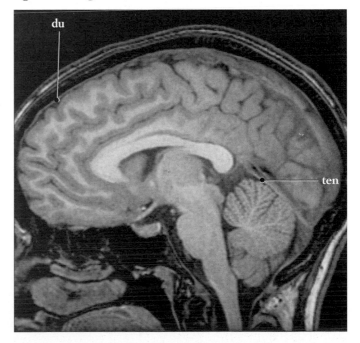

VENTRICULAR SYSTEM

VENTRICLES

The ventricular system provides a pathway for the circulation of the cerebral spinal fluid (CSF) throughout the CNS system. A major portion of the ventricular system is composed of four fluid-filled cavities (**ventricles**), which are located deep within the brain (Figures 2.7 and 2.8). The two most superior cavities are the **right** and **left lateral ventricles.** These ventricles lie within each cerebral hemisphere and are separated at the midline by a thin partition known as the **septum pellucidum.** The lateral ventricles consist of a central portion called the **body** and three extensions: the **anterior, occipital,** and **temporal horns.** The junction of the body and the occipital and temporal horns form the triangular area termed the **trigone (atria).** The lateral ventricles open downward into the **third ventricle** through the paired **interventricular foramen (foramen of Monro)** (Figures 2.9 and 2.10). The third ventricle is located midline just inferior to the lateral ventricles. The anterior wall of the third ventricle is formed by a thin membrane termed the **lamina terminalis.** The third ventricle communicates with the fourth ventricle via a narrow passageway termed the **cerebral aqueduct (aqueduct of Sylvius).** The **fourth ventricle** is a diamond-shaped cavity located anterior to the cerebellum (Figure 2.11). Separating the fourth ventricle from the cerebellum is a thin membrane forming the superior and inferior **medullary velum** (Figure 2.12).

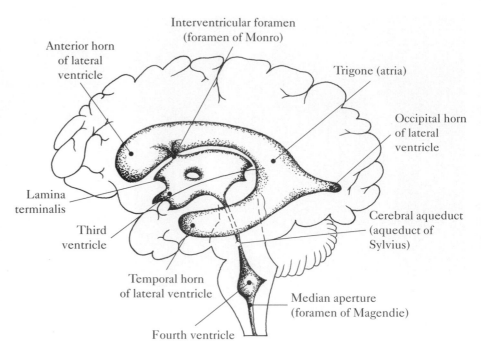

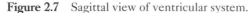

Figure 2.7   Sagittal view of ventricular system.

Figure 2.8   Anterior view of ventricles.

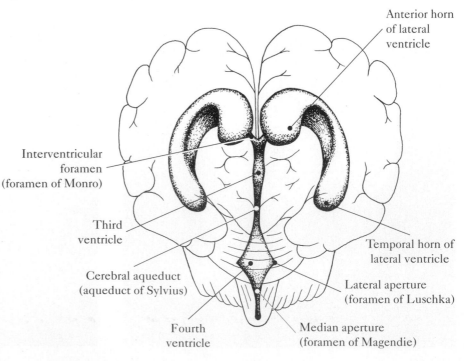

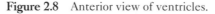

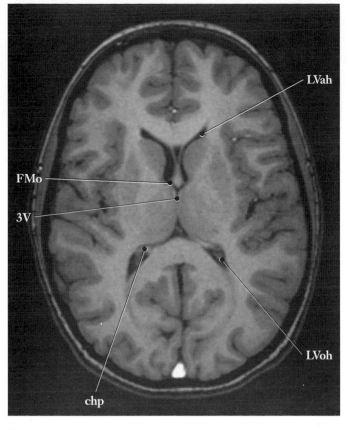

Figure 2.9   Axial MR scan of lateral ventricles.   (R2.A)

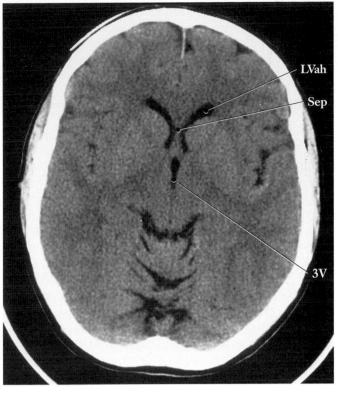

Figure 2.10   Axial CT scan of lateral ventricles.   (R3.C)

Key.   aque cerebral aqueduct; **cer** cerebellum; **chp** choroid plexus; **FMo** foramen of Monroe; **LV** lateral ventricle; **LVah** lateral ventricle, anterior horn; **LVoh** lateral ventricle, occipital horn; **Po** pons; **Sep** septum pellucidum; **smed** superior medullary velum; **3V** third ventricle; **4V** fourth ventricle.

Figure 2.11   Axial CT scan of fourth ventricle.   (R2.J)   **Figure 2.12**   Sagittal MR scan of ventricular system.   (R1.B)

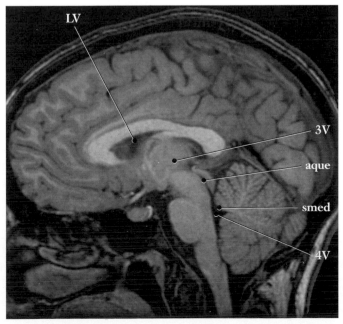

The lateral angles of the fourth ventricle extend to form the **lateral apertures (foramen of Luschka).** The inferior angle of the fourth ventricle has an opening called the **median aperture (foramen of Magendie),** which is continuous with the central canal of the spinal cord (Figures 2.13 and 2.14). The apertures allow for the passage of CSF between the ventricles and the subarachnoid space.

The septum pellucidum is frequently used as a landmark to determine if the midline of the brain has shifted as a result of trauma or pressure.

Located within the ventricular system is a network of blood vessels termed the **choroid plexus,** which produces CSF. The choroid plexus lines the floor of the lateral ventricles, roof of the third ventricle, and inferior medullary velum of the fourth ventricle (Fig. 2.14). Frequently the choroid plexus is partially calcified, making it more noticeable on CT scans (Figure 2.15). There exists a continuous circulation of CSF in and around the brain. Excess CSF is reabsorbed in the dural sinuses by way of **arachnoid villi.** These villi are berrylike projections of arachnoid that penetrate the dura mater. Enlargements of the arachnoid villi are termed granulations. Within the calvaria, these granulations can cause pitting or depressions that are variations of normal anatomy.

CISTERNS

The subarachnoid space is a relatively narrow, fluid-filled space surrounding the brain and spinal cord. There are locations, primarily around the base of the brain, where the subarachnoid space becomes widened. The combined term for these widened areas or pools of CSF is the **subarachnoidal cisterns.** Each cistern is generally named after the brain structure it borders. It is important to recognize the location of these cisterns so they are not misinterpreted as abnormalities.

One of the largest cisterns is the **cisterna magna.** It is located in the lower posterior fossa between the medulla oblongata, cerebellar hemispheres, and occipital bone. It is continuous with the subarachnoid space of the spinal canal (Figures 2.14 and 2.16).

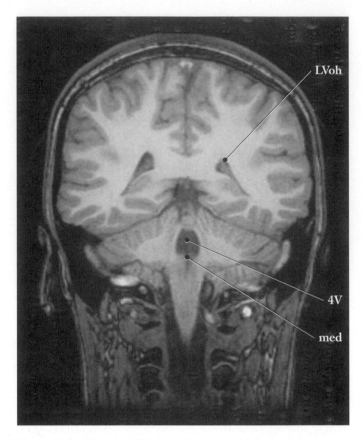

Figure 2.13   Coronal MR scan of lateral and fourth ventricles.   (R3.N)

Key.   LVoh lateral ventricle, occipital horn; **med** median aperture; **4V** fourth ventricle.

Figure 2.14   Sagittal view of choroid plexus and cisterns of ventricular system.

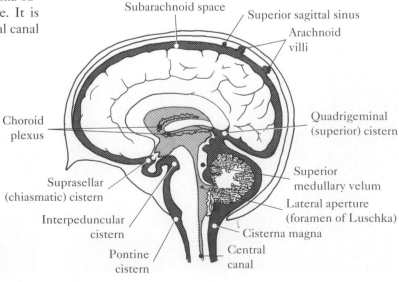

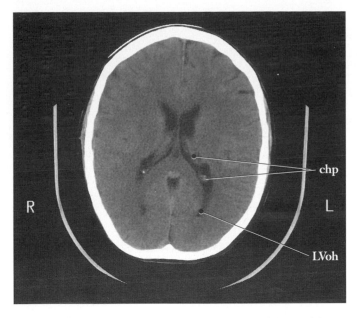

Figure 2.15   Axial CT scan of lateral ventricles with choroid plexus.   (R3.A)

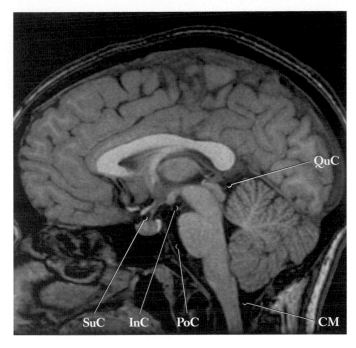

Figure 2.16   Midsagittal MR scan of cisterns.   (R1.B)

Key.   cer cerebellum; **chp** choroid plexus; **CM** cisterna magna; **CPAC** cerebellopontine angle cistern; **InC** interpeduncular cistern; **LVoh** lateral ventricle, occipital horn; **QuC** quadrigeminal cistern; **Po** pons; **PoC** pontine cistern; **SuC** suprasellar cistern; **4V** fourth ventricle.

Figure 2.17   Axial MR scan of cerebellopontine angle cistern.   (R2.K)

Figure 2.18   Axial CT scan of cisterna magna and cerebellopontine angle cistern.   (R2.K)

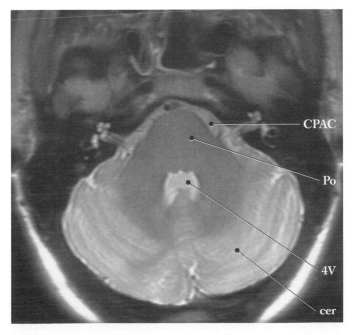

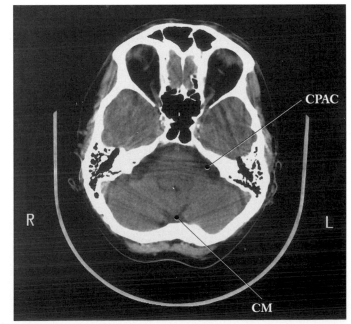

The **interpeduncular cistern** is located between the peduncles of the midbrain and communicates inferiorly with the pontine cistern. The **pontine cistern** is located just anterior and inferior to the pons and communicates laterally with the **cerebellopontine angle (CPA) cistern** (Figures 2.17 and 2.18). Important structures located within the cerebellopontine angle cistern include cranial nerves V, VII, and VIII, and the superior and anterior inferior cerebellar arteries. The **ambient cistern** connects the interpeduncular cistern with the **quadrigeminal (superior) cistern** as it courses around the lateral surface of the midbrain (Figures 2.19 and 2.20). The quadrigeminal cistern lies between the corpus callosum and the superior surface of the cerebellum just posterior to the quadrigeminal plate (Figure 2.21). Located above the sella is the **suprasellar (chiasmatic) cistern,** which contains the optic nerves and chiasm and the circle of Willis (Figures 2.19 and 2.20).

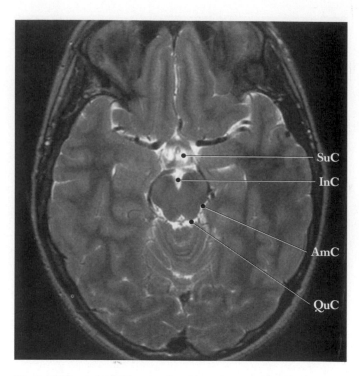

Figure 2.19   Axial MR scan of ambient, interpeduncular, and suprasellar cisterns.
(R2.F)

Key.   AmC ambient cistern; **fa** falx cerebri; **InC** interpeduncular cistern; **LVah** lateral ventricle, anterior horn; **QuC** quadrigeminal cistern; **SuC** suprasellar cistern; **3V** third ventricle.

Figure 2.20   Axial CT scan of ambient and interpeduncular cisterns.
(R2.F)

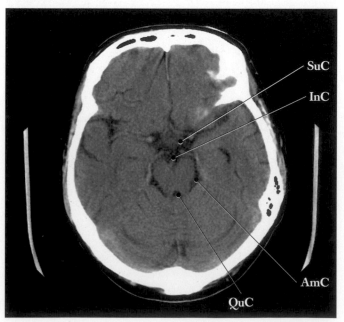

Figure 2.21   Axial CT scan of quadrigeminal cistern.   (R2.E)

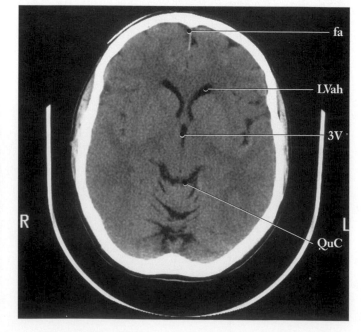

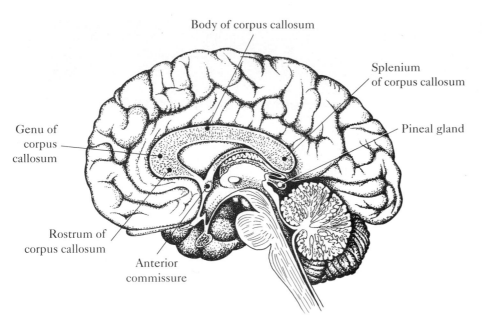

Body of corpus callosum

Splenium
of corpus callosum

Pineal gland

Genu of
corpus
callosum

Rostrum of
corpus callosum

Anterior
commissure

Figure 2.22   Sagittal view of cerebral cortex.

Key.   **CCb** corpus callosum, body; **CCg** corpus callosum, genu;
CCr corpus callosum, rostrum; **CCs** corpus callosum, splenium.

Figure 2.23   Midsagittal MR scan of cerebral cortex.   (R1.B)

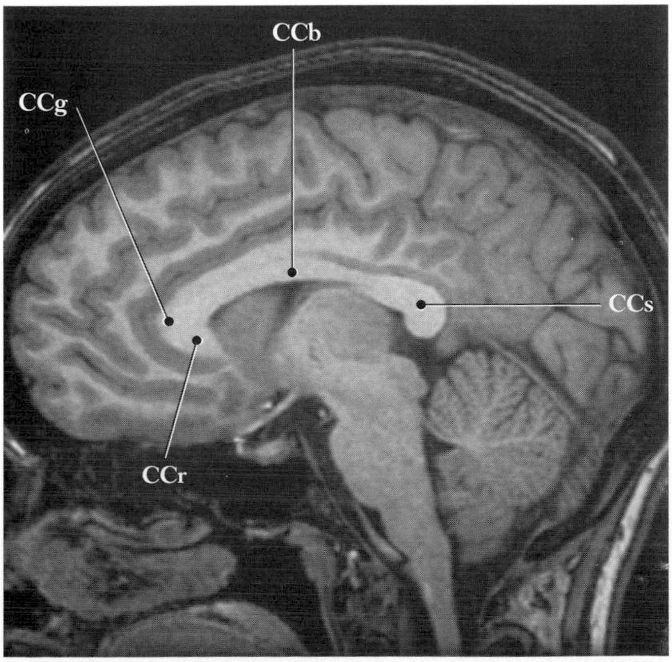

CEREBRUM

CEREBRAL CORTEX

The **cerebrum** is the largest portion of the brain and is divided into **left** and **right cerebral hemispheres.** The cerebrum as a whole has many critically important functions including thought, judgment, memory, and discrimination. The cerebrum consists of **gray matter** (neuron cell bodies) and **white matter** (myelinated axons). The **cerebral cortex,** the outermost portion of the cerebrum, is composed of gray matter approximately 3 to 5 mm thick. The cortex not only receives sensory input but also sends instructions to the muscles and glands for control of bodily movement and activity. Deep to the cortex is the white matter, which contains fibers that create pathways for the transmission of nerve impulses to and from the cortex. The largest and densest bundle of white matter fibers within the cerebrum is the **corpus callosum.** This midline structure forms the roof of the lateral ventricles and connects the right and left cerebral hemispheres. The four parts to the corpus callosum, from anterior to posterior, are the **rostrum, genu, body, and splenium** (Figures 2.22 through 2.25).

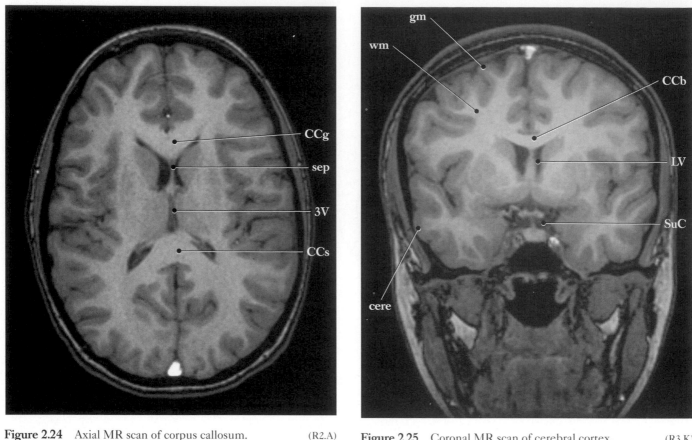

Figure 2.24   Axial MR scan of corpus callosum.   (R2.A)

Figure 2.25   Coronal MR scan of cerebral cortex.   (R3.K)

Key.   CCb corpus callosum, body; **CCg** corpus callosum, genu; **CCs** corpus callosum, splenium; **cere** cerebral cortex; **gm** gray matter; **LV** lateral ventricle; **sep** septum pellucidum; **SuC** suprasellar cistern; **wm** white matter; **3V** third ventricle.

Figure 2.26   Axial view of cerebral cortex and corpus callosum.

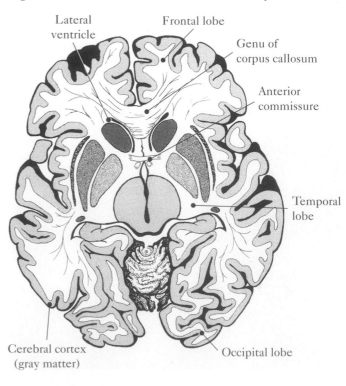

Another important bundle of white matter fibers is the **anterior commissure** (Figure 2.26). This group of fibers crosses the midline within the lamina terminalis and connects the anterior portions of each temporal lobe. The **posterior commissure** is a pathway made of several fibers that transmit nerve impulses for pupillary (consensual) light reflexes. This pathway crosses the midline just inferior to the **pineal gland** (Figure 2.26). The pineal gland, an endocrine structure, secretes the hormone melatonin, which aids in the regulation of day/night cycles and reproductive functions. The pineal gland is located posterior to the third ventricle and is sometimes calcified (Figures 2.22 and 2.27).

CEREBRAL LOBES

The cerebral cortex can be divided into four individual lobes: frontal, parietal, occipital, and temporal. These four lobes correspond in location to the cranial bones with the same name (Figures 2.28 and 2.29). Each lobe has cortical regions with specific functions. The largest of the four lobes is the **frontal lobe,** which is generally concerned with personality and voluntary motor activities. The **parietal lobe** is concerned with peripheral sensations, and the **occipital lobe** is concerned with vision. The **temporal lobe** deals with sensations of smell, taste, and hearing. Another area of cortical gray matter located under the lateral surface of the temporal lobes is the **insula,** frequently referred to as the fifth lobe. The insula mediates motor and sensory function of the organs (Figures 2.30 and 2.31).

Table 2.1   Cerebral lobes

REGION	FUNCTIONS
Frontal lobe	Voluntary motor control; personality
Parietal lobe	Peripheral sensations
Occipital lobe	Vision
Temporal lobe	Sensations of smell, taste, and hearing
Insula	Mediation of motor and sensory functions

Key.   **acom** anterior commissure; **LVoh** lateral ventricle, occipital horn; **pcom** posterior commissure; **PG** pineal gland; **3V** third ventricle.

Figure 2.27   Axial MR scan of anterior and posterior commissures.   (R2.C)

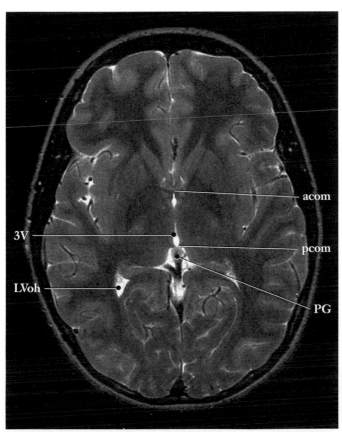

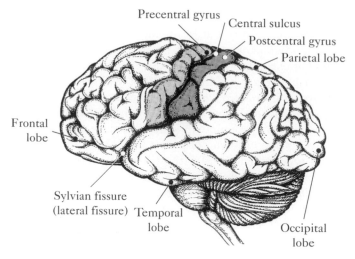

Figure 2.28   Sagittal view of cerebral lobes.

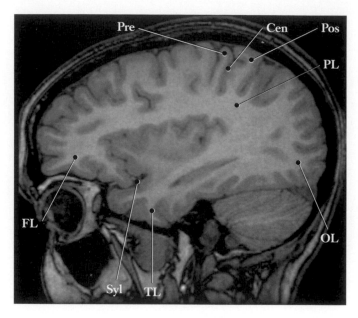

Figure 2.29   Sagittal MR scan of cerebral lobes.   (R1.D)

Key.   Cen central sulcus; **Cer** cerebellum; **FL** frontal lobe; **Ins** insula; **OL** occipital lobe; **PL** parietal lobe; **Pos** postcentral gyrus; **pcom** posterior commissure; **Pre** precentral gyrus; **Syl** Sylvian fissure; **TL** temporal lobe.

Figure 2.30   Axial MR scan of cerebral lobes.   (R2.C)

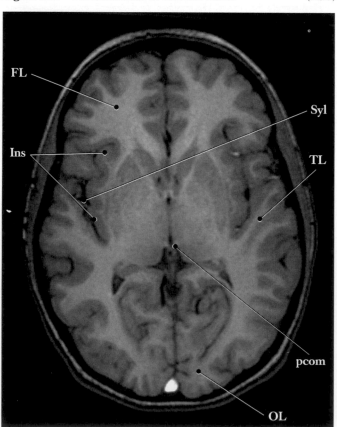

Figure 2.31   Axial CT scan of cerebral lobes.   (R2.D)

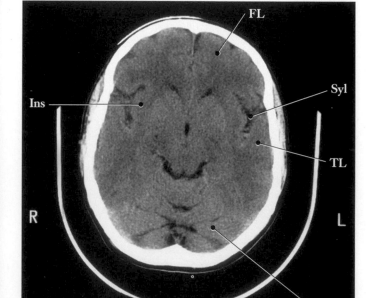

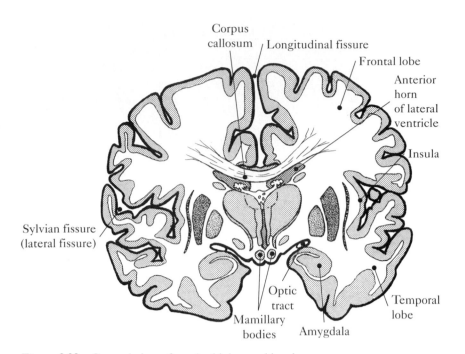

Figure 2.32   Coronal view of cerebral lobes and insula.

The cerebral cortex of each hemisphere is arranged in folds of gray matter called **gyri.** The gyri are separated by shallow grooves called **sulci** and by deeper grooves called **fissures.** The main sulcus that can be identified on CT and MR images of the brain is the **central sulcus,** which divides the **precentral gyrus** of the frontal lobe and **postcentral gyrus** of the parietal lobe (Figures 2.28 and 2.29). These gyri are important to identify because the precentral gyrus is considered the motor strip of the brain and the postcentral gyrus is considered the sensory strip of the brain. Two main fissures of the cerebrum are the **longitudinal fissure** and the **sylvian fissure** (lateral fissure). The longitudinal fissure is a long, deep furrow that divides the left and right cerebral hemispheres. The sylvian fissure separates the frontal and parietal lobes from the temporal lobe (Figures 2.32 and 2.33).

Key. Ins insula; **lon** longitudinal fissure; **PL** parietal lobe; **Syl** Sylvian fissure; **TL** temporal lobe; **3V** third ventricle.

Figure 2.33   Coronal MR scan with cerebral lobes and insula.

(R3.L)

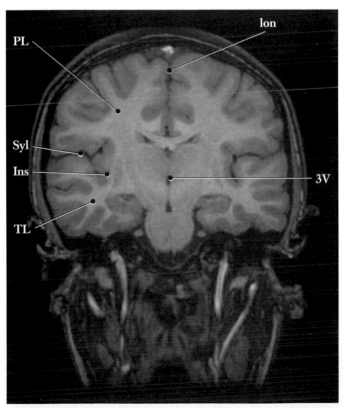

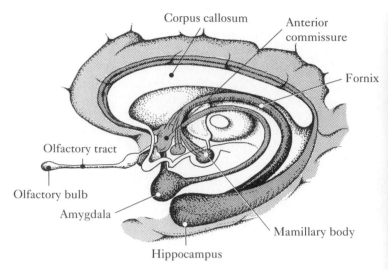

Figure 2.34   Sagittal view of limbic system.

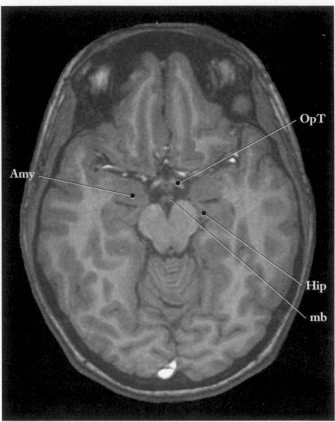

Figure 2.35   Axial MR scan of hippocampus.   (R2.F)

Key.   **AmC** ambient cistern; **Amy** amygdala; **Hip** hippocampus; **mb** mamillary body; **OpT** optic tract.

Figure 2.36   Axial CT scan of hippocampus.   (R3.E)

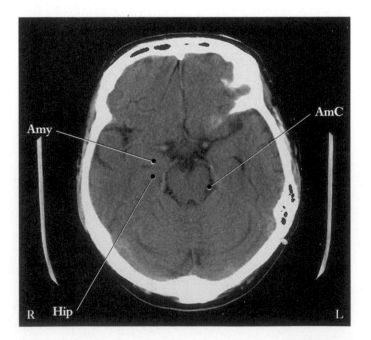

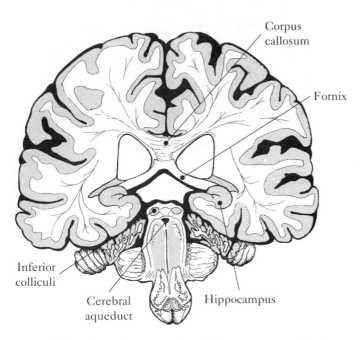

Figure 2.37   Coronal cross section of hippocampus and fornix.

Key.   for fornix; **Hip** hippocampus; **InC** interpeduncular cistern; **3V** third ventricle.

Figure 2.38   Coronal MR scan of hippocampus.   (R3.L)

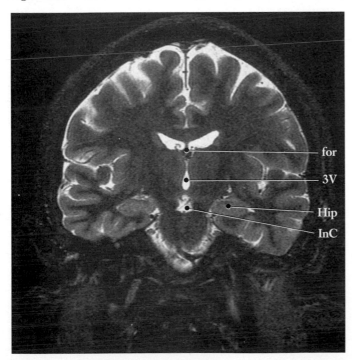

LIMBIC SYSTEM

The **limbic system** is a complex group of brain structures and fiber tracts located within and adjacent to the medial surface of the temporal lobes. They contain critical connecting pathways that extend to other areas deep within the midbrain, basal ganglia, and cerebral hemispheres. These structures have a common functional role in the emotional aspects of behavior. Particularly, the limbic system is involved in aggression, submissive and sexual behavior, memory, learning, and general emotional responses. Structures of the limbic system include the **hippocampus, amygdala, fornix, olfactory bulbs,** and **mamillary bodies** (Figure 2.34). The hippocampus is the inrolled medial border of the temporal lobe that resembles the shape of a sea horse when viewed in the coronal plane. The hippocampus is important for the transition from short-term to long-term memory. The amygdala is a mass of gray matter in the anterior medial portion of the temporal lobe and is concerned with olfactory reflexes and aggressive and sexual behavior (Figures 2.35 and 2.36). The limbic system is integrated with other structures of the brain via limbic tracts. The most frequently identified limbic tract is the **fornix.** The fornix is an arch-shaped structure that lies below the splenium of the corpus callosum and makes up the inferior margin of the septum pellucidum (Figures 2.37 and 2.38). It serves specifically to integrate the hippocampus with other functional areas of the brain. The olfactory tracts run underneath the frontal lobes and connect to the amygdala to bring information on the sense of smell to the limbic system. The mamillary bodies can be found at the anterior end of the fornix. They receive direct input from the hippocampus and give rise to fibers that terminate in the periaqueductal gray matter of the midbrain (Figures 2.34 and 2.35).

Damage to the hippocampus may result in a loss of memory. High-resolution MR images of the hippocampus are useful in evaluating patients with dementia or seizures.

BASAL GANGLIA

The basal ganglia are a collection of subcortical gray matter consisting of the **caudate nucleus, lentiform nucleus, claustrum,** and **thalamus** (Figures 2.39 and 2.40). Collectively, they contribute to the planning and programming of movement. The largest basal ganglia nuclei are the caudate nucleus and lentiform nucleus. Both nuclei serve as relay stations between the thalamus and the cerebral cortex of the same side. The caudate nucleus parallels the lateral ventricle and consists of a head, body, and tail. The head causes an indentation to the frontal horns of the lateral ventricles, and the tail terminates in the amygdala of the temporal lobe. The lentiform nucleus is a biconvex lens–shaped mass of gray matter located between the insula, caudate nucleus, and the thalamus. The lentiform nucleus can be further divided into the globus pallidus and the putamen. The claustrum is a thin linear layer of gray matter lying between the insula and the lentiform nucleus (Figure 2.41).

The thalamus is a pair of large oval gray masses, which are interconnected with most regions of the brain and spinal cord via a vast number of fiber tracts. The thalamus makes up a portion of the walls of the third ventricle and connects through the middle of the third ventricle by adhesions known as the **massa intermedia.**

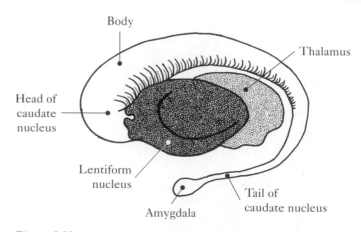

Figure 2.39   Lateral view of basal ganglia with C-shape of caudate nucleus.

Key.   **cl** claustrum; **exc** external capsule; **hcn** head of caudate nucleus; **inc** internal capsule; **ln** lentiform nucleus.

Figure 2.41   Coronal MR scan of basal ganglia.   (R3.J)

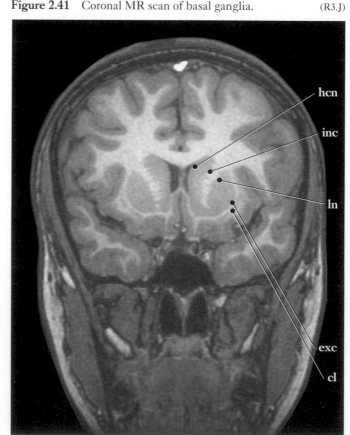

Key.   **Amy** amygdala; **Hip** hippocampus; **LVah** lateral ventricle, anterior horn.

Figure 2.40   Sagittal MR scan with basal ganglia.   (R1.C)

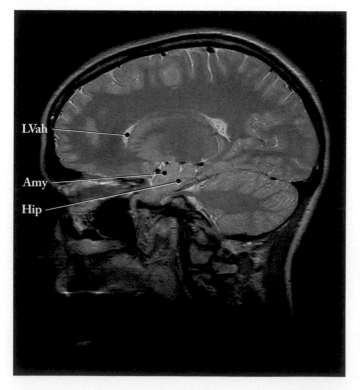

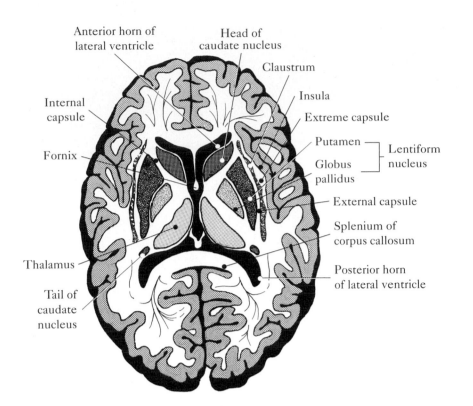

Figure 2.42   Axial view of basal ganglia.

The thalamus serves as a relay station to and from the cerebral cortex for all sensory stimuli with the exception of the olfactory nerves. Tracts of white matter separate the basal ganglia and transmit electrical impulses throughout the brain. The **internal capsule** is shaped like a boomerang and separates the thalamus and caudate nucleus from the lentiform nucleus. The **external capsule** is a thin layer of white matter that separates the claustrum from the lentiform nucleus (Figures 2.42 through 2.44).

> The striate branches of the middle cerebral artery are located within the internal capsule, causing this area to be the most frequent site of strokes.

Key.   cl claustrum; **exc** external capsule; **for** fornix; **gl** globus pallidus; **hcn** head of caudate nucleus; **inc** internal capsule; **Ins** insula; **ln** lentiform nucleus; **pu** putamen; **th** thalamus.

Figure 2.43   Axial MR scan of basal ganglia.   (R2.C)

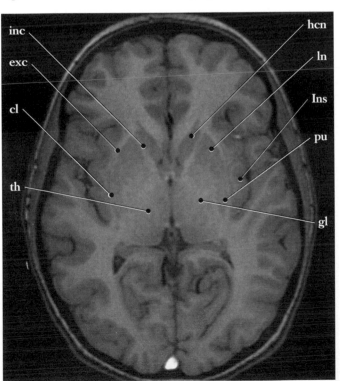

Figure 2.44   Axial CT scan of basal ganglia.   (R3.C)

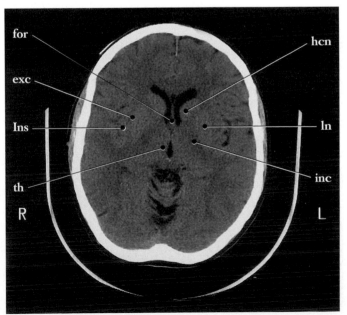

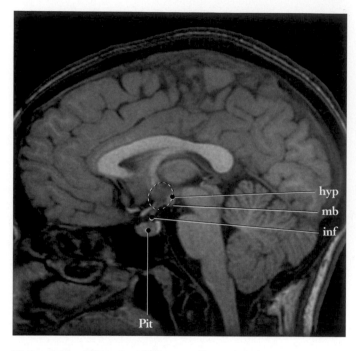

Figure 2.45   Midsagittal MR scan of hypothalamus.   (R1.B)

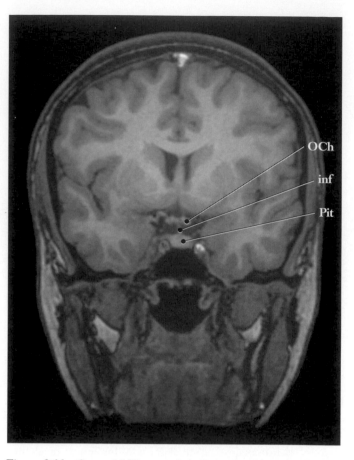

Figure 2.46   Coronal MR scan of pituitary gland and optic chiasm.   (R3.K)

Key.   hyp hypothalamus; **ICA** internal carotid artery; **inf** infundibulum; **mb** mamillary body; **OCh** optic chiasm; **Pit** pituitary gland; **SpS** sphenoid sinus.

Figure 2.48   Axial MR scan of pituitary gland.   (R2.H)

Figure 2.47   Coronal CT scan of pituitary gland.   (R3.J)

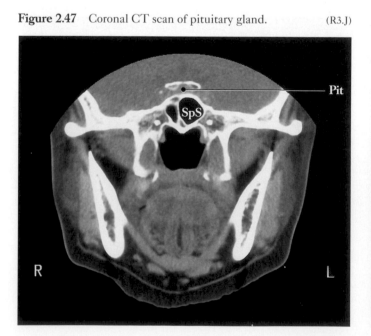

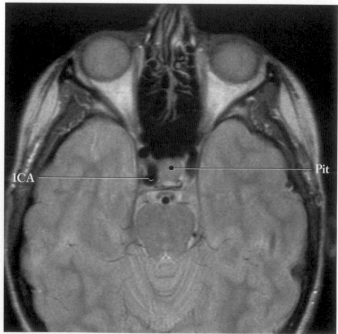

HYPOTHALAMUS

The **hypothalamus** forms the floor of the third ventricle and includes the optic chiasm and mamillary bodies (Figure 2.45). It controls autonomic activity such as the regulation of temperature, appetite, and sleep patterns.

The **pituitary gland (hypophysis)** is an endocrine gland connected to the hypothalamus by the **infundibulum.** The infundibulum is a slender stalk located between the optic chiasm and the mamillary bodies. The pituitary gland is nestled in the sella turcica at the base of the brain. The protected location of this gland suggests its importance. It is known as the *master gland* because it controls and regulates the function of many of the other glands through the action of its six major types of hormones. The pituitary gland can be broken down into an anterior lobe (adenohypophysis) and a posterior lobe (neurohypophysis) (Figures 2.46 through 2.48).

BRAIN STEM

The **brain stem** is a relatively small mass of tissue packed with motor and sensory nuclei, making it vital for normal brain function. Ten of the twelve cranial nerves originate from the brain stem. Its major segments are the **midbrain, pons,** and **medulla oblongata.** The brain stem connects the cerebral hemispheres with the spinal cord (Figure 2.49).

MIDBRAIN

The **midbrain (mesencephalon),** which is located above the pons at the junction of the middle and posterior cranial fossae, is the smallest portion of the brain stem. The midbrain is composed primarily of bundles of nerve fibers and can be divided into two major segments, the **colliculi (quadrigeminal plate)** and the **cerebral peduncles** (Figure 2.50). The midbrain surrounds the **cerebral aqueduct,** which contains CSF and connects the third and fourth ventricles.

Key. **aque** cerebral aqueduct; **cer** cerebellum; **cton** cerebellar tonsils; **iCol** inferior colliculi; **Med** medulla oblongata; **Mid** midbrain; **PG** pineal gland; **Po** pons; **sCol** superior colliculi; **4V** fourth ventricle.

Figure 2.49   Midsagittal MR scan of brain stem.   (R1.B)

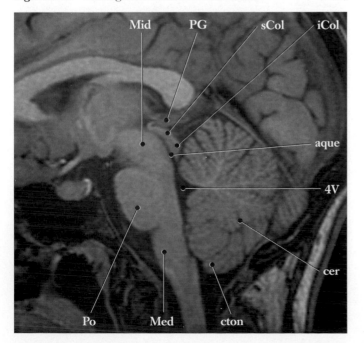

Figure 2.50   Oblique view of brain stem.

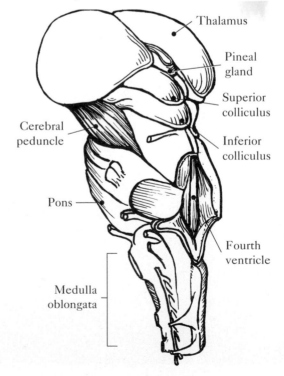

Posterior to the cerebral aqueduct is the **tectum,** which makes up the roof or dorsal surface of the midbrain. The tectum consists of four rounded protuberances termed colliculi (Figures 2.49 and 2.51). The upper pair, **superior colliculi,** are associated with the optic system. The lower pair, **inferior colliculi,** are relay stations associated with the auditory system. Anterior to the cerebral aqueduct are two cerebral peduncles (Figures 2.52 and 2.53). These ropelike bundles, composed predominantly of motor nerve fibers, extend from the cerebral cortex to the spinal cord.

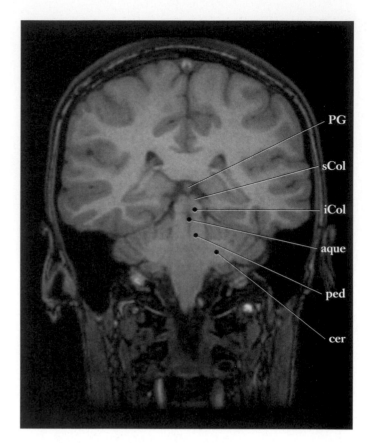

Key. **Amy** amygdala; **aque** cerebral aqueduct; **cer** cerebellum; **Hip** hippocampus; **iCol** inferior colliculi; **InC** interpeduncular cistern; **ped** cerebral peduncle; **PG** pineal gland; **QuC** quadrigeminal cistern; **sCol** superior colliculi.

Figure 2.51   Coronal MR scan of midbrain.   (R3.M)

Figure 2.52   Axial MR scan of cerebral peduncles and inferior colliculi.   (R2.F)

Figure 2.53   Axial CT scan of cerebral peduncles and inferior colliculi.   (R3.D)

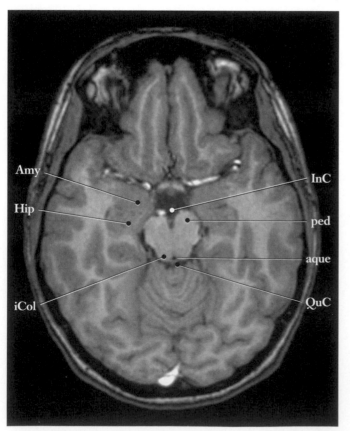

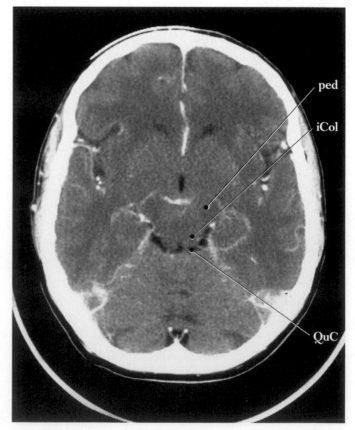

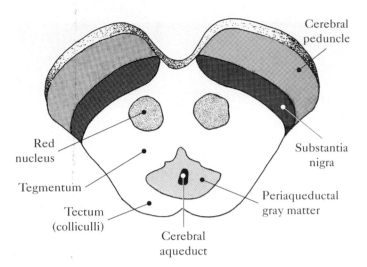

Figure 2.54   Axial view of cerebral peduncles.

The cerebral peduncles are made more noticeable by the presence of the darkly pigmented **substantia nigra,** a broad layer of cells that contain melanin. The substantia nigra is involved with the production of dopamine, a neurotransmitter in the brain that functions in the control of muscular reflexes. Deep within the midbrain, between the cerebral peduncles and the cerebral aqueduct, is the **tegmentum.** Within the tegmentum, at the level of the superior colliculi, is the **red nucleus.** The red nucleus is composed of a tract of motor nerve fibers and serves as a relay station between the cerebellum and the cerebral hemispheres. The red nucleus contributes to the coordination of movements and to the sense of balance. Another portion of the tegmentum is the **periaqueductal gray matter,** which surrounds the cerebral aqueduct. This area receives sensory input that conveys pain and temperature to the brain (Figures 2.54 through 2.56).

> If neurons in the substantia nigra are damaged, dopamine production is decreased, leading to the increased muscle spasticity of Parkinson's disease.

Key.   aque cerebral aqueduct; **ped** cerebral peduncle; **rn** red nucleus; **sub** substantia nigra.

Figure 2.55   Axial MR scan of midbrain and substantia nigra.   (R2.G)

Key.   aque   cerebral aqueduct **QuC** quadrigeminal cistern; **sCol** superior colliculi; **3V** third ventricle.

Figure 2.56   Axial CT scan of superior colliculi.   (R3.C)

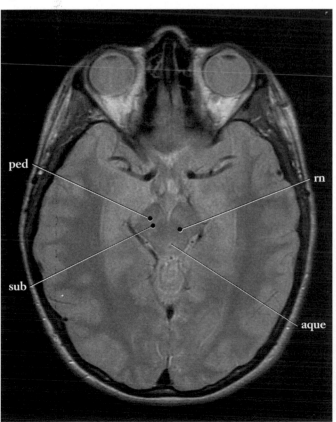

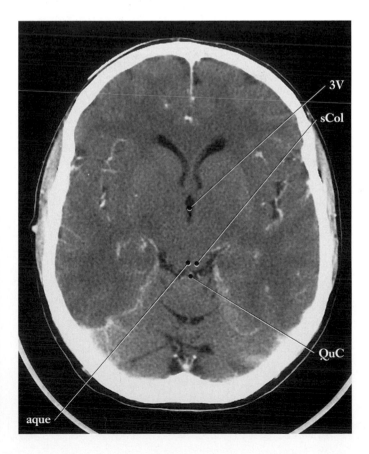

PONS

The **pons** is the large expansion of the brain stem located between the midbrain and medulla oblongata, posterior to the clivus. The term *pons* literally means bridge. This definition is appropriate because the pontine fibers serve to connect the cerebrum and cerebellum (Figures 2.57 through 2.59).

Key. BaA basilar artery; **Ins** insula; **Po** pons; **4V** fourth ventricle.

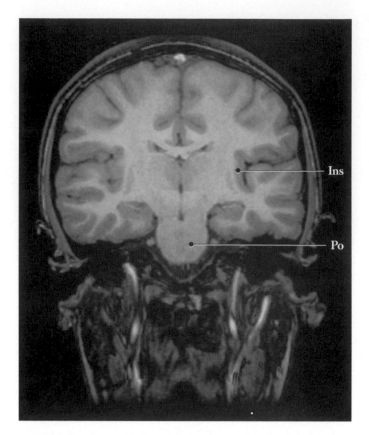

Figure 2.57 Coronal MR scan of pons. (R3.L)

Figure 2.58 Axial MR scan of pons. (R2.I)

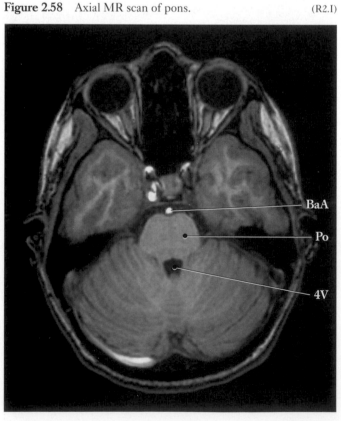

Figure 2.59 Axial CT scan of pons. (R2.J)

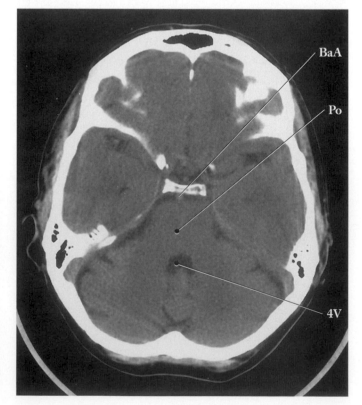

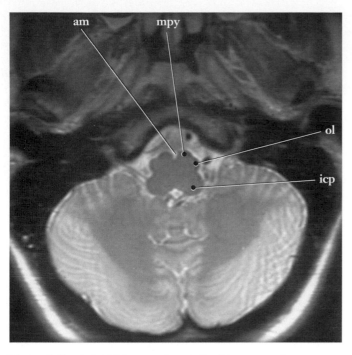

Figure 2.60   Axial MR scan of medulla oblongata and olive.   (R2.M)

Key.   am anterior median fissure; **icp** inferior cerebellar peduncle; **mpy** medullary pyramid; **ol** olive.

MEDULLA OBLONGATA

The **medulla oblongata** extends from the pons to the foramen magnum, where it continues as the spinal cord. The medulla oblongata contains all fiber tracts between the brain and spinal cord, as well as vital centers that regulate internal activities of the body. These centers are involved in the control of heart rate, respiratory rhythm, and blood pressure. The center of the anterior and posterior surfaces of the medulla oblongata are marked by the **anterior** and **posterior median fissures**. These two fissures divide the medulla oblongata into two symmetric halves. Located on either side of the anterior median fissure are two bundles of nerve fibers called **pyramids** (Figure 2.60). The pyramids contain the nerve tracts that contribute to voluntary motor control. At the lower end of the pyramids, some of the nerve tracts cross over (decussate) to the opposite side. This decussation in part accounts for the fact that each half of the brain controls the opposite half of the body. On each lateral surface of the medulla oblongata is a rounded oval prominence termed **olive**. The olives consist of nuclei that are involved in coordination, balance, and modulation of sound impulses from the inner ear (Figures 2.61 and 2.62).

Key.   aque cerebral aqueduct; **ol** olive; **ped** cerebral peduncle; **PG** pineal gland; **sCol** superior colliculi.

Figure 2.62   Coronal MR scan of olive and medulla oblongata.   (R3.M)

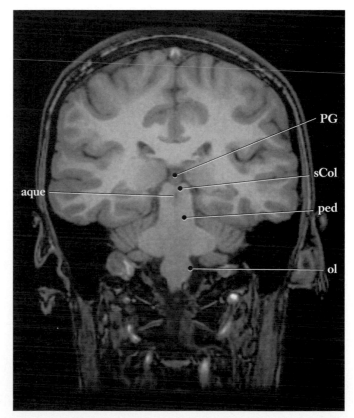

Figure 2.61   Coronal view of medulla oblongata.

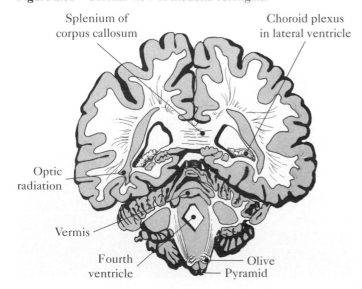

Splenium of corpus callosum

Choroid plexus in lateral ventricle

Optic radiation

Vermis

Fourth ventricle

Olive

Pyramid

CEREBELLUM

The **cerebellum,** which is referred to as the "little brain," attaches posteriorly to the brain stem and occupies the posterior cranial fossa. The cerebellum is the coordination center for motor functions. Although the cerebellum does not initiate actual motor functions, it interacts with many brain stem structures to execute a variety of movements, including maintenance of muscle tone, posture, balance, and coordination of movement.

The cerebellum consists of two **cerebellar hemispheres** (lateral hemispheres). These cerebellar hemispheres have an interesting appearance because the folds of gray matter give the appearance of cauliflower. The **vermis** connects the two cerebellar hemispheres at the midline. On the inferior surface of the cerebellar hemispheres are two rounded prominences called the **cerebellar tonsils** (Figures 2.63 and 2.64). Occasionally, these tonsils can be seen herniating down through the foramen magnum.

A defect involving downward displacement of the brain stem and cerebellum through the foramen magnum is termed Arnold-Chiari malformation (deformity).

Key. **cer** cerebellum; **cton** cerebellar tonsil; **Mid** midbrain; **ten** tentorium cerebelli; **4V** fourth ventricle.

Figure 2.63   Sagittal MR scan of cerebellum.   (R1.B)

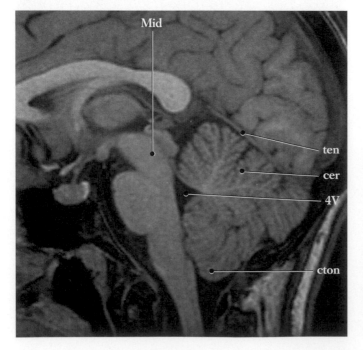

Key. **cer** cerebellum; **dn** dentate nucleus; **StS** straight sinus; **ver** vermis.

Figure 2.64   Coronal MR scan of cerebellum and dentate nucleus.   (R3.P)

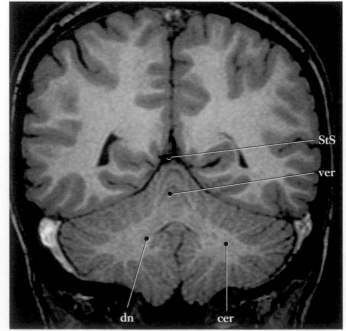

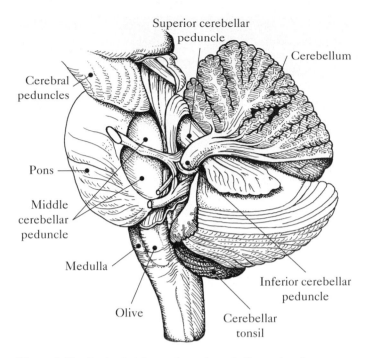

Figure 2.65   Sagittal oblique view of cerebellar peduncles.

Three pairs of nerve tracts, the **cerebellar peduncles,** connect the cerebellum to the brain stem (Figure 2.65). The **superior cerebellar peduncles** connect the cerebellum to the midbrain (Figures 2.66 and 2.67). The **middle cerebellar peduncles** serve as attachments to the pons, and the **inferior cerebellar peduncles** attach to the medulla oblongata (Figures 2.68 and 2.69).

Within each cerebellar hemisphere is a **dentate nucleus,** which is the largest of the deep cerebellar nuclei. Fibers of the dentate nucleus project to the thalamus via the superior cerebellar peduncles (Figure 2.64). From here, the fibers travel to the motor areas of the cerebral cortex, namely the precentral gyrus, thus influencing motor control.

Key.   BaA basilar artery; **Po** pons; **scp** superior cerebellar peduncle; **4V** fourth ventricle.

Figure 2.66   Axial MR scan of superior cerebellar peduncles.   (R2.I)

Key.   AmC ambient cistern; **scp** superior cerebellar peduncle.

Figure 2.67   Axial CT scan of superior cerebellar peduncles.   (R3.E)

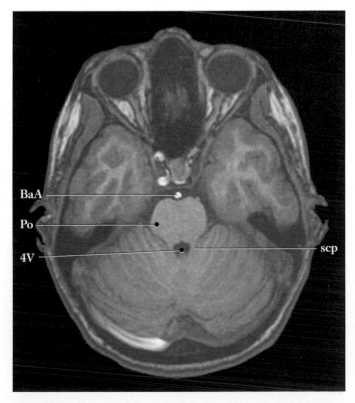

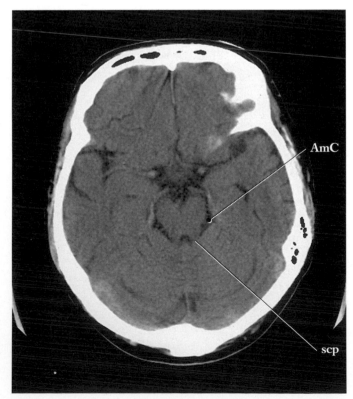

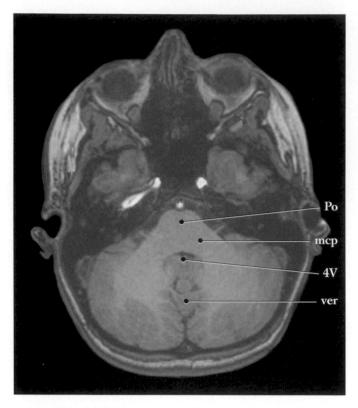

Figure 2.68 Axial MR scan of middle cerebellar peduncles. (R2.K)

Key. mcp middle cerebellar peduncle; **Po** pons; **ver** vermis; **4V** fourth ventricle.

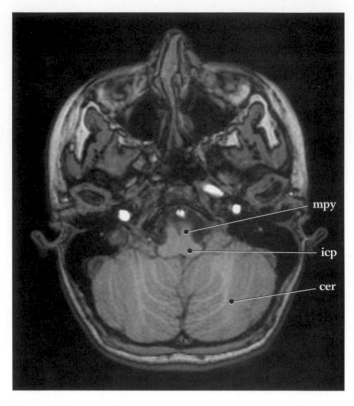

Figure 2.69 Axial MR scan of inferior cerebellar peduncles. (R2.L)

Key. cer cerebellum; **icp** inferior cerebellar peduncle; **mpy** medullary pyramid.

Figure 2.70 Sagittal view of cerebral arterial supply.

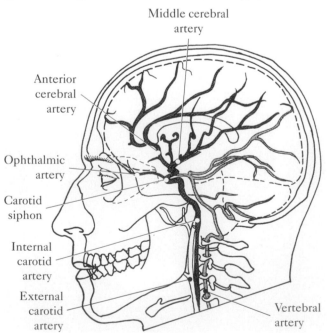

Middle cerebral artery

Anterior cerebral artery

Ophthalmic artery

Carotid siphon

Internal carotid artery

External carotid artery

Vertebral artery

Figure 2.71 Coronal view of cerebral arterial system.

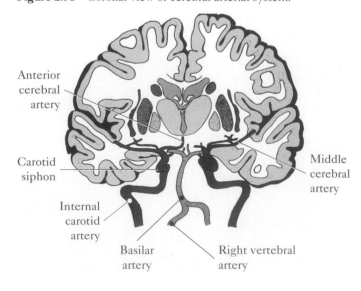

Anterior cerebral artery

Carotid siphon

Internal carotid artery

Basilar artery

Middle cerebral artery

Right vertebral artery

CEREBRAL VASCULAR SYSTEM

The vascular supply to the brain is unique. In comparison to the arteries in the body, the walls of the arteries in the brain are thin and weak, causing them to be susceptible to aneurysms and strokes. The veins of the brain do not contain valves. This lack of valves allows the blood to flow in either direction, creating a route for blood-borne pathogens to pass from the body to the head and vice versa. The capillaries of the brain are unlike those elsewhere in the body in that they do not allow movement of certain molecules from their vascular compartment into the surrounding brain tissue. This unique quality of impermeability is termed the **blood-brain barrier (BBB)**. The presence of a normal blood-brain barrier prevents large amounts of contrast medium from entering the brain. Pathologic conditions can disrupt the integrity of the BBB, allowing contrast to escape from the vessel into the surrounding tissues.

Key. **ACA** anterior cerebral artery; **cav** cavernous portion of internal carotid artery; **ICA** internal carotid artery; **MCA** middle cerebral artery; **PCA** posterior cerebral artery; **PCoA** posterior communicating artery; **siph** carotid siphon; **VA** vertebral artery.

ARTERIAL SUPPLY

The brain receives arterial blood supply from two main pairs of vessels and their branches, the internal carotid arteries and the vertebral arteries. Many normal variations of the arterial blood supply exist. This section focuses on the most common anatomic findings visualized in cross section (Figures 2.70 and 2.71).

INTERNAL CAROTID ARTERIES.   The **internal carotid arteries** supply the frontal, parietal, and temporal lobes of the brain and orbital structures. These arteries arise from the common carotid arteries in the neck and ascend to the base of the skull, where they enter the carotid canals of the temporal bones. The internal carotid artery then turns forward within the cavernous sinus and up and backward through the dura mater, forming an **S**-shape (which is referred to as the **carotid siphon**) before it reaches the base of the brain (Figures 2.72 through 2.74). As the internal carotid artery exits the cavernous sinus, it branches into the **ophthalmic artery** just inferior to the anterior clinoid process. The internal carotid artery runs lateral to the optic chiasm and then branches into a large **middle cerebral artery** and a smaller **anterior cerebral artery**.

Key. **BaA** basilar artery; **car** carotid canal.

Figure 2.74   Axial MR scan with carotid canal.   (R2.L)

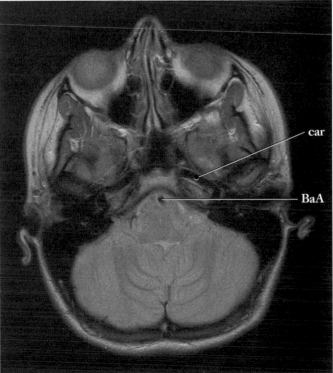

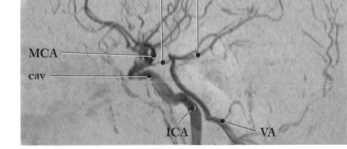

Figure 2.72   Sagittal MRA of cerebral arteries.

Figure 2.73   Coronal MRA of cerebral arteries.

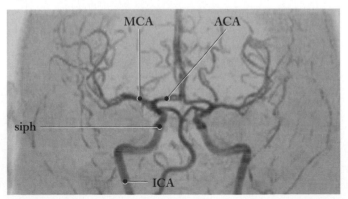

The middle cerebral artery supplies much of the lateral aspect of the cerebrum. It divides into multiple branches that course into the sylvian fissure (Figure 2.75). The anterior cerebral artery and its branches course around the genu of the corpus callosum to supply the anterior frontal lobe and the medial aspect of the cerebral hemispheres. The anterior cerebral arteries meet in the midline to form a short **anterior communicating artery.** This small but important vessel creates an anastomosis between the left and right cerebral hemispheres of the brain. Another small vessel, the **posterior communicating artery,** connects the internal carotid artery to the posterior cerebral artery (Figures 2.76 and 2.77).

Table 2.2 Internal carotid artery branches

ARTERY	REGION SUPPLIED
Ophthalmic artery (OA)	Eyes
Anterior cerebral artery (ACA)	Frontal and parietal lobes
Middle cerebral artery (MCA)	Lateral surfaces of cerebrum

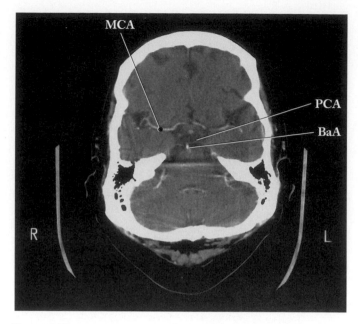

Figure 2.75 Axial CT scan with middle cerebral artery. (R3.F)

Key. ACA anterior cerebral artery; **ACoA** anterior communicating artery; **aque** cerebral aqueduct; **BaA** basilar artery; **MCA** middle cerebral artery; **PCA** posterior cerebral artery; **PCoA** posterior communicating artery; **QuC** quadrigeminal cistern.

Figure 2.76 Axial MR scan with anterior communicating artery. (R2.F)

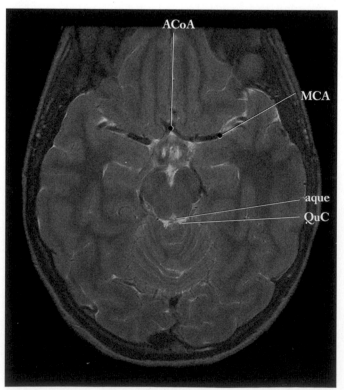

Figure 2.77 Axial CT scan with anterior cerebral artery. (R3.E)

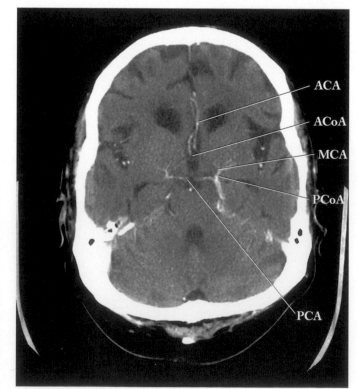

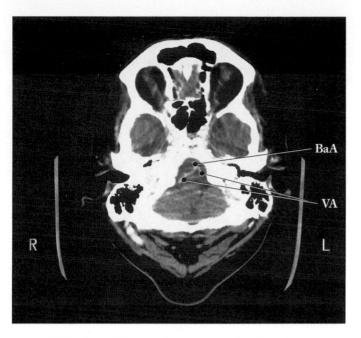

Figure 2.78   Axial CT scan of vertebral and basilar arteries.   (R3.H)

Key.   BaA basilar artery; **VA** vertebral artery.

VERTEBRAL ARTERIES.   The **vertebral arteries** begin in the neck at the subclavian artery and ascend vertically through the transverse foramina of the cervical spine (see Figures 2.70 and 2.71). The vertebral arteries curve around the atlantooccipital joints to enter the cranium through the foramen magnum. The two vertebral arteries course along the medulla oblongata and unite, ventral to the pons, to form the **basilar artery** (Figure 2.78). The vertebral and basilar arteries give rise to several pairs of smaller arteries that supply the cerebellum, pons, and inferior and medial surfaces of the temporal and occipital lobes. The four major pairs of arteries are listed in order from inferior to superior: **posterior inferior cerebellar (PICA), anterior inferior cerebellar (AICA), superior cerebellar (SCA), posterior cerebral (PCA)** (Figures 2.79 through 2.82). Located between the anterior inferior cerebellar artery and the superior cerebellar artery are many tiny perforating **pontine vessels.** The posterior cerebral arteries interconnect with the internal carotid arteries by way of the small posterior communicating artery (Figure 2.83).

Table 2.3   Vertebral and basilar artery branches

ARTERY	REGION SUPPLIED
Posterior inferior cerebellar artery (PICA)	Inferior cerebellum
Anterior inferior cerebellar artery (AICA)	Anterior and inferior cerebellum
Pontine vessels	Pons
Superior cerebellar artery (SCA)	Superior cerebellum and portions of midbrain and pons
Posterior cerebral artery (PCA)	Occipital lobes

Figure 2.79   Sagittal view of vertebral arterial system.

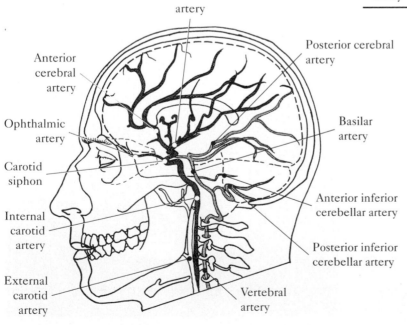

Middle cerebral artery

Anterior cerebral artery

Ophthalmic artery

Carotid siphon

Internal carotid artery

External carotid artery

Posterior cerebral artery

Basilar artery

Anterior inferior cerebellar artery

Posterior inferior cerebellar artery

Vertebral artery

AVMs are the most common type of congenital vascular malformation. They consist of tangles of dilated arteries and veins, usually accompanied by arteriovenous shunting. Approximately 40% of persons with AVMs will bleed by the age of 40 years.

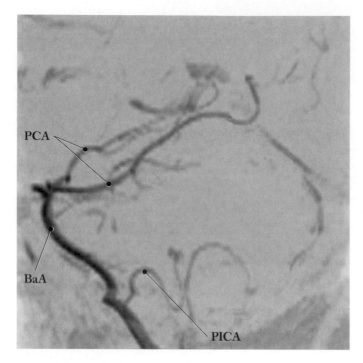

PCA

BaA

PICA

Figure 2.80   Sagittal MRA of vertebral arteries.

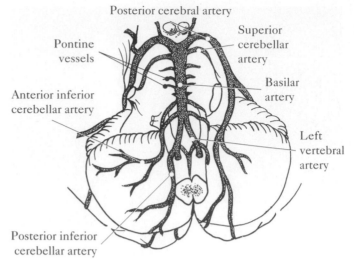

Posterior cerebral artery

Superior cerebellar artery

Pontine vessels

Basilar artery

Anterior inferior cerebellar artery

Left vertebral artery

Posterior inferior cerebellar artery

Figure 2.81   Inferior surface of basilar artery.

Key.   BaA basilar artery; **MCA** middle cerebral artery; **PCA** posterior cerebral artery; **PICA** posterior inferior cerebellar artery; **SCA** superior cerebellar artery.

Figure 2.82   Coronal MRA of vertebral arteries.

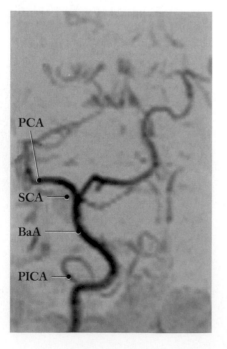

PCA

SCA

BaA

PICA

Figure 2.83   Axial CT scan with posterior cerebral artery.   (R3.F)

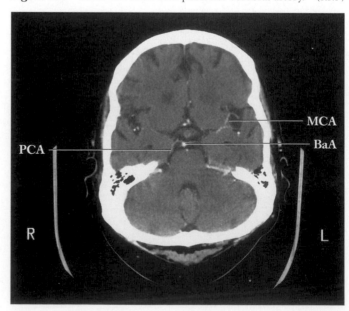

PCA

MCA

BaA

R

L

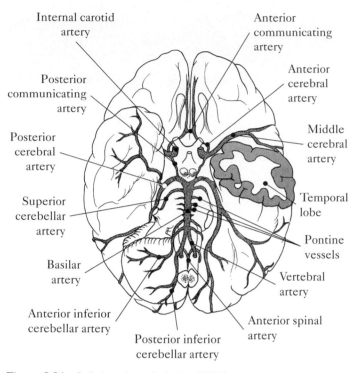

Figure 2.84   Inferior view of circle of Willis.

Internal carotid artery

Anterior communicating artery

Anterior cerebral artery

Posterior communicating artery

Middle cerebral artery

Posterior cerebral artery

Temporal lobe

Superior cerebellar artery

Pontine vessels

Basilar artery

Vertebral artery

Anterior inferior cerebellar artery

Anterior spinal artery

Posterior inferior cerebellar artery

CIRCLE OF WILLIS.   The cerebral arterial circle, or **circle of Willis,** is a critically important anastomosis between the four major arteries (two vertebral and two internal carotid) feeding the brain. The circle of Willis is formed by the anterior and posterior cerebral, anterior and posterior communicating, and the internal carotid arteries. The circle is located mainly in the suprasellar cistern at the base of the brain. Many normal variations of this circle may occur in individuals. The circle of Willis functions as a means of collateral blood flow from one cerebral hemisphere to another in the event of blockage (Figures 2.84 through 2.86).

Key.   ACA anterior cerebral artery; **ACoA** anterior communicating artery; **MCA** middle cerebral artery; **PCA** posterior cerebral artery; **PCoA** posterior communicating artery.

Figure 2.86   Axial CTA of circle of Willis. (Courtesy GE Medical Systems, Milwaukee, Wisc.)

Key.   ACA anterior cerebral artery; **BaA** basilar artery; **ICA** internal carotid artery; **MCA** middle cerebral artery; **PCA** posterior cerebral artery; **PCoA** posterior communicating artery.

Figure 2.85   Axial MRA of circle of Willis.

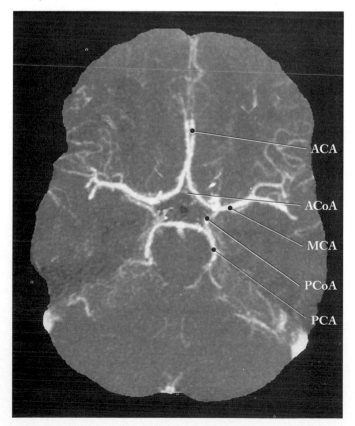

ACA

ACoA

MCA

PCoA

PCA

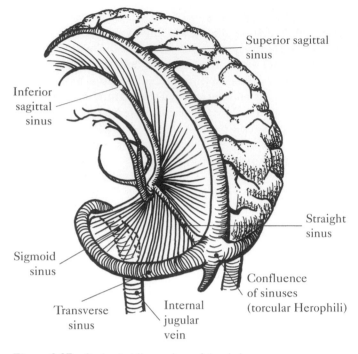

Figure 2.87   Sagittal oblique view of dural sinuses.

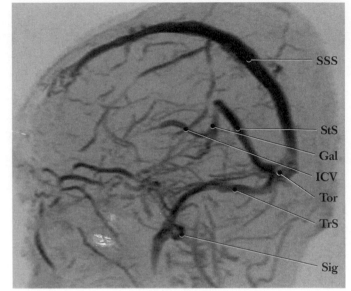

Figure 2.88   Oblique MR venography (MRV) of cerebral venous system.

Key.   ACA anterior cerebral artery; **Gal** vein of Galen; **ICV** internal cerebral veins; **Sig** sigmoid sinus; **SSS** superior sagittal sinus; **StS** straight sinus; **Tor** torcula of Herophili; **TrS** transverse sinus.

Figure 2.89   Midsagittal MR scan of cerebral venous sinuses.

(R1.B)

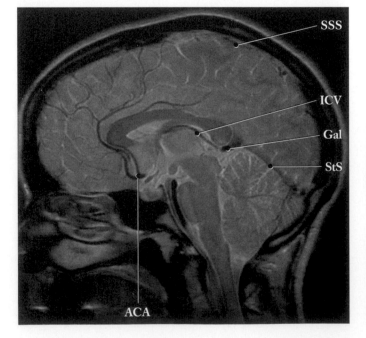

Figure 2.90   Axial CT scan of straight sinus.   (R3.A)

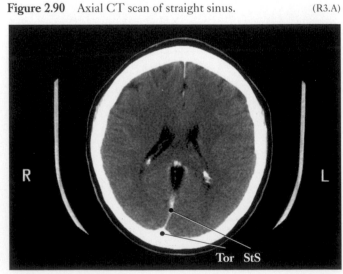

VENOUS DRAINAGE

The venous system of the brain and its coverings is comprised primarily by the dural sinuses, superficial cortical veins, and deep veins of the cerebrum.

DURAL SINUSES. The **dural sinuses** are very large veins located within the dura mater of the brain. All the veins of the head drain into the dural sinuses and ultimately into the **internal jugular veins** of the neck. The major dural sinuses include superior and inferior sagittal, straight, transverse, sigmoid, cavernous, and petrosal (Figures 2.87 and 2.88). The **superior sagittal sinus** lies in the medial plane between the falx cerebri and the calvaria. It begins at the crista galli, runs the entire length of the falx cerebri, and ends at the internal occipital protuberance of the occipital bone. The **inferior sagittal sinus,** which is much smaller than the superior sagittal sinus, runs posteriorly just under the free edge of the falx cerebri. The inferior sagittal sinus converges with the great cerebral vein (vein of Galen) to form the **straight sinus.** The straight sinus extends along the length of the junction of the falx cerebri and the tentorium cerebelli. The junction of the superior sagittal, transverse, and straight sinuses create the large **confluence of the sinuses** or the **torcular Herophili** (Figures 2.89 through 2.90). The **transverse sinuses** extend from the confluence between the attachment of the tentorium and the calvaria. As the transverse sinuses pass through the tentorium cerebelli, they become the **sigmoid sinuses.** The S-shaped sigmoid sinuses continue in the posterior cranial fossa to join the jugular bulbs of the internal jugular veins.

The **cavernous sinuses,** located on each side of the sella and body of the sphenoid bone, are formed by numerous interconnected venous channels. They envelop the internal carotid arteries and several cranial nerves. Each cavernous sinus receives blood from the superior and inferior ophthalmic veins and communicates with the transverse sinuses by way of the **petrosal sinuses** (Figures 2.91 through 2.95).

SUPERFICIAL CORTICAL AND DEEP VEINS. The **superficial cortical veins** are located along the surface of the brain to drain the cortex and some of the white matter. The veins drain into the dural sinuses with numerous anastomoses between the superficial and deep veins.

The deep veins of the cerebrum drain the white matter and include the **thalamostriate, septal, internal cerebral, basal (vein of Rosenthal),** and **great cerebral vein (vein of Galen)** (Figures 2.96 and 2.97). The thalamostriate and septal veins join to create the internal cerebral vein. The internal cerebral veins and the basal veins join to form the great cerebral vein. As mentioned previously, the great cerebral vein joins the inferior sagittal sinus to form the straight sinus, which ultimately drains into the internal jugular veins (Figures 2.98 and 2.99).

Figure 2.91   Sagittal view of cerebral veins and venous sinuses.

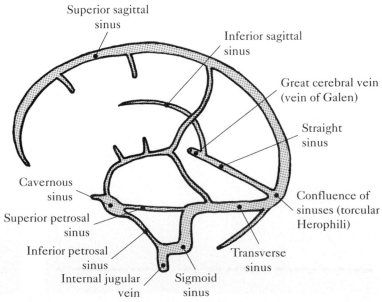

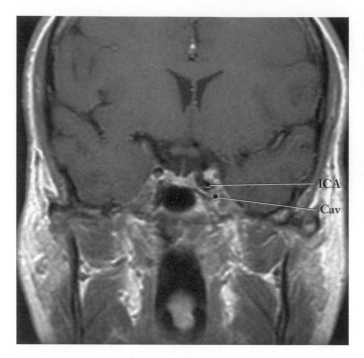

Figure 2.92   Coronal MR scan of cavernous sinus.   (R3.K)

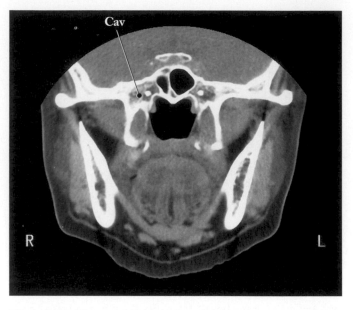

Figure 2.93   Coronal CT scan of cavernous sinus.   (R3.K)

Key.   Cav cavernous sinus; **ICA** internal carotid artery; **Pit** pituitary gland; **SpS** sphenoid sinus.

Figure 2.94   Axial MR scan of cavernous sinus.   (R2.H)

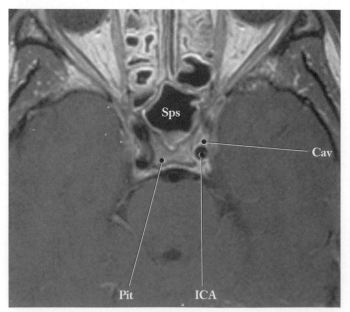

Figure 2.95   Axial CT scan of cavernous sinus.   (R2.I)

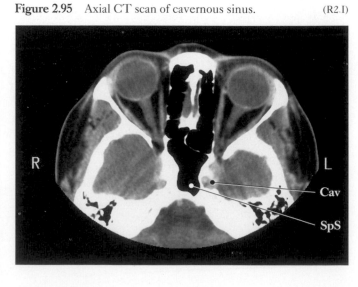

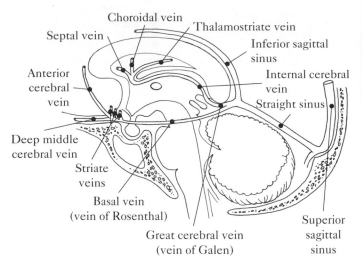

Choroidal vein

Septal vein — Thalamostriate vein

Inferior sagittal sinus

Anterior cerebral vein

Internal cerebral vein

Straight sinus

Deep middle cerebral vein

Striate veins

Basal vein (vein of Rosenthal)

Great cerebral vein (vein of Galen)

Superior sagittal sinus

Figure 2.96 Sagittal view of deep cerebral veins.

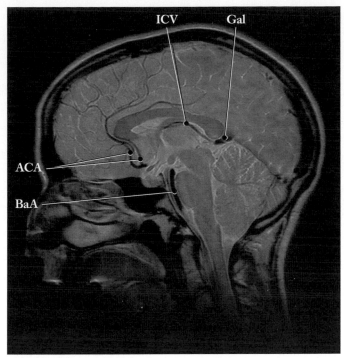

Figure 2.97 Midsagittal MR scan with cerebral veins and venous sinuses.   (R1.B)

Key. **ACA** anterior cerebral artery; **BaA** basilar artery; **BVR** basal vein of Rosenthal; **Gal** vein of Galen; **ICV** internal cerebral vein; **StS** straight sinus; **Tha** thalamostriate veins.

Figure 2.98 Axial CT scan of basal vein of Rosenthal.   (R3.D)

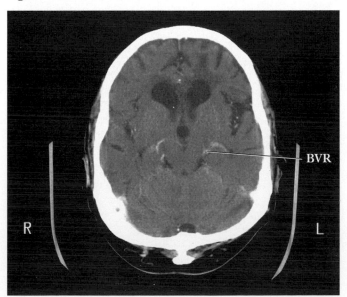

Figure 2.99 Axial CT scan of internal cerebral and thalamostriate veins.   (R3.B)

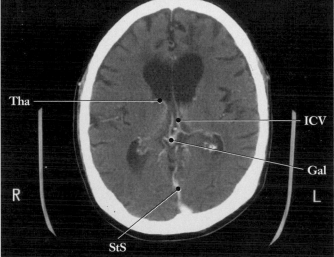

CRANIAL NERVES

There are 12 cranial nerves (CN) numbered from anterior to posterior according to their attachment to the brain. All but the first and second cranial nerves arise from the brain stem. Each of these nerves corresponds to a specific function of the body. It is important to recognize the adjacent brain structures that act as anatomic landmarks to localize the course of the cranial nerves in the head. This section describes the origin of the cranial nerves, because it is not feasible to follow their entire course within the body (Figure 2.100).

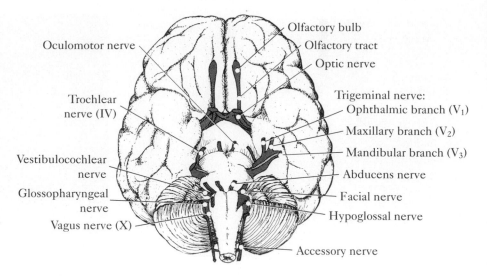

Figure 2.100   Inferior view of brain with cranial nerves.

Figure 2.101   Sagittal view of olfactory nerve.

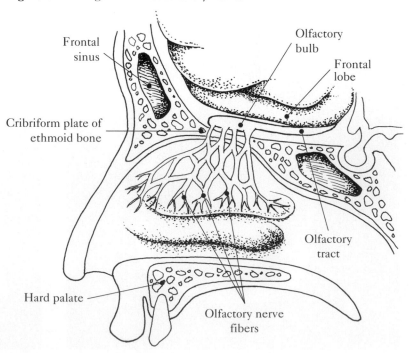

OLFACTORY NERVE (CN I)

The olfactory nerve is the nerve of smell. The olfactory neurosensory cells are located in the covering of the superior nasal concha and the superior part of the nasal septum. The axons of these cells unite to form 18 to 20 small nerve bundles that are known collectively as the olfactory nerve. Each olfactory nerve is surrounded by the three layers of the cranial meninges. The olfactory nerve bundles pass through the olfactory foramina in the cribriform plate of the ethmoid bone to enter the olfactory bulb in the anterior cranial fossa to interact with the limbic system (Figures 2.101 through 2.103).

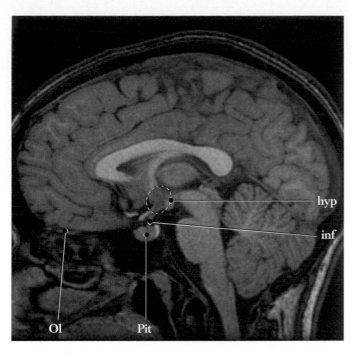

Figure 2.102   Sagittal MR scan of olfactory nerve.   (R1.B)

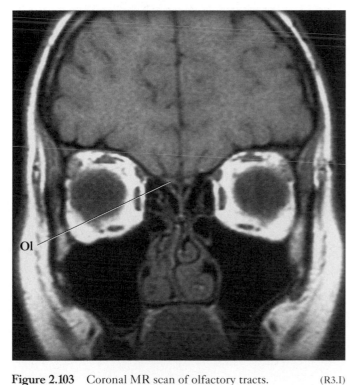

Figure 2.103   Coronal MR scan of olfactory tracts.   (R3.I)

Key.   hyp hypothalamus; **inf** infundibulum; **Ol** olfactory nerve; **Pit** pituitary gland.

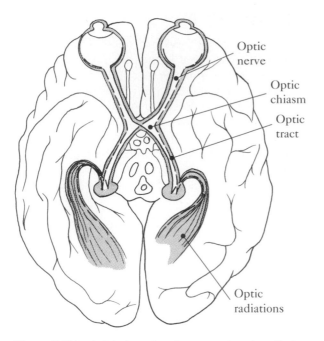

Figure 2.104 Axial view of optic tract and optic radiations.

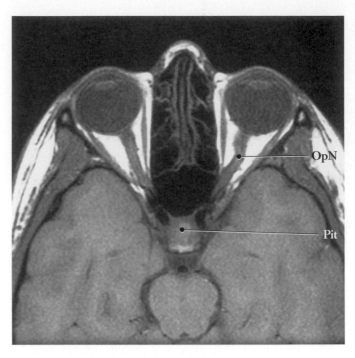

Figure 2.105 Axial MR scan of optic nerves.   (R2.H)

Figure 2.106 Axial MR scan with optic radiations.   (R2.C)

Key. Gal vein of Galen; **mb** mamillary body; **Pit** pituitary gland; **OCh** optic chiasm; **OpN** optic nerve; **OpR** optic radiations; **SpS** sphenoid sinus.

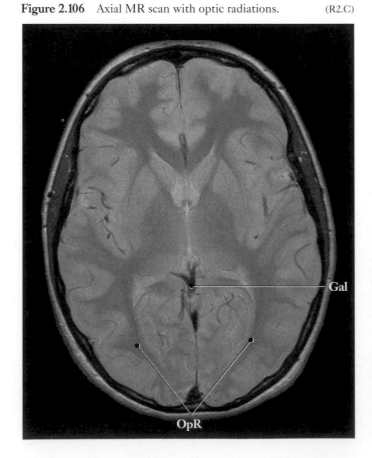

Figure 2.107 Sagittal MR scan of optic nerve.   (R1.B)

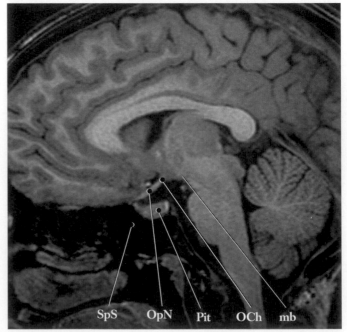

OPTIC NERVE (CN II)

The optic nerve is the nerve of sight. Nerve cells arise from the optic retina and converge toward the posterior aspect of the eye. These fibers unite to form the large optic nerve that passes posteromedially through the optic canal into the middle cranial fossa to join its partner at the **optic chiasm.** In the optic chiasm, the fibers from the medial side of the retina cross to the opposite side, and the fibers from the lateral aspect remain on the same side (Figures 2.104 and 2.105). This decussation of the medial fibers allows for binocular vision. Posterior to the optic chiasm, the optic nerve extends as optic tracts that continue around the midbrain. Most of the fibers of the optic tract terminate in the lateral geniculate bodies of the thalamus. The others form optic radiations that are relayed to the visual cortex on the medial surfaces of the occipital lobe of the brain (Figures 2.106 and 2.107).

OCULOMOTOR NERVE (CN III)

The oculomotor nerve moves the eye by supplying fibers to all extraocular muscles of the eye except the superior oblique and lateral rectus muscles. This nerve emerges from the midbrain and passes anteriorly into the interpeduncular cistern. It runs lateral to the posterior communicating artery into the lateral wall of the cavernous sinus. The nerve enters the orbit through the superior orbital fissure and then breaks into superior and inferior branches, which supply the muscles of the eye (Figures 2.108 through 2.110).

Figure 2.108   Oculomotor and trochlear nerves.

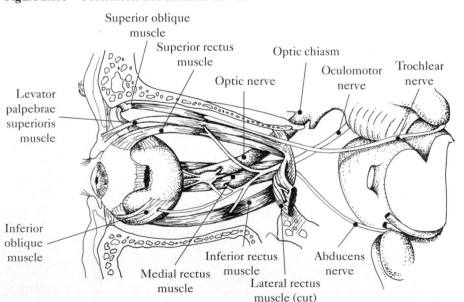

TROCHLEAR NERVE (CN IV)

The trochlear nerve innervates only the superior oblique muscle of the eye. It is the only cranial nerve that emerges from the posterior surface of the brain stem. The nerve originates in the tegmentum of the midbrain, exits the posterior surface of the midbrain, and travels around the brain stem to enter the cavernous sinus. This nerve enters the orbit through the superior orbital fissure, where it finally reaches the superior oblique muscle (Figures 2.108 through 2.110).

TRIGEMINAL NERVE (CN V)

The trigeminal nerve, the largest of the cranial nerves, has three major divisions: **ophthalmic, maxillary,** and **mandibular** (Figure 2.111). It is the major sensory nerve of the face and also contains motor fibers for the muscles of mastication and sensory fibers from the head. The nerve originates at the floor of the fourth ventricle and exits the midlateral portion of the pons. The nerve enters Meckel's cave and forms the gasserian ganglia before trifurcating into three branches. The ophthalmic branch runs through the cavernous sinus and enters the orbit through the superior orbital fissure, where it provides sensation to the cornea, iris, forehead, and nose. The maxillary branch enters the skull through the foramen rotundum, inferior orbital fissure, and infraorbital groove. This branch provides sensation to the cheek, sides of the nose and upper jaw, and maxillary sinuses. The mandibular branch is considered a "motor" nerve, which innervates the muscles of mastication, ear canal, lower jaw and teeth, parotid and sublingual glands, and anterior two thirds of the tongue. The mandibular branch enters the skull through the foramen ovale (Figures 2.112 through 2.114).

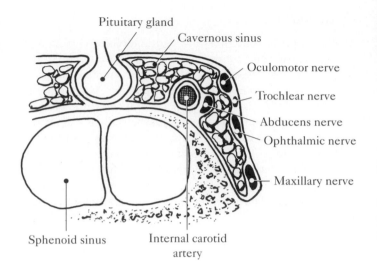

Figure 2.109   Coronal view of cavernous sinus.

Key.   **ICA** internal carotid artery; **inf** infundibulum; **OCh** optic chiasm; **Pit** pituitary gland; **SpS** sphenoid sinus.

Figure 2.110   Coronal MR scan of oculomotor and trochlear nerves.

(R3.K)

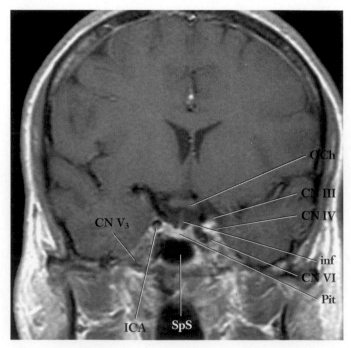

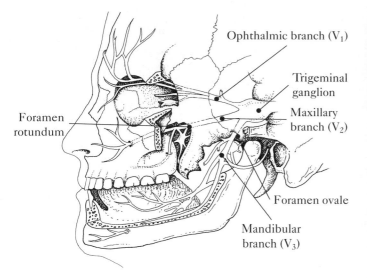

Ophthalmic branch (V₁)

Trigeminal ganglion

Maxillary branch (V₂)

Foramen rotundum

Foramen ovale

Mandibular branch (V₃)

Figure 2.111   Sagittal view of trigeminal nerve.

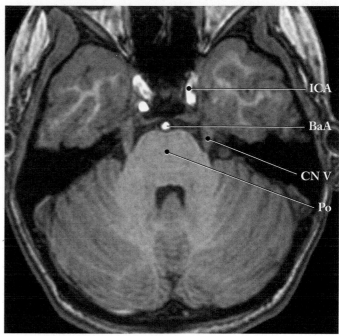

Figure 2.112   Axial MR scan of trigeminal nerve.   (R2.K)

Key.   BaA basilar artery; **CN V** trigeminal nerve; **DS** dorsum sella; **ICA** internal carotid artery; **Mec** Meckel's cave; **Po** pons.

Figure 2.113   Axial CT scan of Meckel's cave.   (R3.G)

Figure 2.114   Coronal MR scan of trigeminal nerve.   (R3.L)

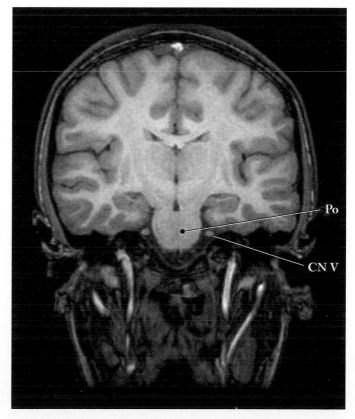

ABDUCENS NERVE (CN VI)

The abducens nerve supplies motor impulses to the lateral rectus muscle of the eye. It originates near the midline of the lower portion of the pons and then passes through the cavernous sinus, entering the orbit through the superior orbital fissure (Figures 2.115 and 2.116).

FACIAL NERVE (CN VII)

The facial nerve emerges from the lower portion of the pons and enters the internal auditory canal. After passing through the petrous bone, the nerve continues along the facial canal, where it finally emerges from the skull through the stylomastoid foramen and runs through the parotid gland. This nerve innervates the facial muscles. In addition, it provides taste sensation to the anterior two thirds of the tongue (Figures 2.117 through 2.120).

VESTIBULOCOCHLEAR NERVE (CN VIII)

The vestibulocochlear nerve has two distinct components, vestibular and cochlear. Both branches pass through the internal auditory canal, behind the facial nerve, and enter the brain stem at the anterior pontomedullary junction. The vestibular branch picks up impulses from the semicircular canals that aid in the maintenance of equilibrium. The cochlear branch receives impulses from the cochlea and separates these impulses into high and low frequencies for the interpretation of sound (Figures 2.117 through 2.120).

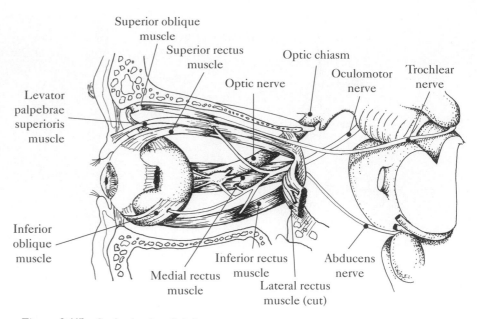

Figure 2.115   Sagittal veiw of abducens nerve.

Key. Cav cavernous sinus; **CN III** oculomotor nerve; **CN V** trigeminal nerve; **CN VI** trochlear nerve; **ICA** internal carotid artery; **OCh** optic chiasm; **Pit** pituitary gland.

Figure 2.116   Coronal MR scan of cavernous sinus.   (R3.K)

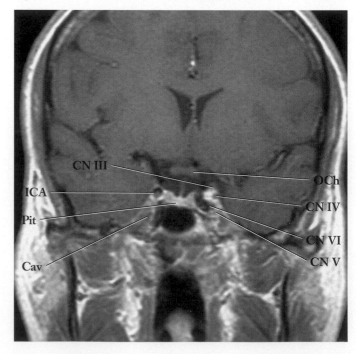

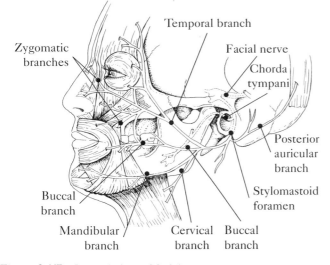

Zygomatic branches

Temporal branch

Facial nerve

Chorda tympani

Buccal branch

Mandibular branch

Cervical branch

Buccal branch

Posterior auricular branch

Stylomastoid foramen

Figure 2.117   Lateral view of facial nerve.

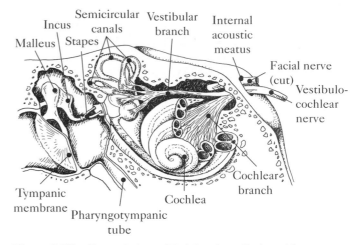

Malleus

Incus

Semicircular canals

Stapes

Vestibular branch

Internal acoustic meatus

Facial nerve (cut)

Vestibulo-cochlear nerve

Tympanic membrane

Pharyngotympanic tube

Cochlea

Cochlear branch

Figure 2.118   Coronal view of facial and vestibulocochlear nerves within internal auditory canal.

Key.   **CN V** trigeminal nerve; **Co** cochlea; **IAC** internal auditory canal; **SC** semicircular canals.

Figure 2.119   Coronal MR scan of facial and vestibulocochlear nerves.   (R3.L)

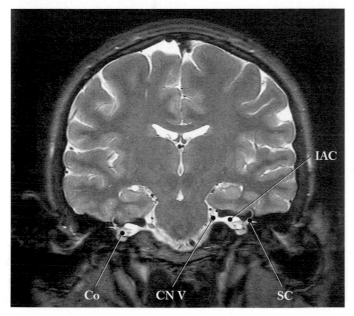

Co   CN V   SC

Key.   **CN VII** facial nerve; **CN VIII** vestibulocochlear nerve; **Co** cochlea; **CPAC** cerebellopontine angle cistern; **SC** semicircular canal.

Figure 2.120   Axial MR scan of facial and vestibulocochlear nerves.   (R2.K)

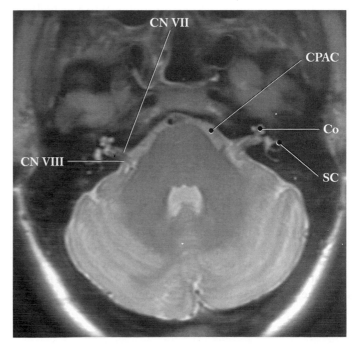

CN VII

CPAC

Co

CN VIII

SC

Chapter 3

1

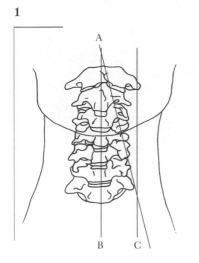

2

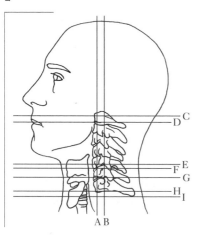

3

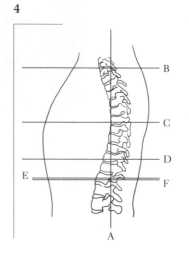

4

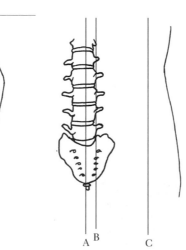

5

6

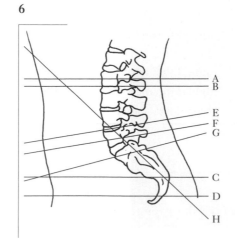

Reference illustrations

Spine

When you suffer an attack of nerves you're being attacked

by the nervous system. What chance has a man got against

a system?

Russell Hoban (1925-)
American writer and illustrator

The spine functions to protect the delicate sensory and motor nerves that allow for peripheral sensations and body movement. Sensory or neurologic loss can be a result of injury or pathologic abnormalities of any of the many areas that comprise the normal anatomy of this region.

Vertebral Column
cervical vertebrae
thoracic vertebrae
lumbar vertebrae
sacrum and coccyx

Ligaments of the Spine

Muscles of the Spine

Spinal Cord
meninges
segments
nerve roots

Plexuses
cervical plexus
brachial plexus
lumbar plexus
sacral plexus

Vasculature of the Spine
spinal arteries
spinal veins

In Figure 3.1, which vertebra is shown and which section is missing? (Answer on p. 109.)

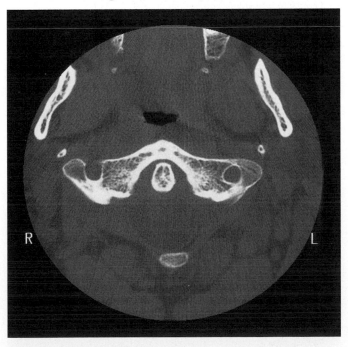

Figure 3.1   Axial CT scan of abnormal cervical vertebra.

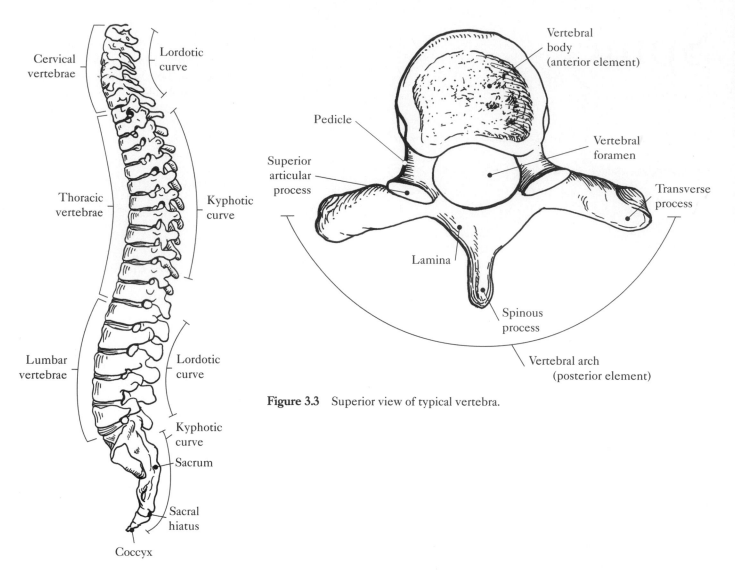

Figure 3.3   Superior view of typical vertebra.

Figure 3.2   Lateral view of the spine.

Key.   b body; **l** lamina; **p** pedicle; **sp** spinous process; **tp** transverse process; **va** vertebral arch; **vf** vertebral foramen or canal.

Figure 3.4   Axial CT scan of lumbar vertebra.   (R6.A)

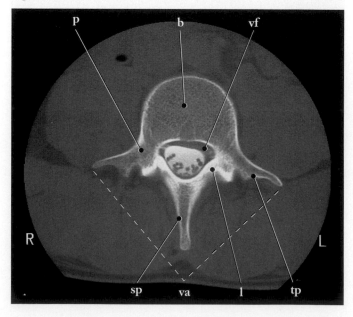

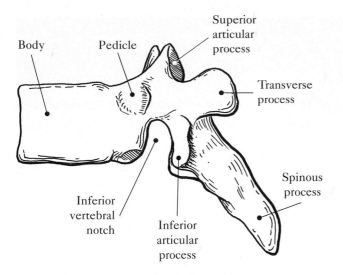

Figure 3.5 Lateral view of typical vertebra.

Key. b body; **d** disk; **iarp** inferior articular process; **sarp** superior articular process.

Figure 3.6 Sagittal MR scan of lumbar vertebra demonstrating articular processes.   (R5.B)

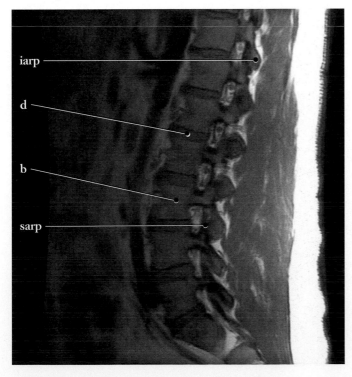

VERTEBRAL COLUMN

The **vertebral column** is a remarkable structure that supports body weight, helps to maintain posture, and protects the delicate spinal cord and nerves. It is made up of thirty-three vertebrae, which can be separated into **cervical, thoracic, lumbar, sacral,** and **coccygeal** sections. There are curvatures associated with the vertebral column. The cervical and lumbar sections convex forward, creating **lordotic curves.** The thoracic and sacral sections convex backward, creating **kyphotic curves** (Figure 3.2).

Vertebrae vary in size and shape from section to section, but a typical vertebra consists of two main parts: the **body** (anterior element) and the **vertebral arch** (posterior element). The cylindric body is located anteriorly and functions to support body weight (Figures 3.3 and 3.4). The compact bone on the superior and inferior surfaces of the body is called the **vertebral end plates.** The vertebral bodies are separated by shock-absorbing cartilaginous disks. These **disks** consist of a central mass of soft semigelatinous material called the **nucleus pulposus** and a firm outer portion termed the **anulus fibrosus.** Located posteriorly is the ringlike arch that attaches to the sides of the body, creating a space called the **vertebral foramen.** The succession of these vertebral foramina forms the **vertebral canal,** which contains and protects the spinal cord. The vertebral arch is formed by **pedicles** (2), **laminae** (2), **spinous process** (1), **transverse processes** (2), and **superior** (2) and **inferior** (2) **articular processes** (Figures 3.5 and 3.6). The two pedicles project from the body to meet with two laminae, which continue posterior and medial to form a spinous process. The transverse processes project laterally from the approximate junction of the pedicle and lamina. On the upper and lower surfaces of the pedicles is a concave surface termed the **vertebral notch.** When the superior and inferior notches of adjacent vertebrae meet, they form **intervertebral foramina,** which allow for the transmission of spinal nerves and blood vessels. Four articular processes, two superior and two inferior, arise from the junctions of the pedicles and laminae to articulate with adjacent vertebrae to form the **apophyseal joints (facet joints).** These joints give additional support and allow movement of the vertebral column (Figures 3.7 through 3.9).

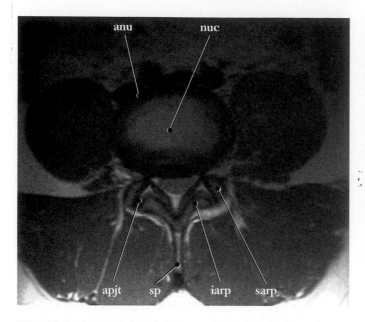

Figure 3.7   Axial MR scan of lumbar spine with intervertebral disk and apophyseal joint.   (R6.E)

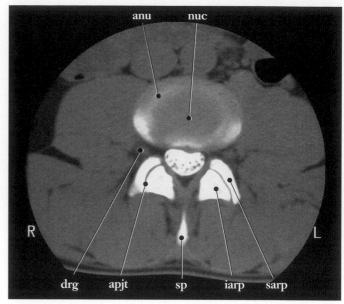

Figure 3.8   Axial CT scan of lumbar spine with intervertebral disk and apophyseal joint.   (R6.E)

Key.   **anu** annulus fibrosus; **apjt** apophyseal joint; **drg** dorsal root ganglion; **iarp** inferior articular process; **nuc** nucleus pulposus; **sarp** superior articular process; **sp** spinous process.

Key.   **b** body; **d** disk; **f** intervertebral foramina; **iarp** inferior articular process; **not** vertebral notch; **sarp** superior articular process; **vep** vertebral endplate.

Figure 3.9   Oblique CT reformat of cervical spine.   (R1.A)

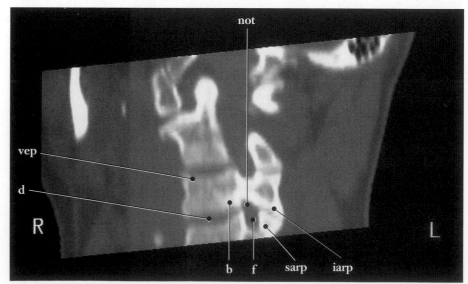

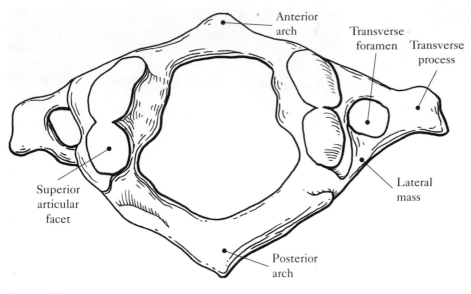

Figure 3.10   Superior view of C1 (atlas).

CERVICAL VERTEBRAE

There are seven cervical vertebrae. The vertebrae vary in size and shape to a large degree. Within the transverse process of each cervical vertebra is a **transverse foramen.** The foramina allow passage of the **vertebral arteries** as they ascend to the head. The first cervical vertebra is termed the **atlas** because it supports the head; its large superior articular processes articulate with the occipital condyles of the head. The atlas is a ringlike structure that has no body and no spinous process. It consists of an **anterior arch, posterior arch,** and two large **lateral masses** (Figures 3.10 and 3.11).

Key.   aa anterior arch; **lm** lateral mass; **od** odontoid process; **pa** posterior arch; **tf** transverse foramen.

Figure 3.11   Axial CT scan of C1 (atlas).   (R2.D)

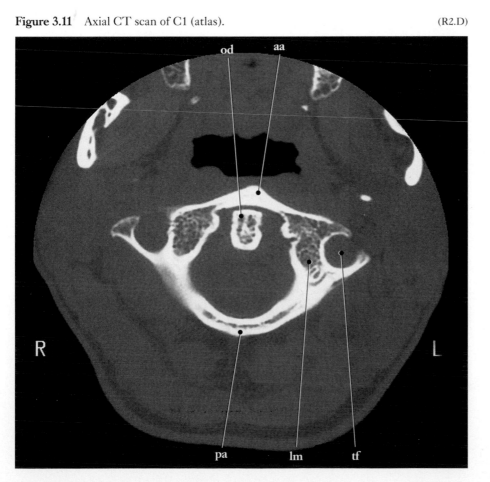

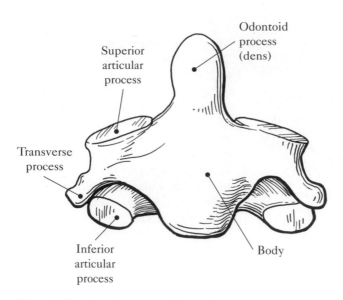

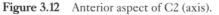

Figure 3.12   Anterior aspect of C2 (axis).

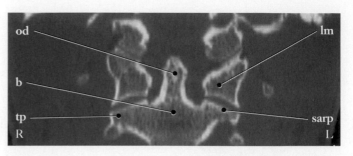

Figure 3.13   Coronal CT reformat of C1 (atlas) and C2 (axis).   (R2.A)

Key.   **b** body; **lm** lateral mass; **od** odontoid process; **sarp** superior articular process; **tp** transverse process.

Figure 3.14   Lateral aspect of C2 (axis).

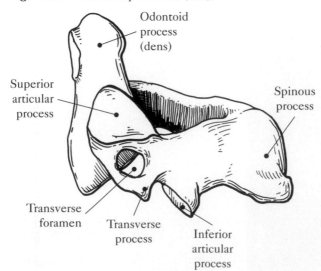

Key.   **aa** anterior arch of C1; **Cl** clivus; **od** odontoid process; **pa** posterior arch of C1; **sp(C2)** spinous process of C2.

Figure 3.15   Sagittal CT reformat of C1 (atlas) and C2 (axis).   (R5.B)

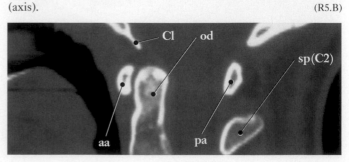

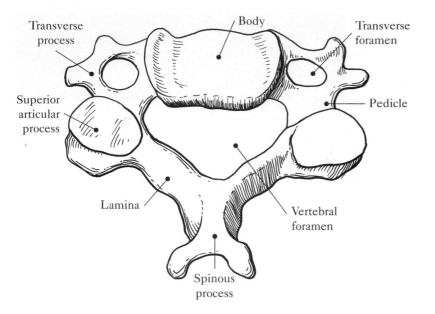

Figure 3.16   Superior aspect of cervical vertebra with bifid spinous process.

The second cervical vertebra, the **axis,** has a large **odontoid process (dens),** which projects upward from the superior surface of the body. The odontoid process projects into the ring of the atlas to act as a pivot for rotational movement of the atlas (Figures 3.12 and 3.13). Lateral to the odontoid process on the upper surface of the body are the **superior articular processes,** on which the atlas rotates (Figures 3.14 and 3.15). The spinous process of the axis is the first projection to be felt in the posterior groove of the neck. The cervical vertebrae C3-6 are considered typical cervical vertebrae with the exception of their bifid spinous process (Figures 3.16 and 3.17). The seventh cervical vertebra (**vertebra prominens**) has a long spinous process that is typically not bifid. This spinous process is easily palpable posteriorly at the base of the neck (Figure 3.18).

Key.   **b** body; **d** disk; **f** intervertebral foramen; **l** lamina; **sp** spinous process.

Figure 3.17   Axial CT scan of cervical vertebra with bifid spinous process.   (R2.G)

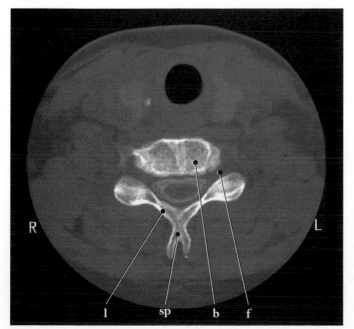

Figure 3.18   Axial CT scan of C7 (vertebra prominens).   (R2.H)

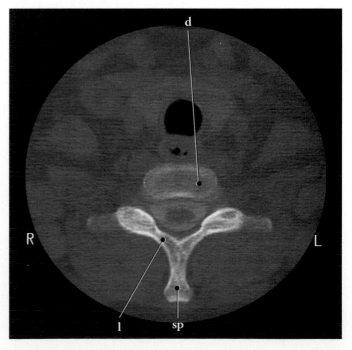

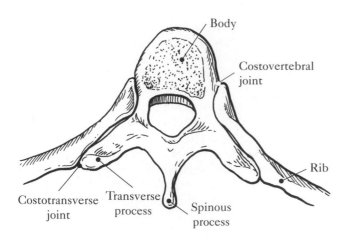

Figure 3.19 Superior view of thoracic vertebra.

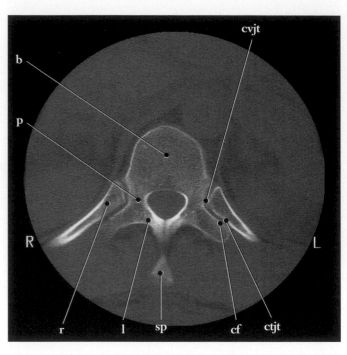

Figure 3.20 Axial CT scan of thoracic vertebra.   (R4.D)

Key. **b** body; **cf** costal facet; **ctjt** costotransverse joint; **cvjt** costovertebral joint; **l** lamina; **p** pedicle; **r** rib; **sp** spinous process; **tp** transverse process.

Figure 3.22 Axial CT scan of lumbar vertebra.   (R6.F)

Figure 3.21 Lateral view of lumbar vertebra.

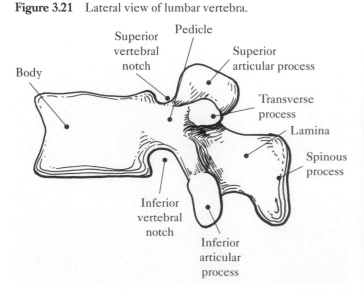

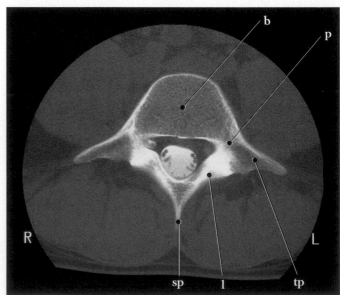

THORACIC VERTEBRAE

Twelve vertebrae make up the thoracic section. They have typical vertebral configurations except for their characteristic **costal facets,** which articulate with the ribs. The head of the rib articulates with the vertebral bodies, while the tubercle of the ribs articulates with the transverse processes. The articulations between the ribs and vertebral bodies are **costovertebral joints,** and the articulations between the ribs and transverse process are **costotransverse joints.** The spinous processes of the thoracic vertebrae are typically long and slender, projecting inferiorly over the vertebral arches of the vertebrae below (Figures 3.19 and 3.20).

LUMBAR VERTEBRAE

The lumbar section typically consists of five vertebrae. Their massive bodies increase in size from superior to inferior. The largest of the lumbar vertebrae, L5, is characterized by its massive transverse processes. The entire weight of the upper body is transferred from the fifth lumbar vertebra to the base of the sacrum across the L5-S1 disk (Figures 3.21 and 3.22).

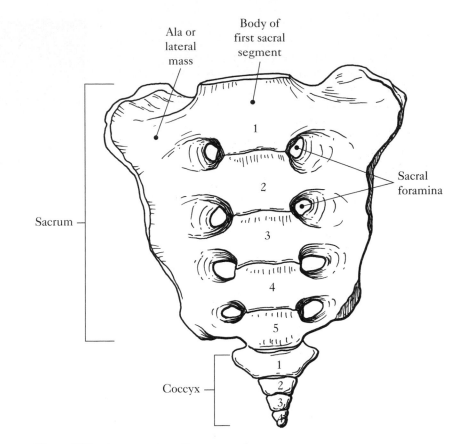

Figure 3.23   Anterior view of sacrum and coccyx.

Key. **b** body of S1; **f** sacral foramina; **lm** lateral mass (ala); **pr** sacral promontory; **SIjt** sacroiliac joint.

Figure 3.24   Coronal CT scan of sacrum and SI joints.   (R6.H)

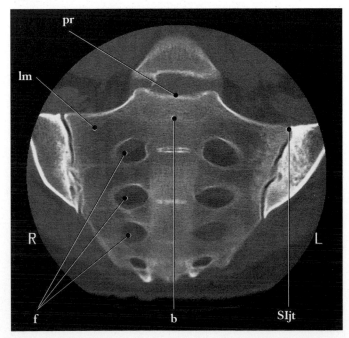

SACRUM AND COCCYX

The sacral section consists of five vertebrae that fuse to form the sacrum. Their transverse processes combine to form the **lateral mass (ala),** which articulates with the pelvic bones at the **sacroiliac joints** (Figures 3.23 and 3.24). Located within the lateral masses are the **sacral foramina,** which allow for the passage of nerves. The first sacral segment has a prominent ridge located on the anterior surface of the body termed the **sacral promontory** (Figures 3.25 and 3.26). This bony landmark is used to separate the abdominal cavity from the pelvic cavity. The spinous process of the fifth sacral segment is absent, leaving an opening termed the **sacral hiatus** (see Figure 3.2). Located inferior to the fifth sacral segment is the coccyx, which consists of three to five small fused bony segments (Figures 3.23 and 3.27). Posterior projections from the first coccygeal segment are called **cornu.** The coccyx represents the most inferior portion of the vertebral column and is commonly called the tailbone.

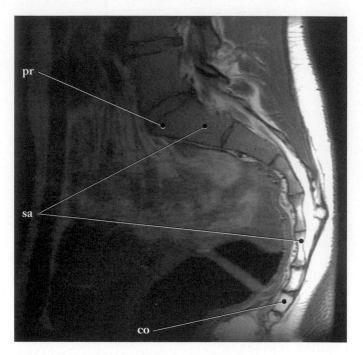

Figure 3.25   Sagittal MR scan of sacrum and coccyx.   (R5.A)

Key.   co coccyx; **pr** sacral promontory; **sa** sacrum.

Key.   ap articular process; **b** body; **lm** lateral mass; **pr** sacral promontory.

Figure 3.26   Axial CT scan of sacrum and sacroiliac joints.   (R6.G)

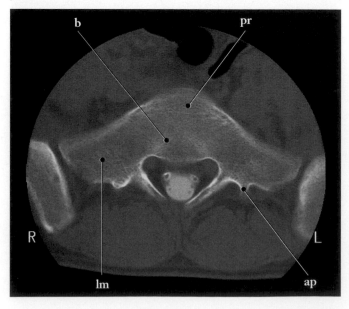

Key.   co coccyx.

Figure 3.27   Axial CT scan of coccyx.   (R6.D)

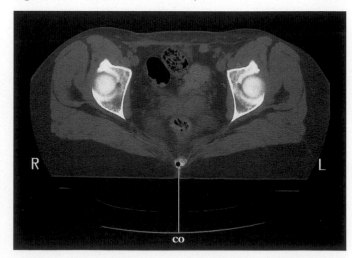

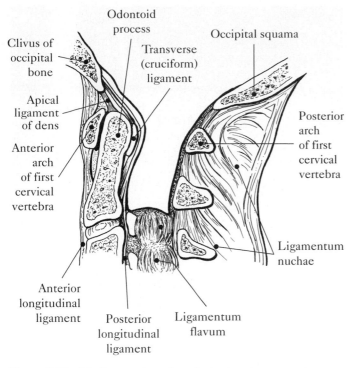

Clivus of occipital bone

Apical ligament of dens

Anterior arch of first cervical vertebra

Odontoid process

Transverse (cruciform) ligament

Occipital squama

Posterior arch of first cervical vertebra

Ligamentum nuchae

Anterior longitudinal ligament

Posterior longitudinal ligament

Ligamentum flavum

Figure 3.28   Median section of cervical spine demonstrating spinal ligaments.

LIGAMENTS OF THE SPINE

Several ligaments enclose the vertebral column to help to protect the spinal cord and maintain stability of the vertebral column. Two of the larger ligaments are the anterior and posterior longitudinal ligaments. The **anterior longitudinal ligament** is a broad fibrous band that extends downward from C1 along the entire anterior surface of the vertebral bodies to the sacrum. This ligament connects the anterior aspects of the vertebral bodies and intervertebral disks to maintain stability of the joints and to help prevent hyperextension of the vertebral column. It is thicker in the thoracic region than in the cervical and lumbar regions. The **posterior longitudinal ligament** is narrower and slightly weaker than the anterior longitudinal ligament. It lies inside the vertebral canal and runs along the posterior aspect of the vertebral bodies (Figures 3.28 through 3.30). The posterior longitudinal ligament runs the entire length of the vertebral column beginning at C2. This ligament helps to prevent posterior protrusion of the nucleus pulposus and hyperflexion of the vertebral column.

Figure 3.29   Midsagittal MR scan of cervical spine demonstrating spinal ligaments.   (R1.B)

Key.   all anterior longitudinal ligament; **ln** ligamentum nuchae; **pll** posterior longitudinal ligament.

pll

ln

all

Figure 3.30   Sagittal CT reformat of upper cervical spine demonstrating spinal ligaments.   (R1.B)

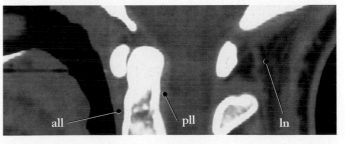

all

pll

ln

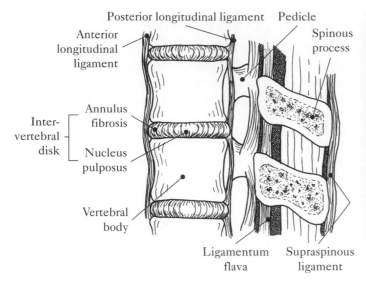

Figure 3.31   Sagittal section of lumbar spine with spinal ligaments.

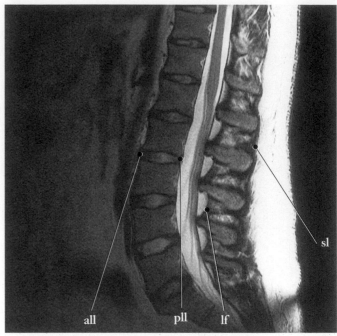

Figure 3.32   Sagittal MR scan of lumbar spine demonstrating spinal ligaments.   (R5.A)

Key.   **all** anterior longitudinal ligament; **lf** ligamentum flava; **pll** posterior longitudinal ligament; **sl** supraspinous ligament.

Figure 3.33   Axial MR scan of thoracic vertebra demonstrating spinal ligaments.   (R4.E)

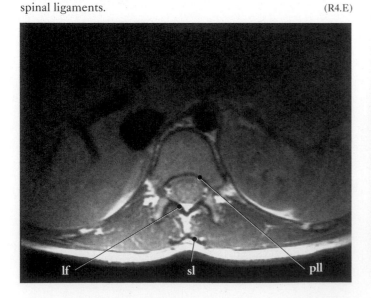

Figure 3.34   Axial CT scan of lumbar vertebra demonstrating spinal ligaments.   (R6.E)

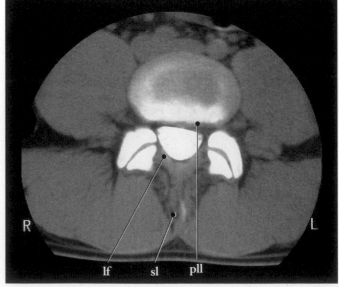

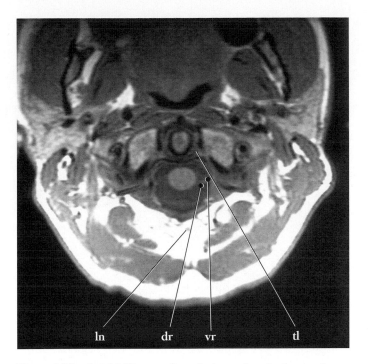

The **ligamentum flava** are strong yellow ligaments (consisting of yellow elastic tissue) present on either side of the spinous process. They join the laminae of adjacent vertebral arches, helping to preserve the normal curvature of the spine (Figures 3.31 and 3.32). The **supraspinous ligament** is a narrow ligament that joins the tips of the spinous processes from the seventh cervical vertebra to the sacrum (Figures 3.33 and 3.34). The supraspinous ligament continues superiorly as the **ligamentum nuchae** of the cervical spine (Figures 3.35 and 3.36).

Figure 3.35   Axial MR scan of cervical vertebra demonstrating spinal ligaments.   (R2.C)

Key. **dr** dorsal root; **ln** ligamentum nuchae; **tl** transverse ligament; **vr** ventral root.

Key. **lf** ligamentum flava; **ln** ligamentum nuchae; **pll** posterior longitudinal ligament.

Figure 3.36   Axial CT scan of cervical vertebra demonstrating spinal ligaments.   (R2.H)

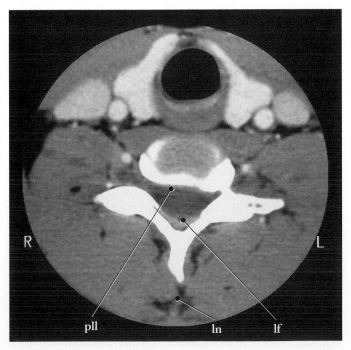

Other ligaments of the spine serve to connect the cervical vertebrae and cranium to provide mobility and protection for the head and neck. The **alar ligaments** are two fibrous cords that extend from the sides of the odontoid process to the lateral margins of the foramen magnum (Figures 3.37 and 3.38). They limit rotation and flexion of the head. The **transverse ligament** extends across the ring of the C1 to form a sling over the posterior surface of the odontoid process. The transverse ligament functions to hold the odontoid process of C2 against the anterior arch of C1 (Figure 3.39). The transverse ligament is sometimes called the *cruciform ligament* because of its crosslike appearance.

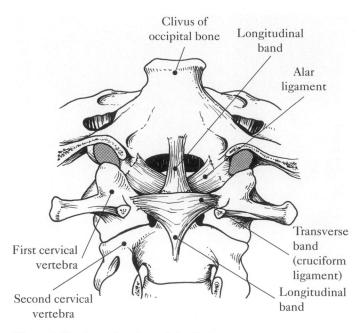

Figure 3.37 Posterior view of alar ligaments.

Key. **aa** anterior arch; **al** alar ligament; **lm** lateral mass; **od** odontoid process; **tl** transverse ligament.

Figure 3.38 Coronal MR scan of cervical spine demonstrating alar ligaments.   (R2.A)

Figure 3.39 Axial CT scan of C1 and C2 demonstrating transverse ligament.   (R2.D)

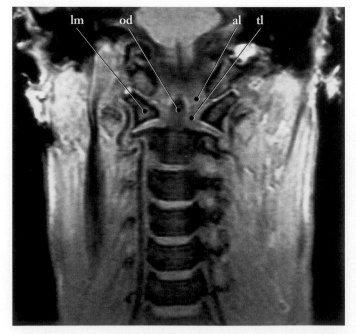

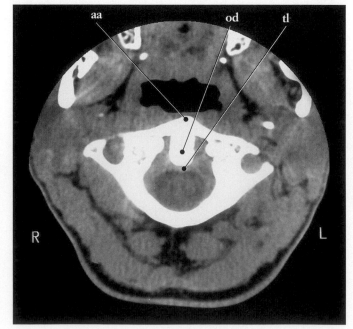

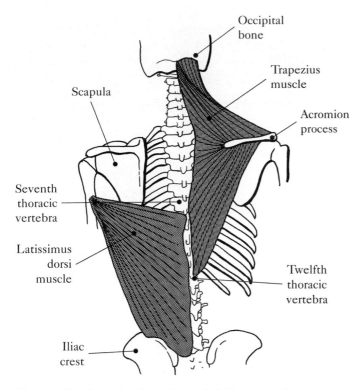

Figure 3.40   Posterior view of superficial back muscles.

Figure 3.41   Posterior view of deep back muscles.

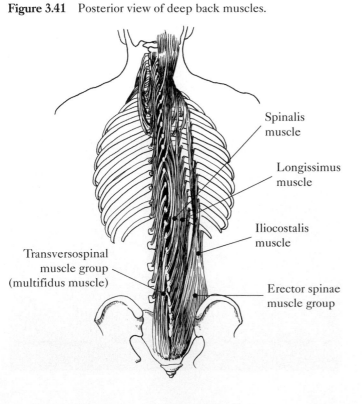

MUSCLES OF THE SPINE

Three main muscle groups on the posterior surface of the spine are concerned with respiration and movement of the vertebral column (Figures 3.40 and 3.41). The first, most superficial muscle group is made up of the **trapezius, latissimus dorsi,** and **serratus posterior muscles** (Figures 3.42 through 3.44). The trapezius muscle extends from the occipital bone and the spinous processes of C7-T12 and attaches to the clavicle, acromion, and spine of the scapula. The latissimus dorsi muscle extends from the spinous processes of the inferior six thoracic vertebrae and the iliac crest. It attaches laterally to the intertubercular groove of the humerus. These two muscles contribute to movement of the upper limbs. The serratus posterior muscle can be broken into superior and inferior sections. The superior section of the serratus posterior muscle arises from the spinous processes of C7-T3 and inserts on the superior borders of the second to fourth ribs. The inferior section of the serratus posterior muscle arises from T12 and L1-L3 and extends laterally to the last three or four ribs. This muscle is involved with respiration.

The second muscle group, the **erector spinae** muscle group, consists of massive muscles that form a prominent bulge on each side of the vertebral column (Figures 3.45 and 3.46). They are arranged in three vertical columns, the **iliocostalis layer** (lateral column), **longissimus layer** (intermediate column), and the **spinalis layer** (medial column). The spinalis layer can be subdivided into the semispinal and splenial muscle groups. The erector spinae muscle group is the chief extensor of the vertebral column.

The third and deepest layer of muscles is the **transversospinal muscle** group, which sits in the grooves between the transverse and spinous processes, providing movements to the vertebral column. The largest of this group is the **multifidus muscle** (Figure 3.41). Another prominent muscle located on the lateral aspect of the lumbar spine is the major **psoas muscle,** which is considered an abdominal muscle (Figures 3.47 and 3.48).

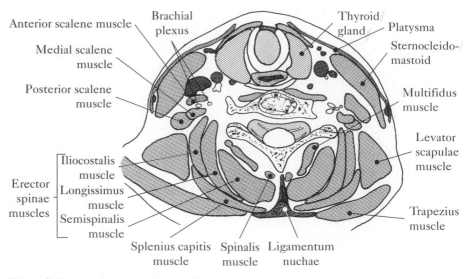

Figure 3.42   Axial section of cervical vertebra with back muscles.

Table 3.1   Muscles of the Spine

MUSCLES	LOCATION	ACTION	MUSCLES	LOCATION	ACTION
SUPERFICIAL GROUP			ERECTOR SPINAE GROUP		
Trapezius	Spinous processes to clavicle, acromion, scapula	Movement of upper limbs	Iliocostalis Longissimus Spinalis	Form prominent bulge on each side of vertebral column	Chief extensor of spine
Latissimus dorsi	Spinous processes and iliac crest to humerus	Movement of upper limbs	TRANSVERSOSPINAL GROUP		
Serratus posterior	Spinous processes to ribs	Respiration	Multifidus	In grooves between transverse and spinous processes	Movement to vertebral column

Key. **le** levator scapula; **mf** multifidus muscle; **spl** splenius capitus muscle; **ssp** semispinalis capitus muscle; **tr** trapezius muscle.

Figure 3.43   Axial MR scan of cervical vertebra with spinal muscles.
(R2.I)

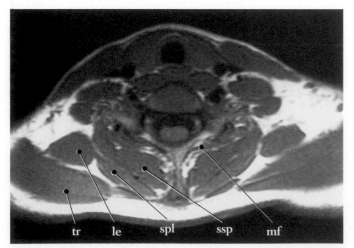

Key. **se** serratus muscle; **tr** trapezius muscle; **ts** transversospinal muscles.

Figure 3.44   Axial CT scan of cervical vertebra with spinal muscles.
(R2.I)

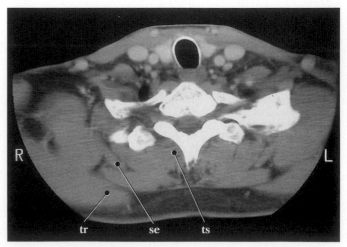

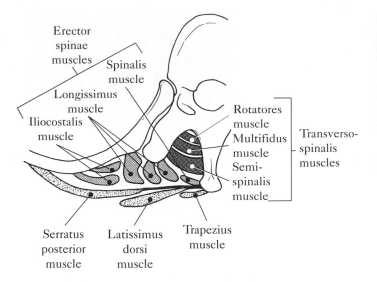

Erector spinae muscles

Spinalis muscle

Longissimus muscle

Iliocostalis muscle

Rotatores muscle

Multifidus muscle

Semi-spinalis muscle

Transverso-spinalis muscles

Serratus posterior muscle

Latissimus dorsi muscle

Trapezius muscle

Figure 3.45   Axial section of thoracic vertebra with back muscles.

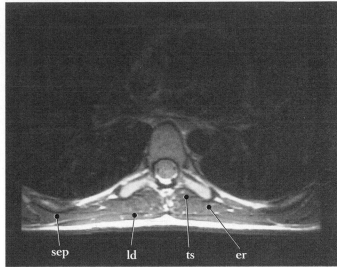

sep   ld   ts   er

Figure 3.46   Axial MR scan of thoracic vertebra with spinal muscles.   (R4.C)

Key.   **er** erector spinae muscles; **il** iliocostalis muscle; **ld** latissimus dorsi; **lo** longissimus muscle; **ps** psoas muscle; **sep** serratus posterior; **ts** transversospinal muscles.

Figure 3.47   Axial MR scan of lumbar vertebra with spinal muscles.   (R6.E)

Figure 3.48   Axial CT scan of lumbar vertebra with spinal muscles.   (R6.A)

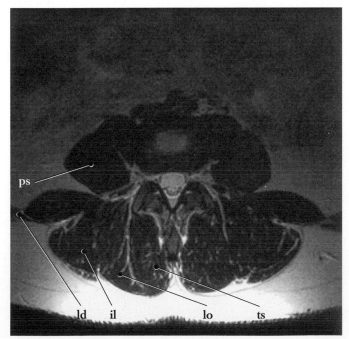

ps

ld   il   lo   ts

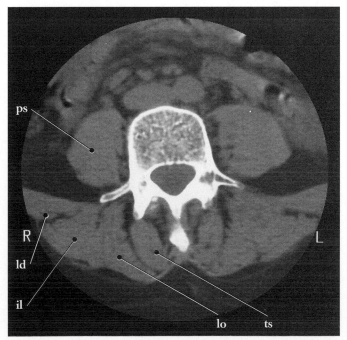

ps

R   L

ld

il

lo   ts

SPINAL CORD

MENINGES

The **spinal cord** functions as a large nerve cable that connects the brain with the body. It begins as a continuation of the medulla at the inferior margin of the brain stem and extends to approximately the first or second lumbar vertebra (Figures 3.49 and 3.50). Throughout its length, the delicate spinal cord is surrounded and protected by cerebrospinal fluid, which is contained in a sac formed by the spinal meninges. Spinal meninges are continuous with the cranial meninges and adhere to the bony vertebral column. Notable amounts of **epidural fat** can be identified surrounding the spinal meninges.

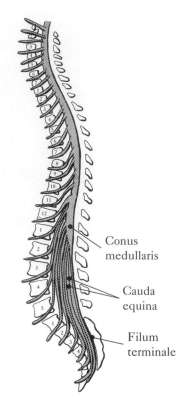

Conus medullaris

Cauda equina

Filum terminale

Figure 3.49 Sagittal section of conus medullaris, cauda equina, and filum terminale.

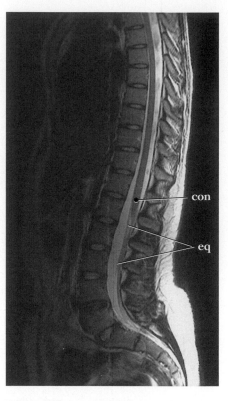

con

eq

Figure 3.50 Sagittal MR scan of conus medullaris and cauda equina.   (R3.A)

Key. **con** conus medullaris; **eq** cauda equina.

Key. **con** conus medullaris; **dr** dorsal root; **ef** epidural fat; **sas** subarachnoid space with contrast; **vr** ventral root.

Figure 3.51 Axial MR scan of conus medullaris.   (R4.F)

Figure 3.52 Axial CT scan of conus medullaris.   (R4.F)

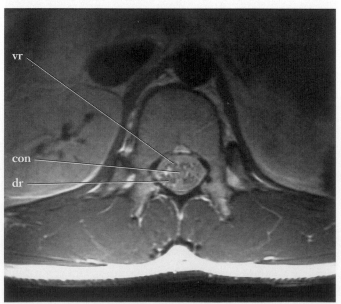

vr

con

dr

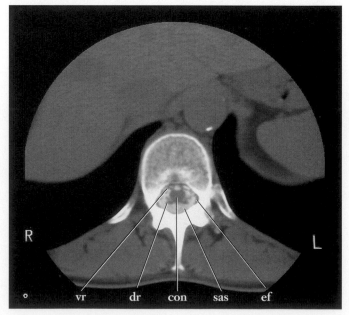

R

L

vr   dr   con   sas   ef

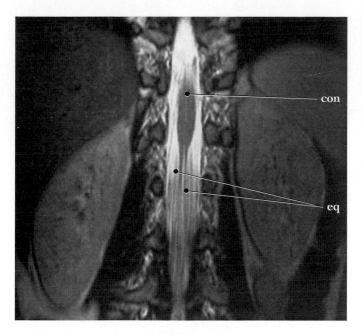

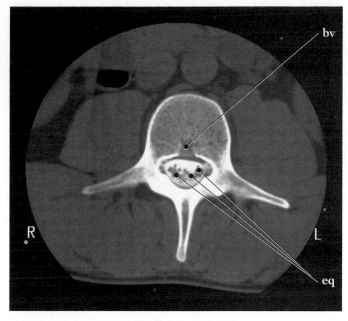

Figure 3.53   Coronal MR scan of spinal cord with conus medullaris.   (R4.A)

Key.   con conus medullaris; **eq** cauda equina.

Figure 3.54   Axial CT scan of cauda equina.   (R6.A)

Key.   bv basivertebral vein; **eq** cauda equina.

Figure 3.55   Axial section of spinal cord.

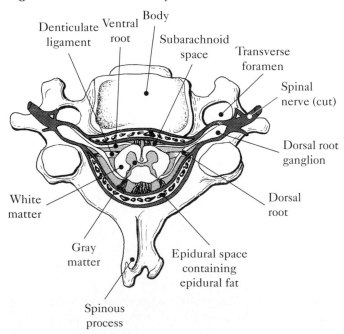

SEGMENTS

The spinal cord is enlarged in two regions by the cell bodies of nerves that extend to the extremities. The **cervical enlargement** extends from the vertebral bodies of approximately C3-C7, and the **lumbosacral enlargement** occurs within the lower thoracic region.

The spinal cord tapers into a cone-shaped segment called the **conus medullaris** (Figures 3.51 through 3.53). The conus medullaris is the most inferior portion of the spinal cord and is located at approximately the level of the first or second lumbar vertebra. At the termination of the spinal cord, nerves continue inferiorly in bundles. This grouping of nerves has the appearance of a horse's tail and is termed the **cauda equina** (Figures 3.53 and 3.54). From the inferior end of the conus medullaris, a slender fibrous strand descends among the cauda equina and passes through the sacral hiatus to attach to the coccyx. This strand is termed the **filum terminale** and functions to anchor the spinal cord to the coccyx (Figure 3.49). In addition, lateral extensions of the pia mater (**denticulate ligaments**) attach to the dura mater to prevent movement of the spinal cord within the vertebral canal (Figure 3.55).

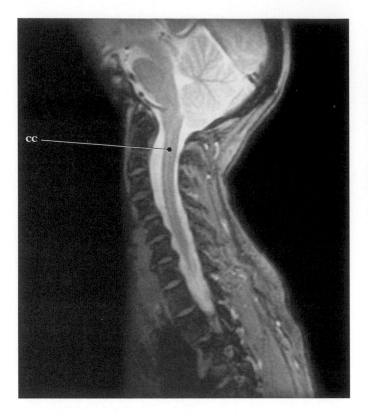

Figure 3.56 Sagittal MR scan of cervical spine with central canal. (R1.B)

Key. **cc** central canal; **dr** dorsal root; **drg** dorsal root ganglion; **eq** cauda equina; **ps** psoas muscle; **sas** subarachnoid space with contrast; **vr** ventral root.

Figure 3.58 Axial CT scan of spinal cord at cervical level with dorsal and ventral horns. (R2.F)

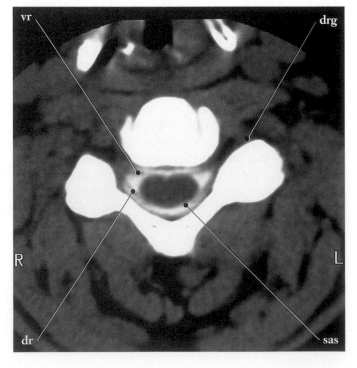

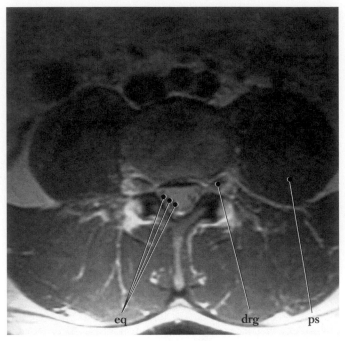

Figure 3.57 Axial MR scan of spinal cord at lumbar level with dorsal root ganglion. (R6.E)

After producing chickenpox, the herpes zoster virus can lie dormant within the ventral horns of the spinal cord for years. When reactivated, the virus attacks the dorsal roots of peripheral nerves, producing a painful rash, with a distribution corresponding to the affected sensory nerve. This condition is termed *shingles*.

Figure 3.59 Sagittal section of spine with neural foramina.

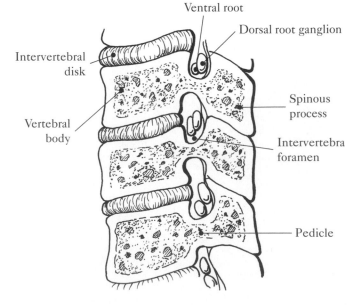

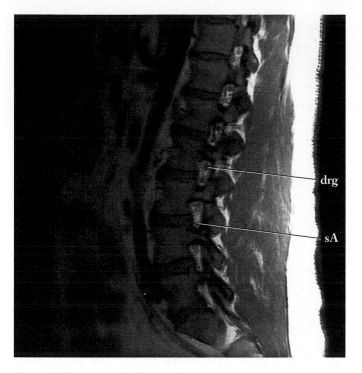

Figure 3.60 Sagittal MR scan of lumbar spine with neural foramina.
(R5.B)

Key. **drg** dorsal root ganglion; **sA** spinal artery.

NERVE ROOTS

The spinal cord is composed of white and gray matter. The white matter comprises the external borders of the cord and is more abundant. The gray matter is composed of nerve cells and runs the entire length of the cord. It is centrally located and surrounds the **central canal,** which contains cerebrospinal fluid and is continuous with the ventricles of the brain (Figure 3.56). In cross section, the gray matter has the appearance of a butterfly. The two posterior projections are the **dorsal horns** and the anterior projections are the **ventral horns** (Figure 3.55). The dorsal horns contain neurons and sensory fibers that enter the cord from the body periphery via the **dorsal roots** (Figures 3.57 and 3.58). These are called the **afferent (sensory) nerve roots.** The **dorsal root ganglion,** an oval enlargement of the dorsal root that contains the nerve cell bodies of the sensory neurons, is located in the intervertebral foramen (Figures 3.59 and 3.60). The ventral horns contain the nerve cell bodies of the efferent (motor) neurons. The **efferent (motor) nerve roots** exit the spinal cord via the **ventral root** and are distributed throughout the body. Just outside the intervertebral foramina, the ventral and dorsal roots unite to form the 31 pairs of **spinal nerves.** Eight of these nerve pairs correspond to the cervical region, twelve belong to the thoracic section, five correspond to the lumbar region, five correspond to the sacrum, and one belongs to the coccyx (Figures 3.61 and 3.62).

Cross-section images of the spinal cord at various levels have considerable differences in size and shape because of the changing proportion of gray and white matter. The gray matter is more abundant in the cervical and lumbar regions.

Key. **eq** cauda equina; **ro** root sleeve; **sa** sacrum.

Figure 3.61 Axial MR scan of sacrum with root sleeve.   (R6.G)

Figure 3.62 Axial CT scan of sacrum with root sleeve.   (R6.G)

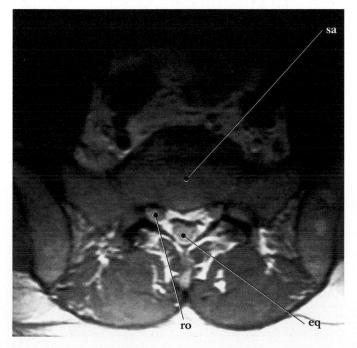

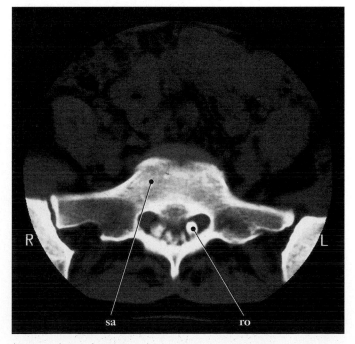

PLEXUSES

Shortly after emerging from the spinal cord, each nerve divides into **dorsal** and **ventral rami.** The rami contain both motor and sensory fibers. The dorsal rami extend posteriorly to innervate the skin and muscles of the posterior trunk. The ventral rami of T2-T12 pass anteriorly as the intercostal nerves to supply the skin and muscles of the anterior and lateral trunk. The ventral rami of all other spinal nerves form complex networks of nerves called plexuses. These plexuses serve the motor and sensory needs of the muscles and skin of the extremities. The four major nerve plexuses are the cervical, brachial, lumbar, and sacral (Figures 3.63 and 3.64).

CERVICAL PLEXUS

The **cervical plexus** arises from the ventral rami of C1-C4 to innervate muscles of the shoulder and neck. The major motor branch of this plexus is the phrenic nerve, which passes into the thoracic cavity in front of the first rib to innervate the diaphragm (Figures 3.65 and 3.66).

> A primary danger of a broken neck in the cervical region is that the phrenic nerve may be severed, leading to paralysis of the diaphragm and difficulty breathing.

BRACHIAL PLEXUS

The **brachial plexus** is large and complex, arising from the ventral rami of C5-C8 and T1 (Figures 3.65 and 3.66). The plexus becomes subdivided into four major peripheral nerves, which form the nerves to the upper extremity. The brachial plexus is located in the lateral part of the neck in the clavicular region, running between the middle and anterior scalene muscles to the axilla (Figures 3.66 through 3.69).

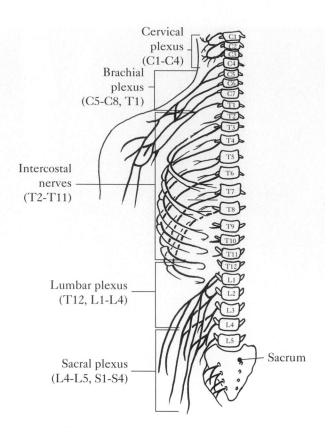

Figure 3.63   Anterior view of nerve plexuses.

Figure 3.64   Distribution of ventral and dorsal rami in transverse section of trunk.

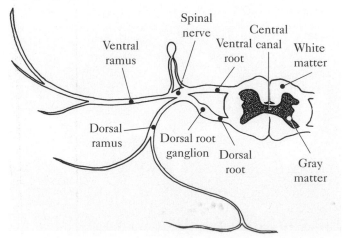

Figure 3.65   Anterior view of cervical and brachial plexuses.

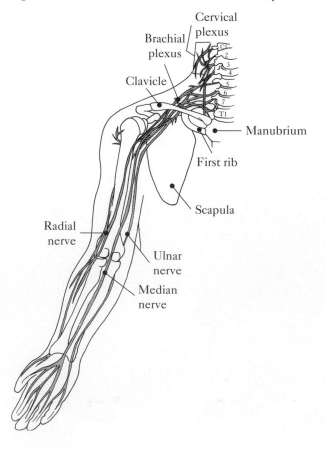

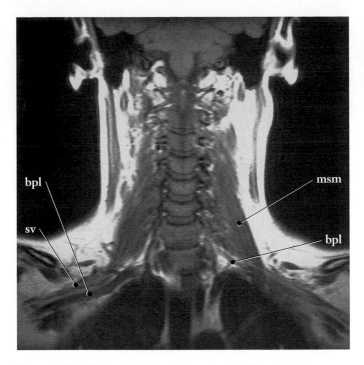

Figure 3.66   Coronal MR scan of cervical and brachial plexuses.

(R2.B)

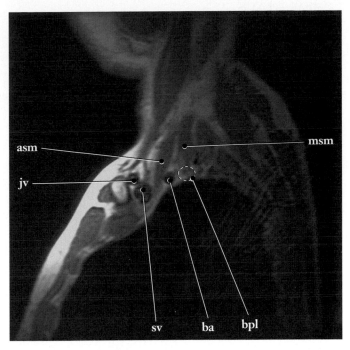

Figure 3.67   Sagittal MR scan of brachial plexus.   (R1.C)

Key. **asm** anterior scalene muscle; **ba** brachiocephalic artery; **bpl** brachial plexus; **cpl** cervical plexus; **jv** jugular vein; **msm** middle scalene muscle; **sv** subclavian vein.

Figure 3.68   Axial MR scan of brachial plexus.   (R4.B)

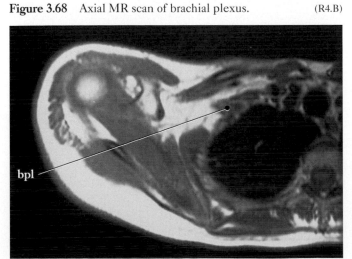

Figure 3.69   Axial CT scan of brachial plexus.   (R2.H)

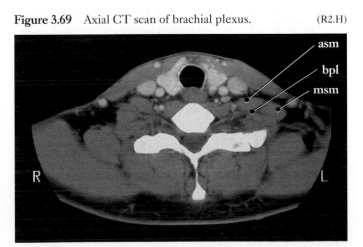

LUMBAR PLEXUS

The **lumbar plexus** arises from the ventral rami of T12 and L1-L4. Its nerves serve the lower abdominopelvic region, buttocks, and anterior thighs. The lumbar plexus is situated on the posterior abdominal wall, between the psoas major muscles and the transverse processes of the lumbar vertebrae (Figure 3.70).

Table 3.2 Spinal Nerve Plexuses

PLEXUS	ARISE	INNERVATION
Cervical	C1-C4	Muscles of the shoulder and neck
Brachial	C5-C8 and T1	Upper extremity
Lumbar	T12 and L1-L4	Lower abdominopelvic region, buttocks, and anterior thighs
Sacral	L4-L5 and S1-S4	Lower trunk, posterior thigh, and feet

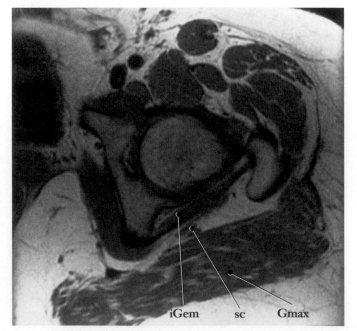

Figure 3.70 Anterior and posterior views of lumbar and sacral plexuses.

Key. **Gmax** gluteus maximus muscle; **iGem** inferior gemellus muscle; **Qfem** quadratus femoris; **sc** sciatic nerve.

Figure 3.71 Sagittal MR scan of sciatic nerve. (R5.C)

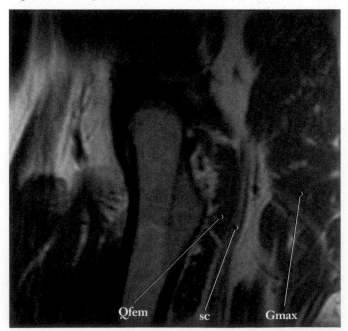

Figure 3.72 Axial MR scan of sciatic nerve. (R6.C)

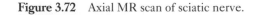

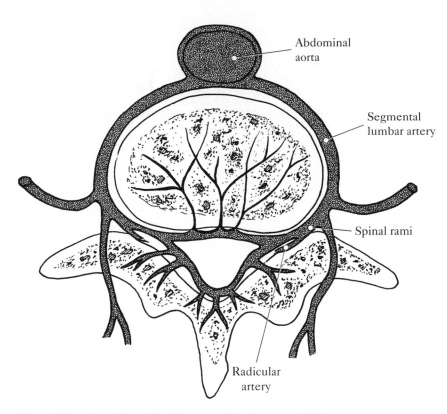

Figure 3.73 Arterial supply of lumbar spine (cross section).

Key. **VA** vertebral arteries.

Figure 3.74 Axial CT scan of cervical vertebra with vertebral artery. (R2.E)

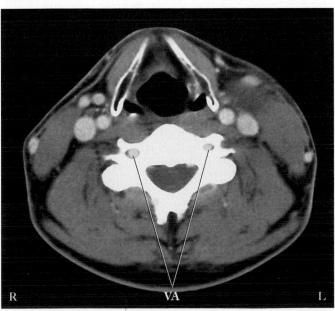

SACRAL PLEXUS

Arising from L4-L5 and S1-S4, the nerves of the **sacral plexus** innervate the lower trunk, posterior thigh, and feet (Figure 3.70). These nerves converge toward the inferior sacral foramina to unite into a large flattened band. Most of this nerve network continues into the thigh as the **sciatic nerve,** which is the largest nerve in the body. The sacral plexus lies against the posterior and lateral wall of the pelvis between the piriformis muscle and internal iliac vessels (Figures 3.71 and 3.72).

VASCULATURE OF THE SPINE

SPINAL ARTERIES

The spinal cord receives its blood supply from two sources: the **vertebral arteries,** which run through the transverse foramina of the cervical vertebrae, and the **segmental arteries,** which are formed by the horizontal portions of the intercostal and lumbar arteries (Figures 3.73, and 3.74). The vertebral arteries form channels that extend longitudinally along the entire spinal cord and are divided into a single **anterior spinal artery** and a pair of **posterior spinal arteries.** The anterior spinal artery is located in the anterior median fissure, and the paired posterior spinal arteries run adjacent to the dorsal roots. Because of the small size of the spinal arteries, they are difficult to visualize with cross-section imaging. The segmental arteries give rise to the **spinal rami,** which pass through the intervertebral foramina along with the spinal nerve roots. The spinal rami divide into ventral and dorsal branches called the **radicular arteries,** which are the main blood supply of the spinal nerve roots.

Spinal veins

The veins of the vertebral column form an extensive network of internal and external venous plexuses. The **internal venous plexus** surrounds the spinal cord while the **external venous plexus** is located at the outer surfaces of the vertebral column (Figures 3.75 and 3.76). The internal and external venous plexuses communicate via the **basivertebral veins,** which drain the bodies of the vertebra (Figures 3.77 to 3.79).

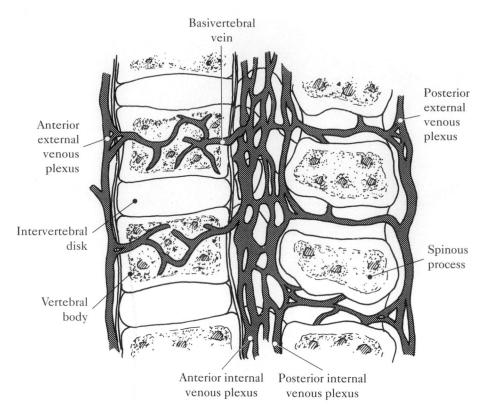

Figure 3.75 Sagittal view of venous plexuses of the spine.

Key. pll posterior longitudinal ligament; **vpl** venous plexus.

Figure 3.76 Sagittal MR scan of lumbar spine showing internal venous plexus.

(R5.A)

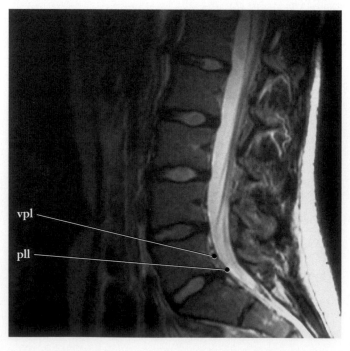

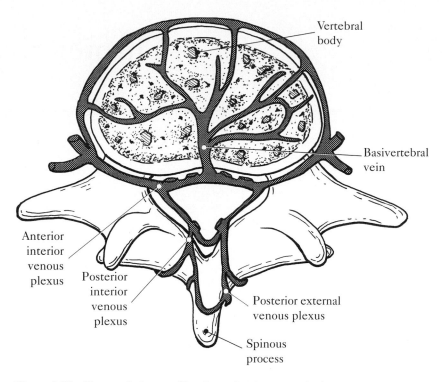

Figure 3.77   Venous drainage of lumbar spine (cross section).

ANSWER TO FIGURE 3.1

The image is an axial CT scan of C1 (atlas). The posterior ring of this vertebra is almost completely missing because of a congenital anomaly.

Key.   **bv** basivertebral vein.

Figure 3.78   Axial CT scan of lumbar spine demonstrating basivertebral vein.   (R6.A)

Key.   **vpl** venous plexus.

Figure 3.79   Axial CT scan of sacrum with internal venous plexus.   (R6.G)

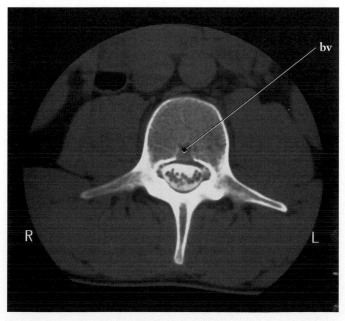

Chapter 4

1

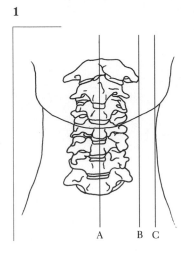

A B C

2

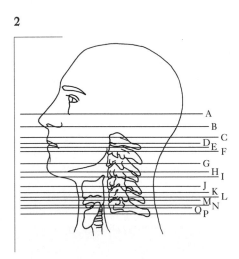

A
B
C
D
E
F
G
H
I
J
K
L
M
N
O
P

3

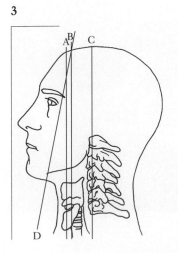

A B C

D

Reference illustrations

Neck

A sharp tongue and a dull mind are usually found in the same head.

Proverb

In Figure 4.1, there is an abscess within this neck. Can you tell which structures are involved? (Answer on p. 135.)

The neck has a large amount of complex anatomy situated in a relatively small area. Recent advances in medical imaging have enhanced the ability to differentiate between the structures of the neck. This chapter demonstrates sectional anatomy of the following structures:

Organs
pharynx
larynx
esophagus and trachea
salivary glands and thyroid gland
lymph nodes

Muscles
muscles of facial expression
muscles of mastication
muscles within the anterior triangle
muscles within the posterior triangle

Vascular Structures
carotid arteries
vertebral arteries
jugular veins
carotid sheath

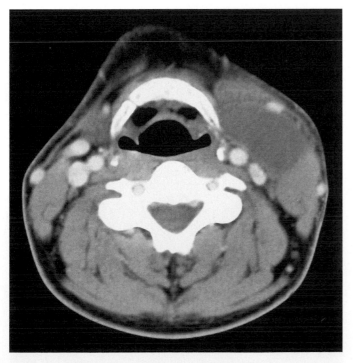

Figure 4.1 Axial CT scan of abnormal neck.

ORGANS

The organs of the neck are attached to one another by connective tissue. They are located primarily in the anterior and middle portion of the neck and include the pharynx, larynx, esophagus, trachea, thyroid gland, and salivary glands.

PHARYNX

The **pharynx,** a funnel-shaped muscular tube that acts as an opening for both the respiratory and digestive systems, can be subdivided into three sections: nasopharynx, oropharynx, and the laryngopharynx (Figures 4.2 through 4.4). The **nasopharynx,** the most superior portion of the pharynx, is an extension of the nasal cavities. It is bordered inferiorly by the **soft palate** and extends down to the level of the **uvula,** which is a soft process on the posterior edge of the soft palate (Figures 4.5 and 4.6).

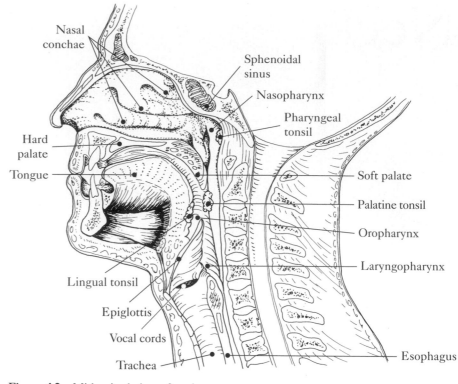

Figure 4.2   Midsagittal view of neck.

Key.   la laryngopharynx; **na** nasopharynx; **or** oropharynx.

Figure 4.3   Midsagittal MR scan of pharyngeal divisions.   (R1.A)

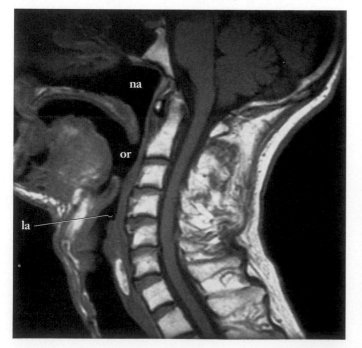

Figure 4.4   Lateral CT scout of neck.

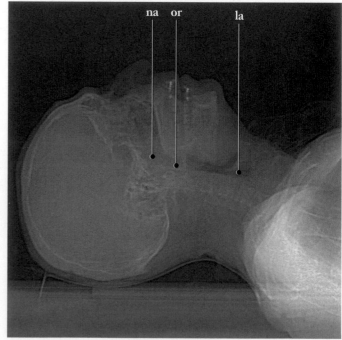

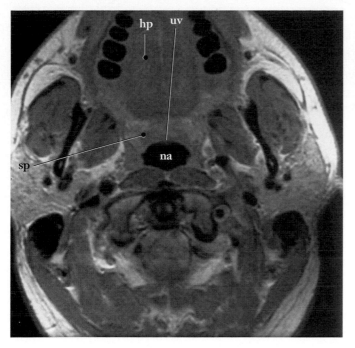

Figure 4.5   Axial MR scan of nasopharynx.   (R2.B)

Key.   **hp** hard palate; **na** nasopharynx; **sp** soft palate; **uv** uvula.

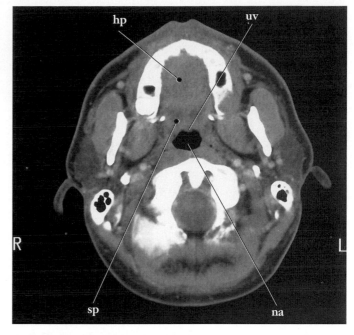

Figure 4.6   Axial CT scan of nasopharynx.   (R2.B)

Key.   **or** oropharynx; **pal** palatine tonsils; **uv** uvula.

Figure 4.7   Axial MR scan of oropharynx.   (R2.E)

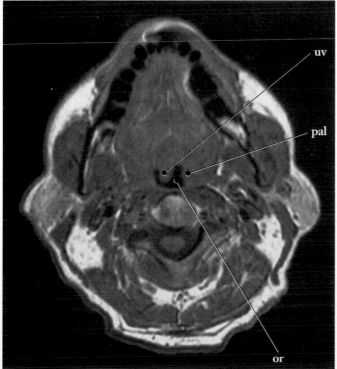

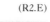

Key.   **ep** epiglottis; **or** oropharynx; **va** vallecula.

Figure 4.8   Axial CT scan of oropharynx.   (R2.I)

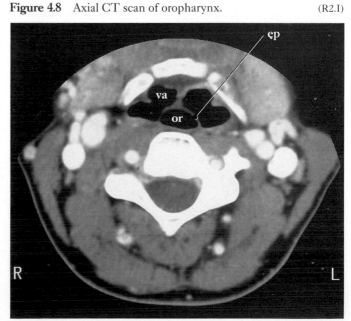

The nasopharynx has a respiratory function: it allows for the passage of air from the nasal cavity to the trachea. Located in the roof of the nasopharynx are the **pharyngeal tonsils,** which aid the immune system by filtering bacteria. The **oropharynx** is a posterior extension of the oral cavity and extends from the soft palate to the level of the hyoid bone. Two pairs of tonsils are found within the oropharynx: the **palatine tonsils,** which are located on the lateral walls, and the **lingual tonsils,** which are situated on the base of the tongue. Located inferior to the tongue and superior to the epiglottis are two depressions called **valleculae,** which are common sites for foreign objects to become lodged (Figures 4.7 and 4.8). The **laryngopharynx** extends from the oropharynx to the esophagus, immediately posterior to the larynx (Figures 4.9 and 4.10).

> The pharyngeal tonsils, when enlarged, are frequently referred to as the *adenoids.*

LARYNX

The **larynx** marks the beginning of the lower respiratory pathway by allowing for the passage of air into the **trachea.** The larynx consists of an outer skeleton made up of nine cartilages that extend from C3 to C6 (Figure 4.11). These cartilages are connected to each other by muscles and ligaments. Six of the cartilages are paired, and three are unpaired. Those that are easily identifiable in cross section are the **thyroid cartilage, epiglottis, cricoid cartilage,** and **arytenoid cartilage** (Figures 4.12 through 4.14). The largest and most superior is the thyroid cartilage. It consists of a right and a left lamina that unite anteriorly to form a shield-like structure. Located between the larynx and the thyroid cartilage are two pear-shaped cavities called the **piriform sinuses (recesses).**

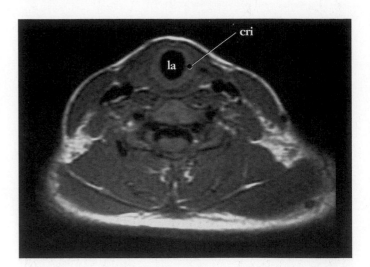

Figure 4.9 Axial MR scan of larynx. (R2.N)

Key. **cri** cricoid cartilage; **la** larynx.

Key. **la** larynx; **pir** piriform sinus.

Figure 4.10 Axial CT scan of laryngopharynx. (R2.J)

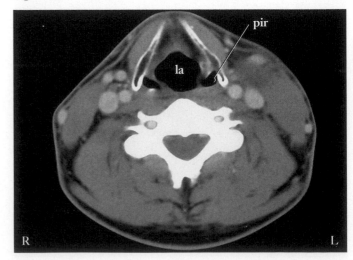

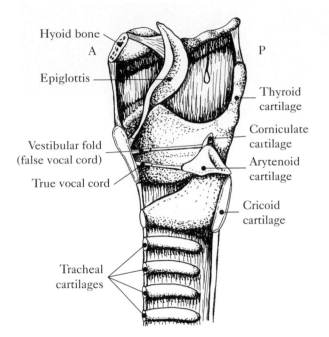

Figure 4.11   Midsagittal view of the larynx.

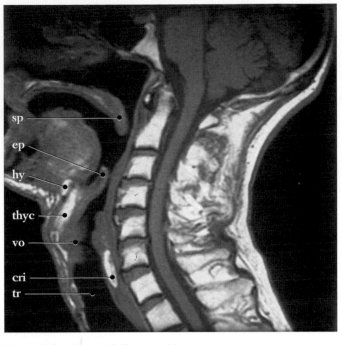

Figure 4.12   Sagittal MR scan of larynx.   (R1.A)

Key.   **ary** arytenoid cartilage; **aryf** arytenoid fold; **cri** cricoid cartilage; **ep** epiglottis; **hy** hyoid bone; **sp** soft palate; **thyc** thyroid cartilage; **to** tongue; **tr** trachea; **vo** vocal cords.

Figure 4.13   Sagittal CT reformat of larynx.   (R1.A)

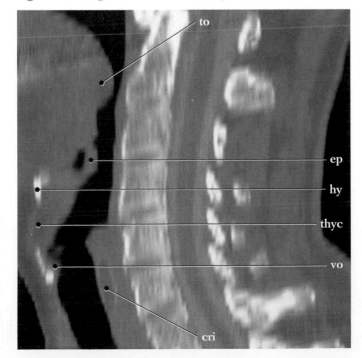

Figure 4.14   Coronal MR scan of larynx.   (R3.B)

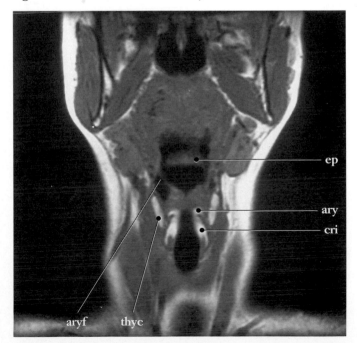

Attached to the posterior aspect of the thyroid cartilage at the junction of the right and left lamina is the epiglottis (Figures 4.11, 4.15 and 4.16). The epiglottis differs from the other cartilages in that it is elastic and allows for movement. It acts as a flap that covers the opening of the larynx during swallowing. The paired arytenoid cartilages are shaped like pyramids and sit on top of the posterior element of the cricoid cartilage (Figure 4.17). The cricoid cartilage is a complete ring that forms the base of the larynx on which the rest of the cartilages rest (Figure 4.18). The cricoid cartilage marks the junction between the larynx and the trachea, which extends inferiorly. All of these cartilages act together as a skeleton to protect the inner structures of the larynx.

Resultant swelling of the epiglottis because of bacterial or viral infection can be very dangerous (acute epiglottitis). This condition can result in closure of the glottis and suffocation.

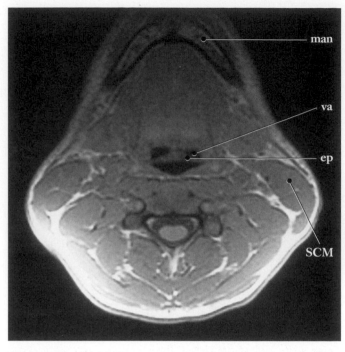

Figure 4.15   Axial MR scan of neck with epiglottis.   (R2.H)

Key. **ep** epiglottis; **man** mandible; **SCM** sternocleidomastoid muscle; **va** vallecula.

Key. **aryf** arytenoid fold; **ep** epiglottis; **pir** piriform sinus; **thyc** thyroid cartilage.

Figure 4.16   Axial CT scan with thyroid cartilage.   (R2.J)

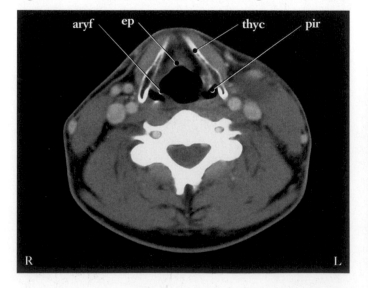

Key. **ary** arytenoid cartilage; **rim** rima glottis; **thyc** thyroid cartilage; **vo** vocal cords.

Figure 4.17   Axial CT scan of larynx with vocal cords and arytenoid cartilage.   (R2.K)

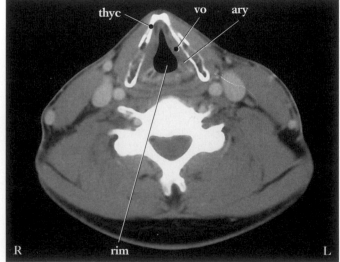

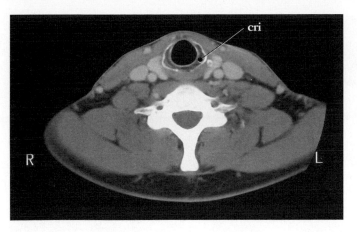

Figure 4.18 Axial CT scan of larynx with cricoid cartilage.

(R2.N)

Key. **cri** cricoid cartilage.

The inner structures of the larynx include the true and false vocal cords, the aryepiglottic folds, and the piriform sinuses (Figures 4.2, 4.11, and 4.12). Two pair of ligaments extend from the arytenoid cartilages to the posterior surface of the thyroid cartilage. The superior pair are the **vestibular folds** or **false vocal cords,** and the inferior pair are the **true vocal cords.** With quiet respiration, the true vocal cords are in a relaxed position, creating an opening between them called the **glottis (rima glottidis)** (Figures 4.19 and 4.20). The glottis is the part of the larynx most directly involved with voice production. The vocal cords are best imaged during quiet breathing in the axial plane. The **aryepiglottic folds** consist of tissue projecting off the arytenoid cartilages to the inferior margin of the epiglottis (Figures 4.14 and 4.16). These folds form the lateral margins of the entrance to the larynx. Located lateral to these folds are the piriform sinuses, which are triangular-shaped spaces that divert food away from the entrance of the larynx into the esophagus (see Figure 4.16). These spaces are common sites for foreign objects to become lodged.

Key. **rim** rima glottis; **thyc** thyroid cartilage; **vo** vocal cord.

Figure 4.19 Axial MR scan of larynx with vocal cords.   (R2.K)

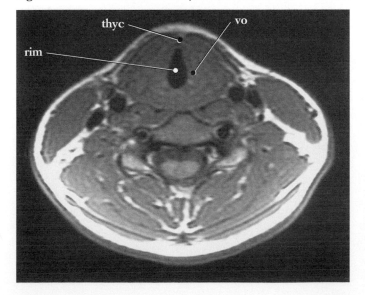

Key. **vo** vocal cord (closed).

Figure 4.20 Axial CT scan of larynx with closed vocal cords.

(R2.K)

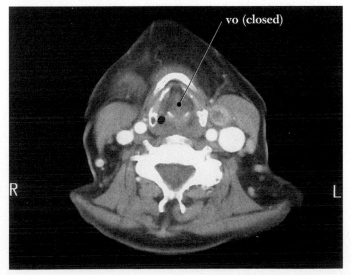

ESOPHAGUS AND TRACHEA

At the level of the cricoid cartilage, the laryngopharynx divides into the **esophagus** and the **trachea** (Figure 4.21; see also Figure 4.2). The esophagus is a muscular tube that extends down to the cardiac orifice of the stomach. It is located between the trachea and anterior longitudinal ligament of the vertebrae and follows the curve of the vertebral column as it descends through the neck and posterior mediastinum. The trachea, considered the airway, lies immediately anterior to the esophagus. This muscular tube is reinforced by many C-shaped pieces of cartilage that maintain an open passageway for air. At approximately the level of T5, the trachea bifurcates into the left and right mainstem bronchi. This location is termed the carina (Figures 4.22 and 4.23).

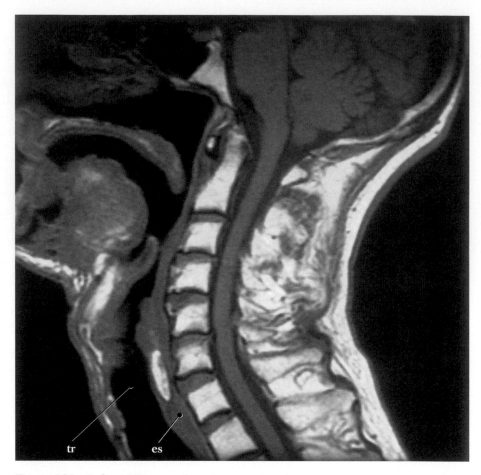

Figure 4.21   Sagittal MR scan of esophagus and trachea.   (R1.A)

Key.   **es** esophagus; **tr** trachea.

Figure 4.22   Axial MR scan of esophagus and trachea.   (R2.P)

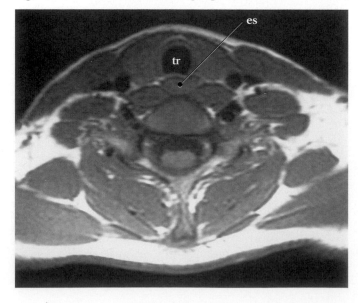

Figure 4.23   Axial CT scan of esophagus and trachea.   (R2.P)

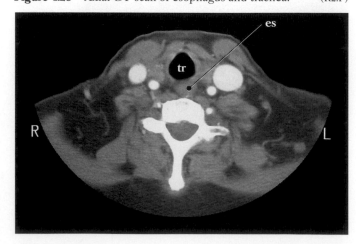

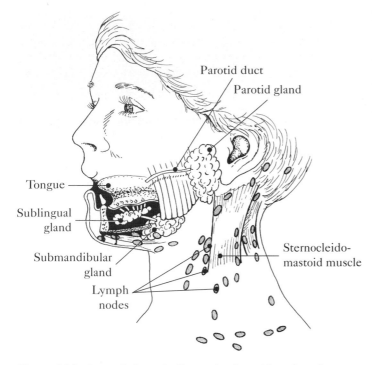

Figure 4.24   Lateral view of salivary glands and lymph nodes.

SALIVARY GLANDS AND THYROID GLAND

The three large paired salivary glands are the **parotid, submandibular,** and **sublingual glands** (Figure 4.24). The largest of the pairs are the parotid glands, which are wedged between the ramus of the mandible and the sternocleidomastoid muscle. The parotid glands extend inferiorly from the level of the external auditory meatus to the angle of the mandible. Their appearance may differ from the other salivary glands because of the amount of fat they contain (Figures 4.25 through 4.27). The submandibular glands border the posterior half of the mandible, extending from the angle of the mandible to the level of the hyoid bone (Figures 4.28 through 4.29). The sublingual glands are the smallest of the salivary glands and lie under the tongue on the floor of the mouth. Each pair of glands produces saliva with a slightly different property that ultimately aids in digestion.

Key.   man mandible; **par** parotid gland; **SCM** sternocleidomastoid muscle.

Figure 4.25   Axial MR scan of neck with parotid gland.   (R2.D)

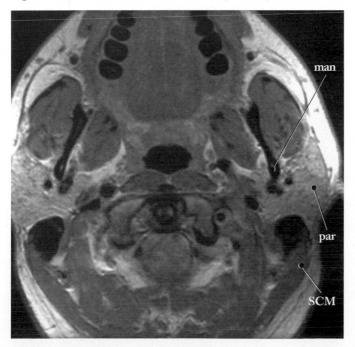

Figure 4.26   Axial CT scan of neck with parotid gland.   (R2.D)

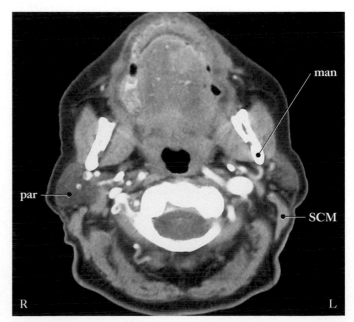

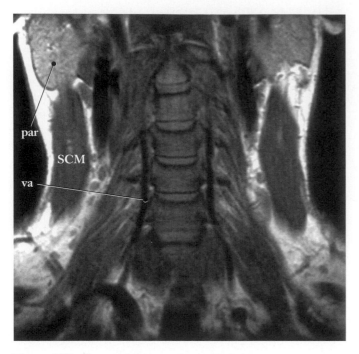

Figure 4.27   Coronal MR scan of parotid glands.   (R3.C)

The mumps virus often targets the salivary glands, most commonly the parotid gland. Infection usually occurs between 5 and 9 years of age. Because of an effective mumps vaccine, the incidence of this disease has been reduced dramatically.

The **thyroid gland** is a bilobed endocrine gland located at the level of the cricoid cartilage (Figures 4.30 and 4.31). In the axial plane, the thyroid gland appears as a wedge-shaped structure, hugging both sides of the trachea (Figures 4.32 and 4.33). The thyroid gland produces hormones that are concerned with the regulation of metabolic rates. Located on the posterior surface of the thyroid lobes are the small **parathyroid glands,** which are typically four in number (Figure 4.30). They are involved primarily with metabolism of calcium and phosphorus.

Key.   par parotid gland; **SCM** sternocleidomastoid muscle; **slin** sublingual gland; **sman** submandibular gland; **va** vallecula.

Figure 4.28   Axial CT scan of neck with submandibular and sublingual glands.   (R2.H)

Figure 4.29   Axial MR scan of neck with submandibular and sublingual glands.   (R2.H)

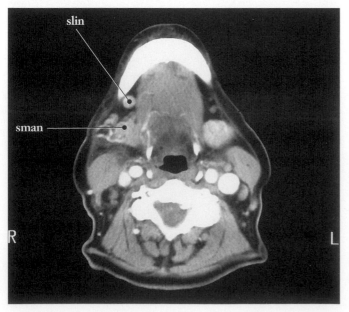

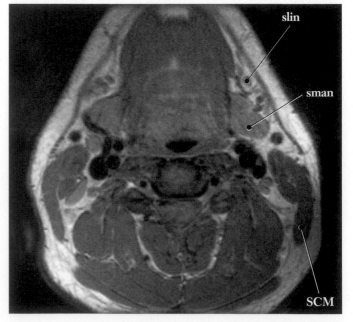

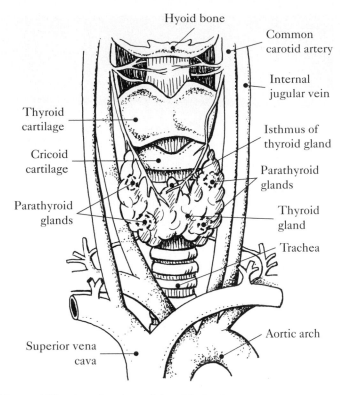

Figure 4.30   Anterior view of thyroid gland.

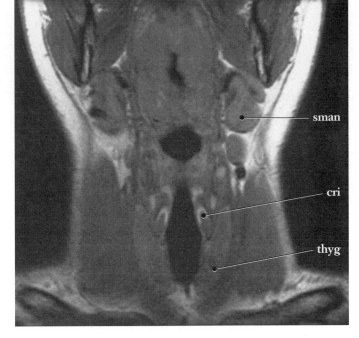

Figure 4.31   Coronal MR scan of thyroid gland.   (R3.B)

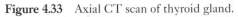

Key.   cri cricoid cartilage; **es** esophagus; **sman** submandibular gland; **thyg** thyroid gland.

Figure 4.32   Axial MR scan of thyroid gland.   (R2.P)

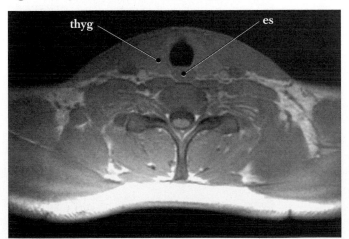

Figure 4.33   Axial CT scan of thyroid gland.   (R2.P)

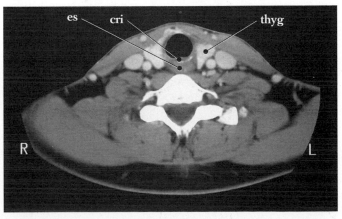

LYMPH NODES

Several chains of lymph nodes are located in the neck to drain the lymph in this area. They are primarily clustered along the vascular and muscular structures of the neck (Figure 4.34; see also Figure 4.24).

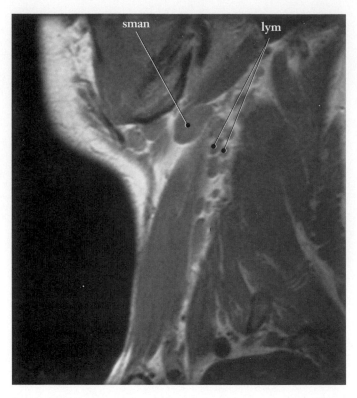

Figure 4.34   Sagittal MR scan of lymph nodes.   (R1.B)

Key.   lym lymph nodes; **sman** submandibular gland.

Key.   alv alveolar process of maxilla; **bu** buccinator muscle; **mass** masseter muscle; **tem** temporalis muscle.

Figure 4.36   Coronal MR scan of facial muscles.
(R3.D)

Figure 4.35   Lateral view of facial muscles.

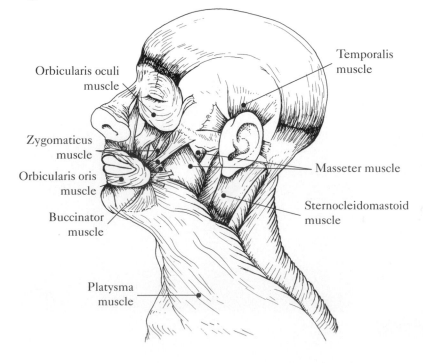

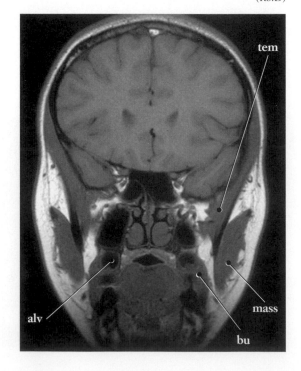

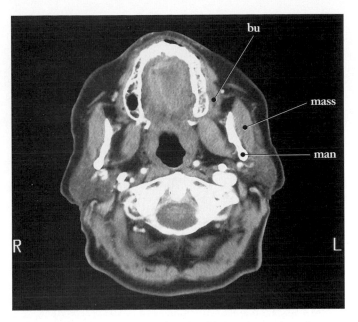

Figure 4.37   Axial CT scan of neck with buccinator muscle.

(R2.D)

Key. bu buccinator muscle; **man** mandible; **mass** masseter muscle.

MUSCLES

Numerous muscles are located within the neck. Each muscle can be difficult to identify individually because the margins seem to blend together in cross-section images. This section of text addresses only the largest and most significant muscles of the neck region. These muscles can be divided into the muscles of facial expression, muscles of mastication, and muscles within the anterior and posterior triangles. In addition, two prominent muscle groups of the spine, erector spinae and transversospinal, are visualized in this region.

MUSCLES OF FACIAL EXPRESSION

There are many muscles involved with facial expression. Two of the muscles located within the neck region are the **buccinator** and **platysma muscles,** which are innervated by the facial nerve (CN VII) (Figure 4.35). The buccinator muscle is located on the lateral surface of the face between the alveolar processes of the maxilla and mandible (Figures 4.36 and 4.37). This muscle acts to compress the cheeks when blowing. The platysma muscle is a wide sheath of muscle that covers almost the entire anterior surface of the neck (Figures 4.38 and 4.39). It extends from the mandible and crosses the clavicles to insert in the cervical fascia. Compression of the platysma muscle causes depression of the mandible and creates ridges in the neck.

Key. plat platysma muscle.

Figure 4.39   Axial CT scan of neck with platysma muscle.

(R2.G)

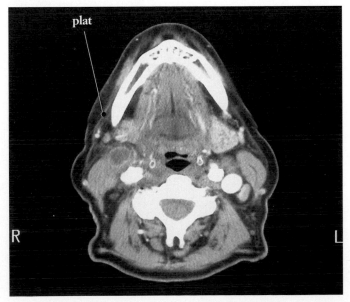

Key. cars carotid sheath; **plat** platysma muscle.

Figure 4.38   Axial MR scan of neck with platysma muscle. (R2.K)

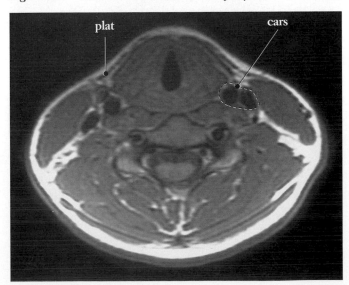

MUSCLES OF MASTICATION

The muscles of mastication are innervated by the trigeminal nerve (CN V). Together they aid in chewing by acting on the temporomandibular joint to move the mandible. This group of muscles are easily identified in cross section and include the **temporalis, masseter,** and **lateral** and **medial pterygoid muscles** (Figures 4.40 and 4.41). The temporalis muscle, named as such because it originates on the temporal bone, inserts on and acts to elevate the mandible. The masseter muscle, the primary muscle of chewing, also acts to elevate the mandible and is located on the lateral ramus of the mandible (Figure 4.42). The pterygoid muscles (medial and lateral) originate from the pterygoid processes of the sphenoid bone and insert on the mandible. The medial pterygoid muscle acts to close the jaw, whereas the lateral pterygoid muscle opens the jaw, protrudes the jaw, and moves the mandible from side to side (Figures 4.43 and 4.44).

MUSCLES WITHIN THE ANTERIOR TRIANGLE

The neck is frequently divided into two areas called the **anterior** and **posterior triangles** by the **sternocleidomastoid muscle (SCM)** (Figures 4.45 and 4.46). Everything anteromedial to the SCM is considered part of the anterior triangle, and everything posterior to the SCM is considered part of the posterior triangle. The SCM is a broad, straplike muscle that originates on the sternum and clavicle and inserts on the mastoid tip of the temporal bone. It functions to turn the head from side to side and to flex the neck.

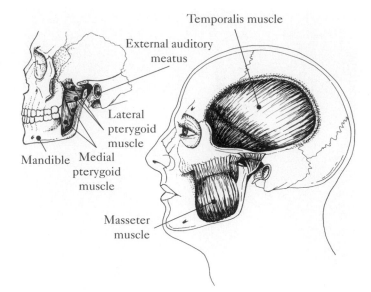

Figure 4.40   Lateral view of medial and lateral pterygoid muscles.

Key.   **lpt** lateral pterygoid muscle; **mass** masseter muscle; **mpt** medial pterygoid muscle; **par** parotid gland.

Figure 4.41   Sagittal MR scan of pterygoid muscles.   (R1.C)

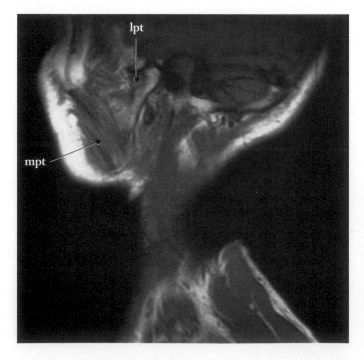

Figure 4.42   Axial MR scan of neck with masseter and medial pterygoid muscles.   (R2.D)

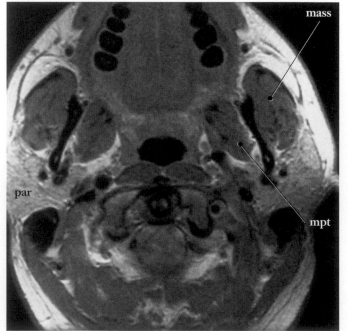

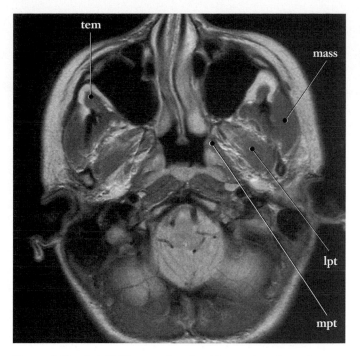

Figure 4.43   Axial MR scan of neck with muscles of mastication.   (R2.A)

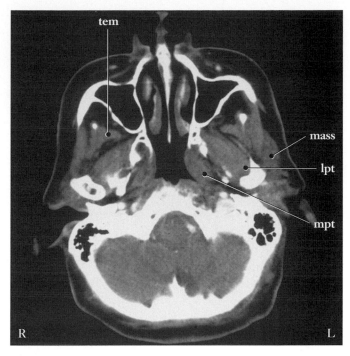

Figure 4.44   Axial CT scan of neck with muscles of mastication.   (R2.A)

Key. lpt lateral pterygoid muscle; **mass** masseter muscle; **mpt** medial pterygoid muscle **tem** temporalis muscle.

Figure 4.45   Anterior view of neck muscles.

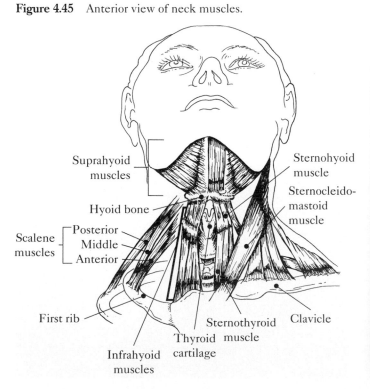

Key. cri cricoid cartilage; **hy** hyoid bone; **ihy** infrahyoid muscle; **SCM** sternocleidomastoid muscle; **suhy** suprahyoid muscles; **sman** submandibular gland; **thyc** thyroid cartilage; **thyg** thyroid gland; **to** tongue.

Figure 4.46   Coronal MR scan of anterior neck muscles.   (R3.B)

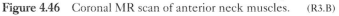
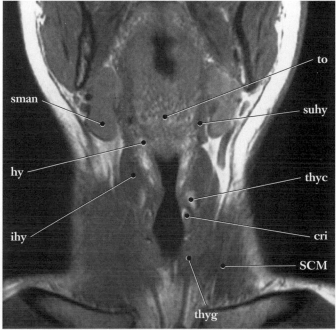

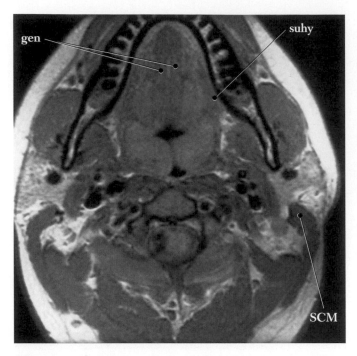

Figure 4.47   Axial MR scan of neck with SCM and suprahyoid
muscles.   (R2.G)

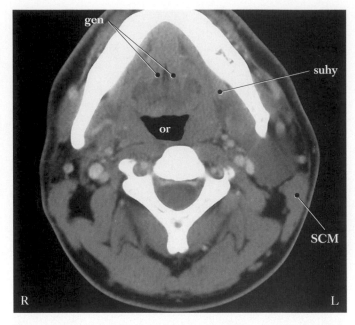

Figure 4.48   Axial CT scan of neck with SCM and suprahyoid
muscles.   (R2.G)

Key.   cri cricoid cartilage;   **gen** genioglossus muscle;   **inhy** infrahyoid muscle;   **or**
oropharynx;   **SCM** sternocleidomastoid muscle;   **suhy** suprahyoid muscle;   **thyc** thyroid
cartilage.

Figure 4.49   Axial MR scan of neck with SCM and infrahyoid
muscles.   (R2.L)

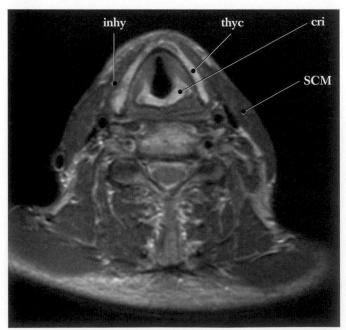

Figure 4.50   Axial CT scan of neck with SCM and infrahyoid
muscles.   (R2.L)

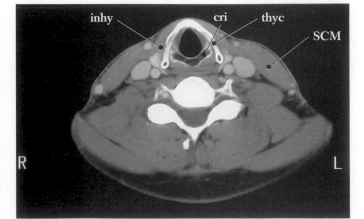

The muscles of the anterior triangle are referred to as the muscles of the throat and can be divided into the **suprahyoid** and **infrahyoid muscle groups.** These muscle groups are named according to their location in relation to the horseshoe-shaped **hyoid bone** (Figures 4.45 and 4.46). The hyoid bone lies in the anterior surface of the neck superior to the thyroid cartilage and below the mandible; it forms a base for the tongue. The suprahyoid and infrahyoid muscles aid in the movement of the hyoid bone and larynx. The suprahyoid muscles connect the hyoid bone to the temporal bone and mandible and elevate the hyoid and floor of the mouth and tongue during swallowing and speaking (Figures 4.47 and 4.48). The infrahyoid muscles are often called strap muscles because of their ribbonlike appearance (Figure 4.45). They act primarily to depress the hyoid bone and extend inferiorly to insert on the sternum, thyroid cartilage, and scapula (Figures 4.49 and 4.50).

MUSCLES WITHIN THE POSTERIOR TRIANGLE

The muscles of the posterior triangle include the **trapezius, splenius capitis, levator scapulae,** and the **anterior, middle,** and **posterior scalene muscles** (Figures 4.51 and 4.52). The trapezius muscle, a superficial muscle located on the posterior portion of the neck, acts to elevate the scapula. It originates from the occipital bone and spinous processes of C7-T12 to insert on the clavicle, acromion, and spine of the scapula. Located just anterior to the trapezius muscle, the splenius capitis muscle arises from the lower cervical and upper thoracic vertebrae to insert on the occipital bone and acts to extend the head. The levator scapulae muscle is located in the posterolateral portion of the neck. It arises from the transverse processes of the upper four cervical vertebrae to insert on the vertebral border of the scapula and acts to raise the scapula. The scalene muscle group (anterior, middle, and posterior scalene muscles) is located in the anterolateral portion of the neck (see Figure 4.45 and 4.52). The muscles originate from the transverse processes of the cervical vertebrae to insert on the first two ribs. Together, the scalene muscles act to elevate the upper two ribs and flex the neck. The anterior and middle scalene muscles can serve as a landmark for the brachial plexus because it courses between them (Figures 4.53 and 4.54).

Figure 4.51   Posterior view of trapezius and levator scapulae muscles.

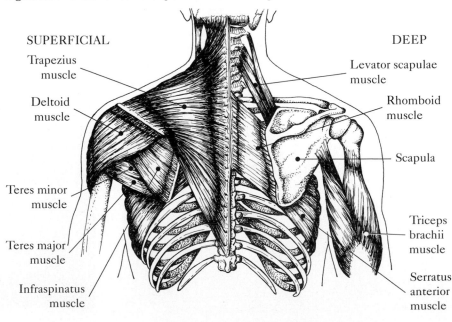

SUPERFICIAL

DEEP

Trapezius muscle

Deltoid muscle

Teres minor muscle

Teres major muscle

Infraspinatus muscle

Levator scapulae muscle

Rhomboid muscle

Scapula

Triceps brachii muscle

Serratus anterior muscle

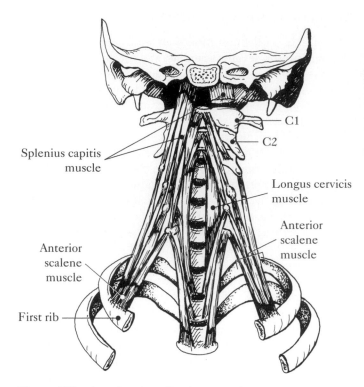

Figure 4.52   Anterior view of scalene muscles.

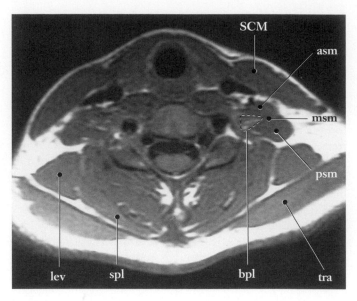

Figure 4.53   Axial MR scan of neck with posterior triangle muscles.   (R2.P)

Key.   asm anterior scalene muscle; **bpl** brachial plexus; **lev** levator scapula; **msm** middle scalene muscle; **psm** posterior scalene muscle; **SCM** sternocleidomastoid muscle; **spl** splenius capitus muscle; **tra** trapezius muscle.

Figure 4.54   Axial CT scan of neck with posterior triangle muscles.   (R2.M)

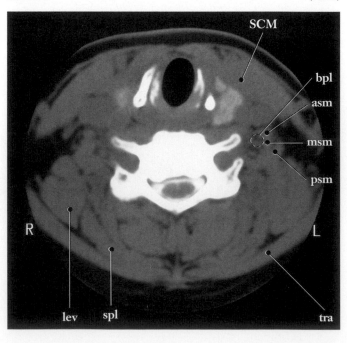

Table 4.1   Muscles associated with the neck

MUSCLE	LOCATION	ACTION
MUSCLES OF FACIAL EXPRESSION		
Buccinator	Between alveolar process of maxilla and mandible	Compress cheeks when blowing
Platysma	Anterior surface of neck extends from mandible to cervical fascia	Depress mandible, create ridges in neck
MUSCLES OF MASTICATION		
Temporalis	Extends from temporal bone to mandible	Elevate mandible
Masseter	Lateral ramus, extends from zygomatic arch to mandible	Elevate mandible
Medial pterygoid	Extends from pterygoid processes of sphenoid bone to mandible	Close jaw
Lateral pterygoid	Extends from pterygoid processes of sphenoid bone to mandible	Open jaw and move mandible from side to side
STERNOCLEIDOMASTOID		
	Extends from sternum and clavicle to mastoid tip and divides neck into anterior and posterior triangles	Turn head from side to side and flex neck
MUSCLES OF ANTERIOR TRIANGLE		
Suprahyoid muscle group	Extends from hyoid bone to temporal bone and mandible	Elevate hyoid bone, floor of mouth, tongue during swallowing
Infrahyoid muscle group	Extends from hyoid bone to sternum, thyroid cartilage, and scapula	Depress hyoid bone
MUSCLES OF POSTERIOR TRIANGLE		
Trapezius	Occipital bone and C7-T12 spinous processes to clavicle, acromion, and spine of scapula	Elevate scapula
Splenius capitis	Extends from lower cervical and upper thoracic vertebrae to occipital bone	Extend head
Levator scapulae	C1-C4 to scapula	Elevate scapula
Scalene (anterior, middle, and posterior)	Transverse processes of cervical vertebrae to first two ribs	Elevate upper two ribs

VASCULAR STRUCTURES

The vascular structures are located primarily in the lateral portions of the neck. The main vessels of the neck include the carotid and vertebral arteries and the jugular veins.

CAROTID ARTERIES

The **right common carotid artery** arises from the **brachiocephalic artery** posterior to the sternoclavicular joint (Figures 4.55 through 4.57). The **left common carotid artery** arises directly from the aortic arch (Figure 4.58). The common carotid arteries lie medial to the internal jugular vein and bifurcate into the internal and external carotid arteries at approximately the level of the thyroid cartilage (C3-C4). The **internal carotid artery** continues to ascend vertically to enter the base of the skull through the carotid canal, where it supplies blood to the brain (Figures 4.59 and 4.60). As the **external carotid artery** ascends the neck, it passes through the parotid gland to the level of the temporomandibular joint, where it bifurcates into its terminal branches to supply blood to the face. The external carotid artery changes position in relation to the internal carotid artery as it ascends the neck. At its lower level, the external carotid artery is anterior and medial to the internal carotid artery and becomes anterior and lateral to the internal carotid artery at its higher levels (Figures 4.60 through 4.62).

Figure 4.55 Oblique view of carotid and vertebral arteries.

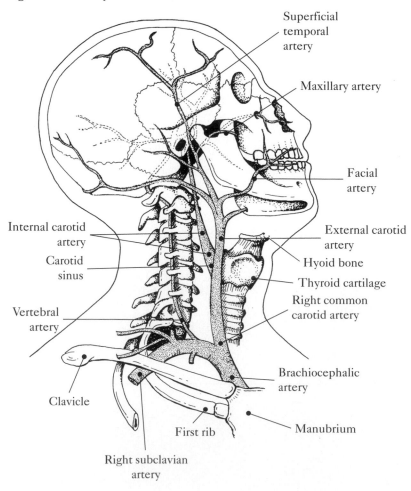

Superficial temporal artery

Maxillary artery

Facial artery

Internal carotid artery

Carotid sinus

External carotid artery

Hyoid bone

Thyroid cartilage

Right common carotid artery

Vertebral artery

Brachiocephalic artery

Clavicle

First rib

Manubrium

Right subclavian artery

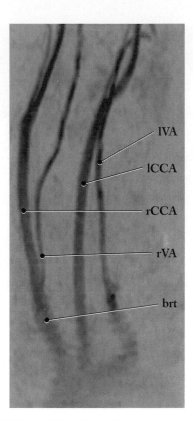

Figure 4.56   Oblique MRA of carotid and vertebral arteries.

Key.   brT brachiocephalic trunk; **CCA** common carotid artery; **ECA** external carotid artery; **ICA** internal carotid artery; **lCCA** left common carotid artery; **lSA** left subclavian artery; **lVA** left vertebral artery; **rCCA** right common carotid artery; **rVA** right vertebral artery.

Figure 4.57   Oblique CTA of carotid artery. (Courtesy GE Medical Systems, Milwaukee, Wisc.)

Figure 4.58   Anterior MRA of carotid and vertebral arteries. (Courtesy GE Medical Systems, Milwaukee, Wisc.)

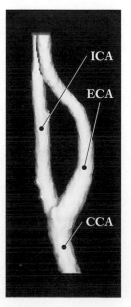

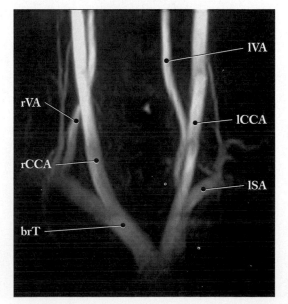

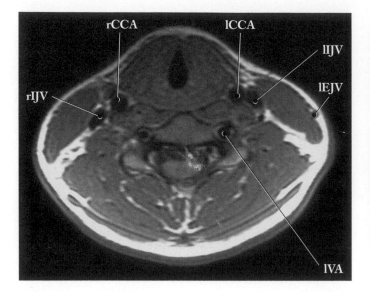

Figure 4.59 Axial MR scan of neck with carotid and vertebral arteries. (R2.K)

Key. **lCCA** left common carotid artery; **lEJV** left external jugular vein; **lIJV** left internal jugular vein; **lVA** left vertebral artery; **rCCA** right common carotid artery; **rIJV** right internal jugular vein.

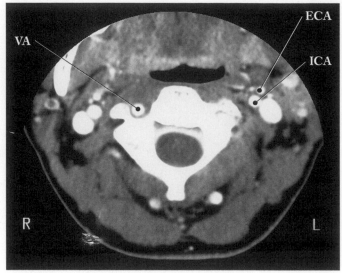

Figure 4.60 Axial CT scan of neck with carotid and vertebral arteries. (R2.G)

Key. **ECA** external carotid artery; **ICA** internal carotid artery; **VA** vertebral artery.

Key. **ECA** external carotid artery; **ICA** internal carotid artery; **VA** vertebral artery.

Figure 4.61 Axial MR scan of neck with bifurcation of carotid arteries and vertebral arteries. (R2.G)

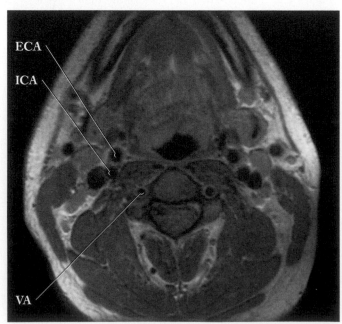

Figure 4.62 Axial CT scan of neck with bifurcation of carotid arteries and vertebral arteries. (R2.I)

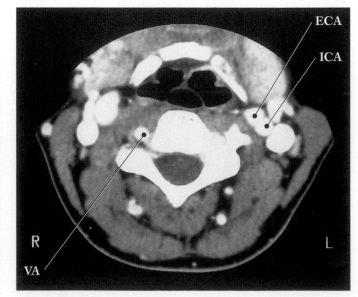

VERTEBRAL ARTERIES

The **vertebral arteries** begin as a branch of the **subclavian artery** and ascend the neck through the transverse foramina of C6-C1, where the arteries enter the foramen magnum to supply blood to the brain (Figures 4.55, 4.58, and 4.60).

JUGULAR VEINS

The **internal jugular veins** are typically the largest of the vascular structures of the neck (Figures 4.63 through 4.65). Commonly, the right internal jugular vein is larger than the left because it is the continuation of the sigmoid sinus from the head. The internal jugular veins typically run lateral to the common carotid artery. At the upper levels of the neck, they run posterior to the internal carotid artery; as they course inferiorly toward the subclavian vein, they become anterior in relation to the common carotid arteries. Blood from the lateral region of the face is drained by the **retromandibular vein,** which courses inferiorly through the parotid gland, where it continues as the external jugular vein (Figures 4.66 and 4.67). The **external jugular veins** begin near the angle of the mandible and cross the SCM just beneath the skin to empty into the subclavian vein. The **anterior jugular vein** begins at approximately the level of the hyoid bone and drains blood from the lower lip. This vessel enters the external jugular vein just below the SCM (Figures 4.68 and 4.69).

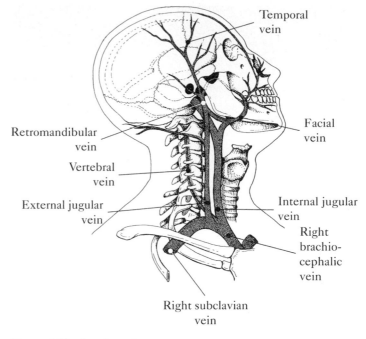

Figure 4.63   Jugular veins.

Key.   rCCA right common carotid artery; **rJV** right jugular vein.

Figure 4.64   Axial MR scan of neck with internal jugular vein.
(R2.P)

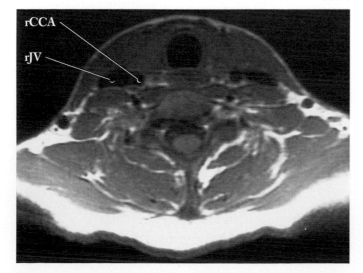

Key.   rCCA right common carotid artery; **rJV** right jugular vein.

Figure 4.65   Axial CT scan of neck with internal jugular vein.
(R2.P)

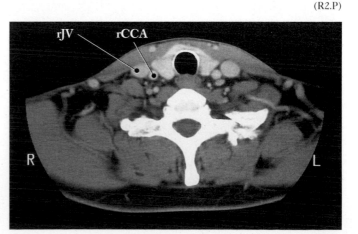

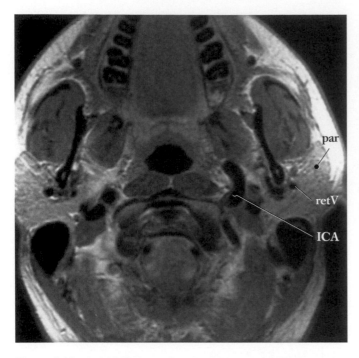

Figure 4.66 Axial MR scan of neck with retromandibular vein. (R2.D)

Key. **ICA** internal carotid artery; **par** parotid gland; **retV** retromandibular vein.

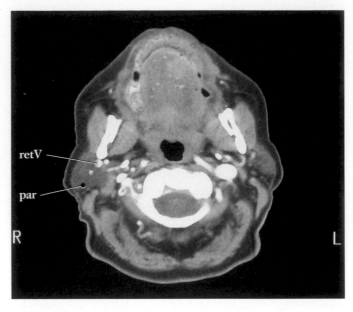

Figure 4.67 Axial CT scan of neck with retromandibular vein. (R2.D)

Key. **par** parotid gland; **retV** retromandibular vein.

Key. **AJV** anterior jugular vein; **cars** carotid sheath; **lCCA** left common carotid artery; **lEJV** left external jugular vein; **lIJV** left internal jugular vein; **lVA** left vertebral artery; **rCCA** right common carotid artery; **rIJV** right internal jugular vein.

Figure 4.68 Axial MR scan of neck with carotid sheath and anterior and external jugular veins. (R2.K)

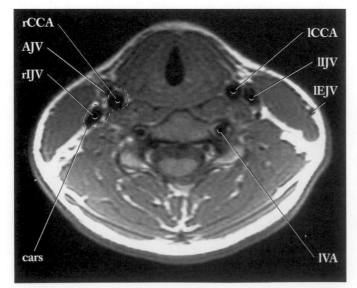

Key. **AJV** anterior jugular vein; **cars** carotid sheath; **CCA** common carotid artery; **EJV** external jugular vein; **IJV** internal jugular vein.

Figure 4.69 Axial CT scan of neck with carotid sheath and anterior and external jugular veins. (R2.K)

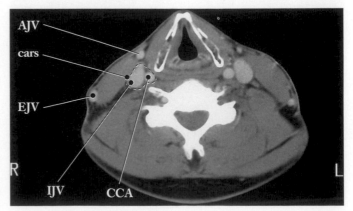

CAROTID SHEATH

The **carotid sheath** is a compartment composed of cervical fascia that encloses the common and internal carotid arteries, the internal jugular vein and associated lymph nodes, and the **vagus** nerve (Figures 4.68 through 4.70). The vagus nerve (CN X) exits the skull through the jugular foramen along with the jugular vein and descends posteriorly in the carotid sheath between the carotid artery and internal jugular vein.

ANSWER TO FIGURE 4.1

The left internal jugular vein is thrombosed because of the erosion of the large abscess. The abscess has also eroded into the esophagus.

Figure 4.70   Axial view of neck with carotid sheath.

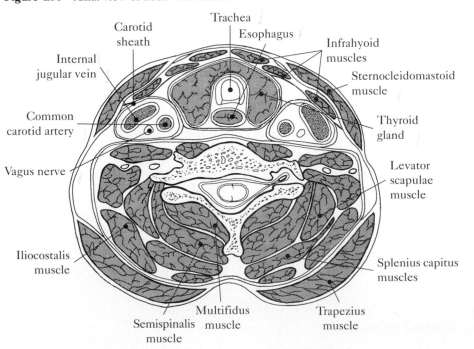

Carotid sheath

Trachea

Esophagus

Infrahyoid muscles

Internal jugular vein

Sternocleidomastoid muscle

Common carotid artery

Thyroid gland

Vagus nerve

Levator scapulae muscle

Iliocostalis muscle

Splenius capitus muscles

Multifidus muscle

Trapezius muscle

Semispinalis muscle

Chapter 5

1

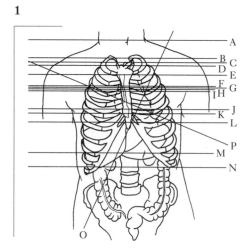

A
B
D
F
IH
C
E
G
J
K
L
P
M
N
O

2

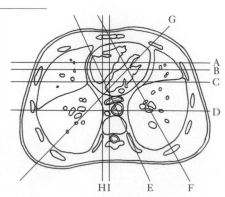

G
A
B
C
D
HI   E   F

Reference illustrations

Thorax

Life is an incurable Disease.

Abraham Cowley (1618–1667)
English poet

In Figure 5.1, the chest mass is in contact with which mediastinal structures? (Answer on p. 163.)

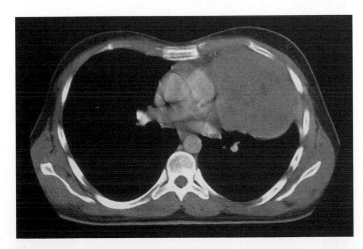

Figure 5.1 Axial CT scan of chest.

Many structures of the chest are in constant motion. Although physiologic motion can make imaging difficult, a thorough knowledge of chest anatomy and physiology can improve diagnostic imaging of this area. This chapter demonstrates sectional anatomy of the following structures:

Bony Thorax
thoracic vertebrae
sternum
ribs
costal cartilages
thoracic apertures

Lungs
apex
diaphragm
angles
hilum
lobes

Pleural Cavities
parietal pleura
visceral pleura

Bronchi
mainstem bronchi
secondary bronchi
tertiary bronchi
carina

Mediastinum
thymus gland
heart
branches of the aortic arch
tributaries of the superior vena cava
trachea
esophagus
thoracic duct
lymph nodes

Azygos Venous System

Muscles of the Thorax
pectoralis muscles
serratus muscles
rhomboid muscles
trapezius muscle
intercostal muscles
diaphragm

Breast
subcutaneous layer
mammary layer
retromammary layer

BONY THORAX

THORACIC VERTEBRAE, STERNUM, RIBS, AND COSTAL CARTILAGES

The bony thorax functions to protect the organs of the thorax and to aid in respiration. It consists of the **thoracic vertebrae, sternum, ribs,** and **costal cartilages** (Figure 5.2). The twelve thoracic vertebrae make up the posterior boundary of the thoracic cage. The anterior boundary is created by the sternum, located midline. The sternum has three components: **manubrium, body,** and **xiphoid process** (Figure 5.3). The triangular-shaped manubrium is the most superior portion. The manubrium articulates with the first two pairs of ribs and the clavicles. The articulations between the manubrium and clavicles are termed the **sternoclavicular joints.** A common landmark, the **jugular notch,** is located on the superior border of the manubrium. The manubrium and body of the sternum come together at an angle to form a ridge known as the **sternal angle.** The sternal angle is another important landmark located at approximately the level of T4-T5. The slender body of the sternum has several indentations along its sides where it articulates with the third through seventh ribs. The small xiphoid process is located on the inferior border of the sternum and is a site for muscle attachments.

Forming the lateral borders of the thoracic cage are the twelve pairs of ribs. All twelve pairs of ribs articulate posteriorly with the thoracic spine. As stated earlier, the first seven pairs of ribs (true ribs) articulate anteriorly with the sternum by costal cartilage. The lower five pairs of ribs are considered false ribs because they do not attach directly to the sternum.

Key. **b** body; **ma** manubrium; **sta** sternal angle; **tho** thoracic outlet.

Figure 5.3 Sagittal MR scan of thoracic cage. (Courtesy Anne Marie Sawyer, Radiologic Sciences Laboratory, Stanford University School of Medicine, Stanford, Calif.) (R2.H)

Figure 5.2 Anterior view of thoracic cage.

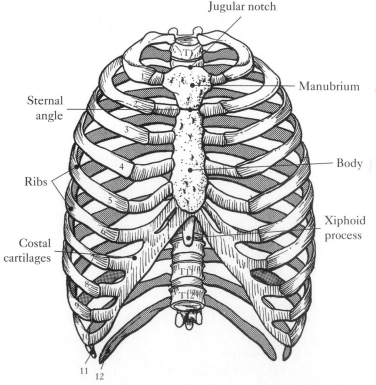

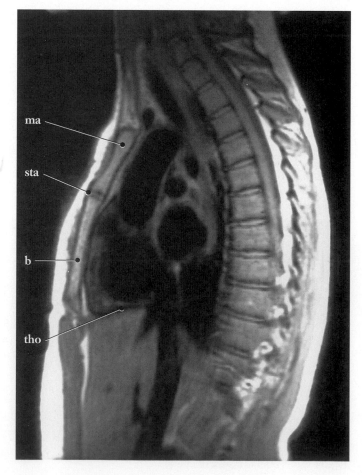

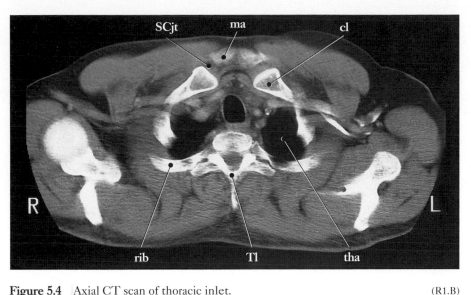

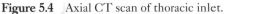

Figure 5.4 Axial CT scan of thoracic inlet.   (R1.B)

Key. **cl** clavicle; **ma** manubrium; **rib** first rib; **SCjt** sternoclavicular joint; **tha** thoracic aperture; **T1** first thoracic vertebra.

THORACIC APERTURES

There are two openings or **apertures** associated with the bony thorax. The **superior aperture** is formed by the first thoracic vertebra, first pair of ribs and their costal cartilages, and manubrium. This aperture, known as the **thoracic inlet,** allows for the passage of nerves, vessels, and viscera from the neck into the thoracic cavity. The **inferior aperture** is much larger and is made up of the twelfth thoracic vertebra, twelfth pair of ribs and costal margins, and xiphoid sternal junction. This aperture is known as the **thoracic outlet** (Figures 5.4 and 5.5).

Key.   **T12** twelfth thoracic vertebra; **x** xiphoid process.

Figure 5.5 Axial CT scan of thoracic outlet.   (R1.L)

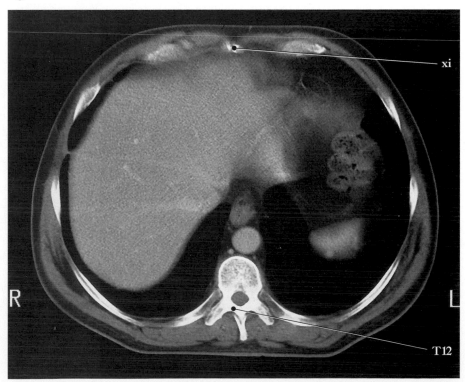

Lungs

Apex, diaphragm, angles, hilum, and lobes

The **lungs** are the organs of respiration. They are large, conical-shaped structures that extend up to or slightly above the level of the first rib at their **apex** and down to the dome of the **diaphragm** at their wide concave-shaped bases. Two prominent angles can be identified at the medial and lateral edges of the lung bases. The **medial angle** is termed the **cardiophrenic sulcus,** and the **lateral angle** is termed the **costophrenic sulcus** (Figures 5.6 and 5.7). The lungs are divided into lobes by thin structures called **fissures** (Figure 5.8). The right lung has three lobes (superior [upper], middle, and inferior [lower]), whereas the left lung has just superior (upper) and inferior (lower) lobes. The left lung has a large notch on its medial surface called the **cardiac notch.** On the medial surface of the lungs is an opening termed the **hilum** (Figures 5.9 and 5.10). This opening acts as a passage for mainstem bronchi, blood vessels, lymph vessels, and nerves to enter the lung.

Figure 5.6   Anterior view of lungs.

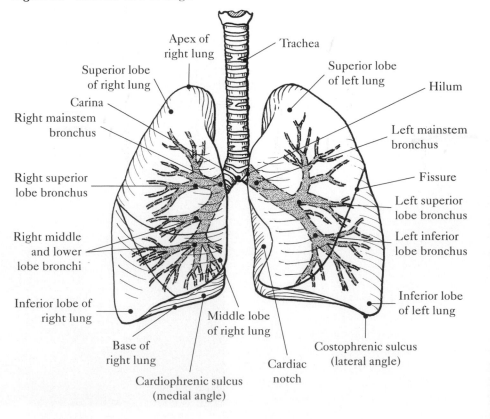

Apex of
right lung

Trachea

Superior lobe
of right lung

Superior lobe
of left lung

Hilum

Carina

Right mainstem
bronchus

Left mainstem
bronchus

Right superior
lobe bronchus

Fissure

Left superior
lobe bronchus

Left inferior
lobe bronchus

Right middle
and lower
lobe bronchi

Inferior lobe of
right lung

Inferior lobe
of left lung

Base of
right lung

Middle lobe
of right lung

Cardiac
notch

Costophrenic sulcus
(lateral angle)

Cardiophrenic sulcus
(medial angle)

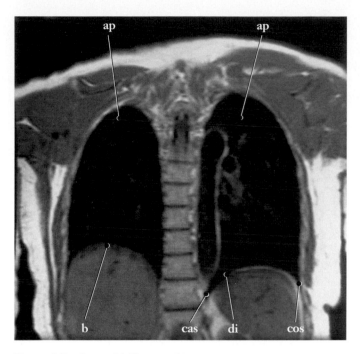

Figure 5.7   Coronal MR scan of lungs.   (R2.D)

Key.   **ap** apex of lung; **b** base of lung; **cas** cardiophrenic sulcus; **cos** costophrenic sulcus; **di** diaphragm.

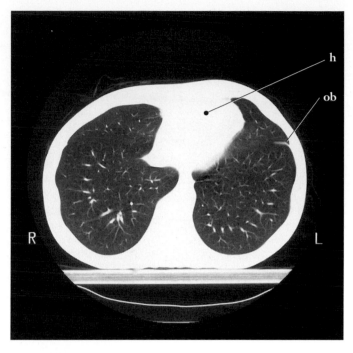

Figure 5.8   Axial CT scan of lungs with fissure.   (R1.H)

Key.   **h** heart; **ob** oblique fissure of left lung.

Key.   **hi** hilum.

Figure 5.9   Axial MR scan of lungs at hilum. (Courtesy Anne Marie Sawyer, Radiologic Sciences Laboratory, Stanford University School of Medicine, Stanford, Calif.)   (R1.G)

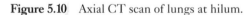

Key.   **hi** hilum; **mbr** mainstrem bronchi.

Figure 5.10   Axial CT scan of lungs at hilum.   (R1.G)

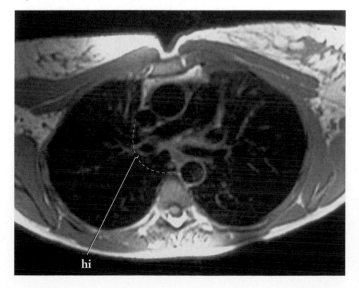

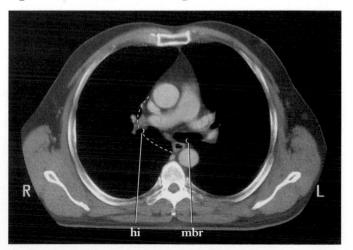

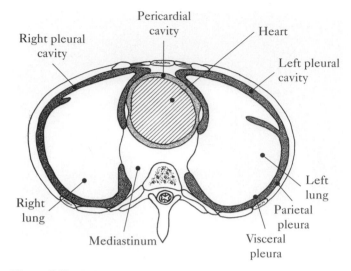

Figure 5.11   Axial cross section of pleural cavity.

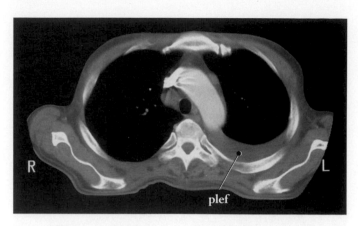

Figure 5.12   Axial CT scan with pleural effusion.   (R1.E)

Key.   plef pleural effusion.

Figure 5.13   Anterior view of bronchial tree.

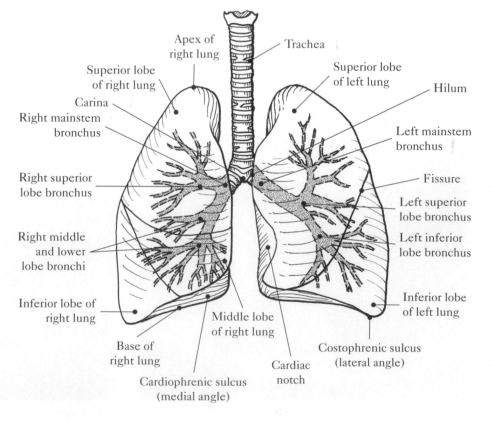

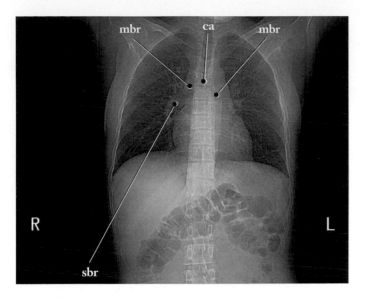

Figure 5.14 CT anterior scout of chest.

Key. **ca** carina; **mbr** mainstem bronchi; **sbr** secondary bronchi; **tbr** tertiary bronchi.

PLEURAL CAVITIES

PARIETAL AND VISCERAL PLEURAE

Each lung lies within a single **pleural cavity** that is lined by a serous membrane or **pleura.** The pleura can be divided into two portions. The **parietal pleura** is continuous with the thoracic wall and diaphragm and moves with these structures with respiration. The **visceral pleura** is the inner layer that closely covers the outer surface of the lung and continues into the fissures to cover the individual lobes as well. Both membranes secrete a small amount of pleural fluid that provides lubrication between the surfaces during breathing (Figures 5.11 and 5.12).

BRONCHI

MAINSTEM, SECONDARY, AND TERTIARY BRONCHI AND CARINA

The **trachea** bifurcates into the **left** and **right mainstem (primary) bronchi** at approximately the level of T5. This location is commonly referred to as the **carina.** At the hilum the mainstem bronchi enter the lung and divide into **secondary bronchi** (Figures 5.13 through 5.15). Secondary bronchi are associated with each lobe of the lungs. There is further division of the secondary bronchi into **tertiary bronchi,** which extend into the lobes (Figure 5.16). The bronchial tree continues to divide many times until it reaches the terminal end as alveoli, which are the functional units of the respiratory system.

Figure 5.15 Axial MR scan at carina. (Courtesy Anne Marie Sawyer, Radiologic Sciences Laboratory, Stanford University School of Medicine, Stanford, Calif.)   (R1.F)

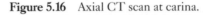

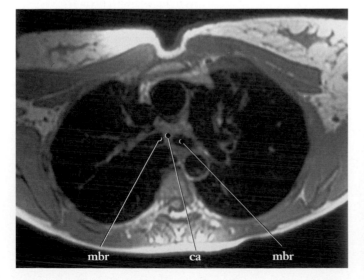

Figure 5.16 Axial CT scan at carina.   (R1.F)

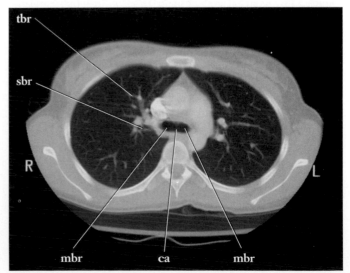

MEDIASTINUM

The **mediastinum** is the midline region located between the two lungs. This region is composed of the thymus gland, heart and great vessels, trachea and esophagus, thoracic duct, lymph nodes, and other structures.

THYMUS GLAND

The **thymus gland** is a triangular-shaped, bilobed gland located in the superior portion of the mediastinum behind the manubrium. The thymus gland produces lymphocytes and plays an important role in the maintenance and development of the immune system (Figures 5.17 through 5.19).

> The thymus gland is large in children. It gradually decreases in size with increasing age and is replaced by mediastinal fat.

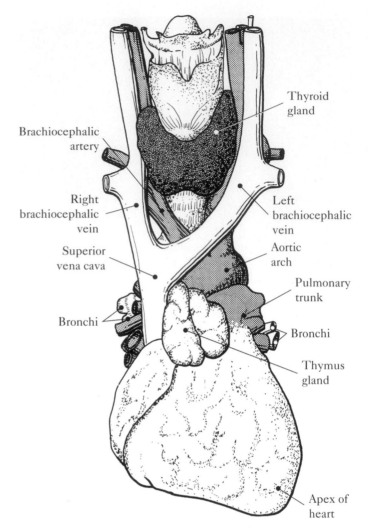

Figure 5.17   Anterior view of thymus gland.

Key.   thym thymus gland.

Figure 5.18   Axial CT scan of pediatric chest with thymus gland (Courtesy Mercy Medical Center, Computed Tomography Department, Nampa, Idaho.).   (R1.B)

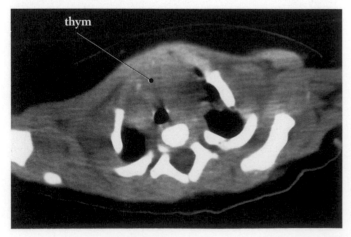

Key.   ma manubrium; **thym** thymus gland.

Figure 5.19   Axial CT scan of adult chest with thymus gland.   (R1.E)

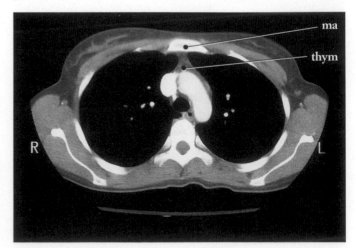

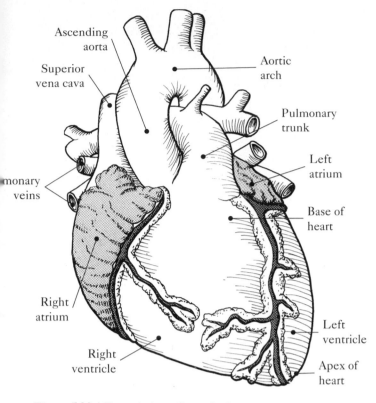

Figure 5.20 Frontal view of anterior heart.

HEART

The **heart** is a muscular organ located within the mediastinum. Its function is to pump deoxygenated blood to the lungs and oxygenated blood to the vessels and tissues. Surrounding the heart is a serous membrane called the **pericardium,** which lubricates the heart as it beats. Located between the pericardium and the heart wall is a layer of **epicardial fat,** which is typically more prominent near the venous inflow and arterial outflow of the heart (Figures 5.20 through 5.22). The heart lies at a 45-degree angle within the thorax. The inferior point of the heart, the **apex,** projects anteriorly and to the left of the midline at the level of the fifth intercostal space. The broad superior portion of the heart is termed the **base,** which gives rise to the great vessels. The walls of the heart consist of three layers: (1) **epicardium,** the thin outer layer that is in contact with the pericardium; (2) **myocardium,** the thick middle layer consisting of strong cardiac muscle; and (3) **endocardium,** the thin layer lining the inner surface (Figure 5.23).

Key. **epif** epicardial fat.

Figure 5.21 Axial MR scan of heart with epicardial fat. (Courtesy Anne Marie Sawyer, Radiologic Sciences Laboratory, Stanford University School of Medicine, Stanford, Calif.) (R1.I)

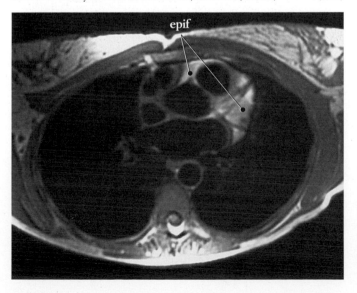

Key. **epif** epicardial fat; **myo** myocardium; **per** pericardium.

Figure 5.22 Axial CT scan of heart with epicardial fat. (R1.K)

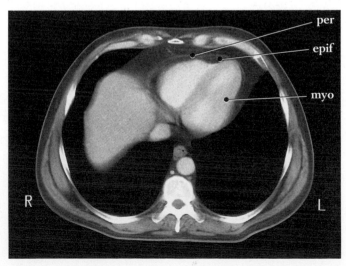

The heart is divided into four **chambers** (Figures 5.23 and 5.24). The two superior collecting chambers called **atria** are divided by the **interatrial septum** (Figures 5.25 through 5.27). The two inferior pumping chambers called **ventricles** are divided by the **interventricular septum** (Figures 5.28 and 5.29). The myocardium of the ventricles is thicker than that of the atria because of the strong muscular contractions necessary to force blood through the body. The left ventricle makes up the apex of the heart and has a particularly thick myocardium to enable it to pump blood to the peripheral tissues of the body (Figures 5.30 through 5.32).

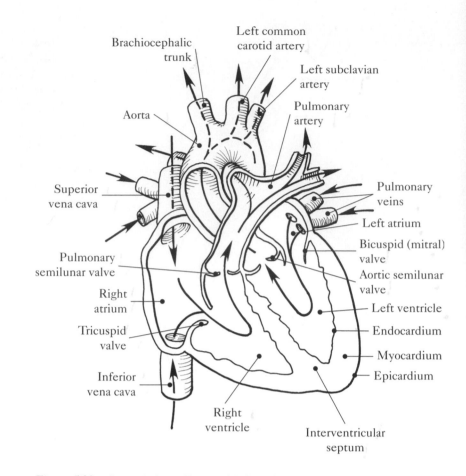

Figure 5.23   Coronal view of heart with four chambers.

Key.   asa ascending aorta; **asv** aortic semilunar valve; **lv** left ventricle; **PA** pulmonary arteries; **ra** right atrium.

Figure 5.24   Coronal MR scan of heart. (Courtesy GE Medical Systems, Milwaukee, Wisc.)   (R2.A)

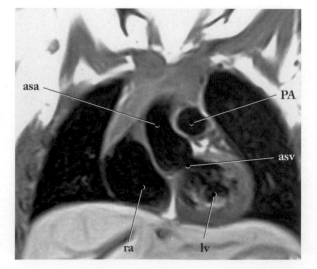

Figure 5.25   Axial view of heart with four chambers.

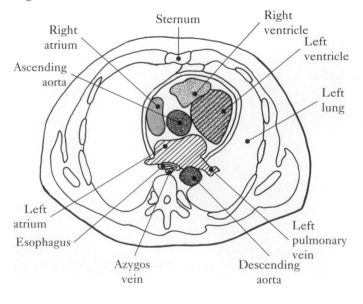

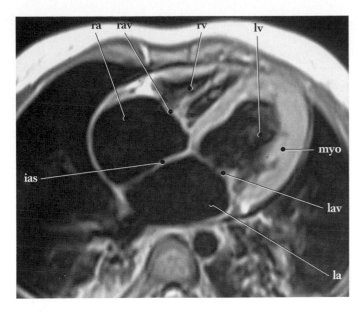

Figure 5.26   Long-axis MR scan of heart with four chambers. (Courtesy GE Medical Systems, Milwaukee, Wisc.)   (R1.P)

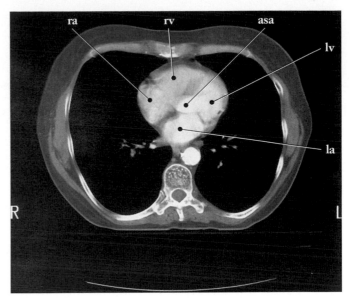

Figure 5.27   Axial CT scan of heart with four chambers.   (R1.I)

Key. **asa** ascending aorta; **ias** intraatrial septum; **ivs** interventricular septum; **la** left atrium; **lav** left atrioventricular valve; **lv** left ventricle; **myo** myocardium; **ra** right atrium; **rav** right atrioventricular valve; **rv** right ventricle.

Figure 5.28   Axial MR scan of heart with ventricles. (Courtesy Anne Marie Sawyer, Radiologic Sciences Laboratory, Stanford University School of Medicine, Stanford, Calif.)   (R1.J)

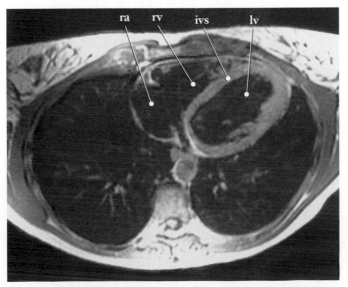

Figure 5.29   Axial CT scan of heart with ventricles.   (R1.K)

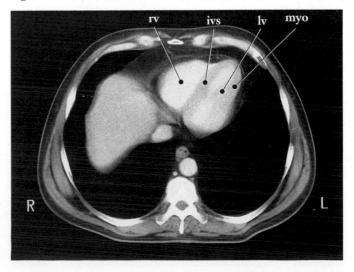

Four **valves** are located in the heart that function to maintain one-way directional blood flow throughout the heart (Figure 5.23). The valves can be divided into two groups: **atrioventricular** and **semilunar**. The atrioventricular valves prevent backflow of blood between the atria and ventricles. The right atrioventricular valve is called the **tricuspid valve,** and the left atrioventricular valve is called the **bicuspid (mitral) valve.** Semilunar valves are located at the junction where the ventricles meet the great vessels. The **pulmonary semilunar valve** is associated with the right ventricle, and the **aortic semilunar valve** is associated with the left ventricle.

Carditis, an inflammation of the heart, can often lead to valvular heart disease. When infection damages or destroys the heart valves, valve leakage, heart failure, and death can ensue.

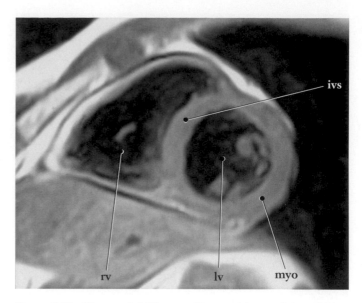

Figure 5.30   Short-axis MR scan of heart with ventricles. (Courtesy GE Medical Systems, Milwaukee, Wisc.)   (R1.O)

Key.   **ivs** interventricular septum; **la** left atrium; **lv** left ventricle; **mv** mitral valve; **myo** myocardium; **rv** right ventricle.

Figure 5.31   RAO MR scan of two-chamber view of the heart. (Courtesy Anne Marie Sawyer, Radiologic Sciences Laboratory, Stanford University School of Medicine, Stanford, Calif.)   (R2.G)

Figure 5.32   RAO MR scan of heart with right ventricle. (Courtesy GE Medical Systems, Milwaukee, Wisc.)   (R2.F)

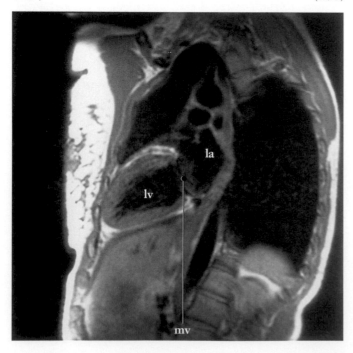

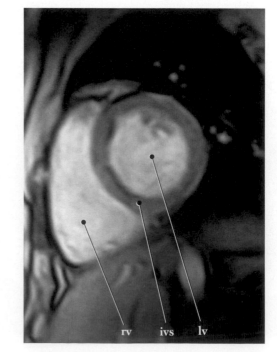

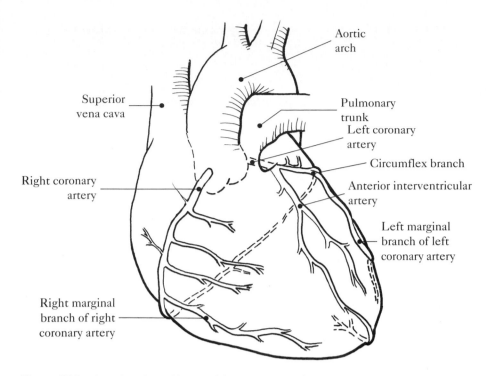

Figure 5.33   Anterior view of heart with coronary arteries.

CORONARY ARTERIES.   The **coronary arteries** supply oxygenated blood to the heart muscle. The two main coronary arteries are the first vessels to branch off the ascending aorta, arising from its anterior surface (Figure 5.33). These arteries provide the myocardium with a constant supply of blood. The **right coronary artery** adheres closely to the right surface of the heart as it branches to supply primarily the right atrium, right ventricle, and interatrial septum. The **left coronary artery** extends transversely between the pulmonary trunk and the left atrium and then branches to supply the left atrium, left ventricle, and interventricular septum (Figure 5.34).

Key.   **a** aorta; **la** left atrium; **lCA** left coronary artery; **lv** left ventricle; **ra** right atrium; **rCA** right coronary artery; **rv** right ventricle.

Figure 5.34   Axial CT scan of heart with left and right coronary arteries.   (R1.I)

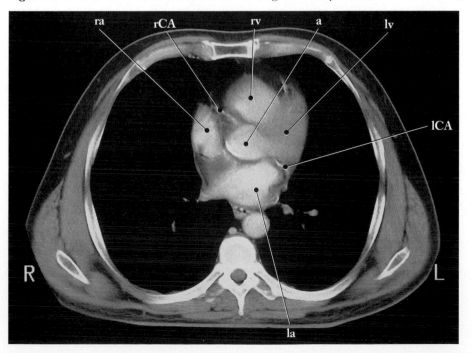

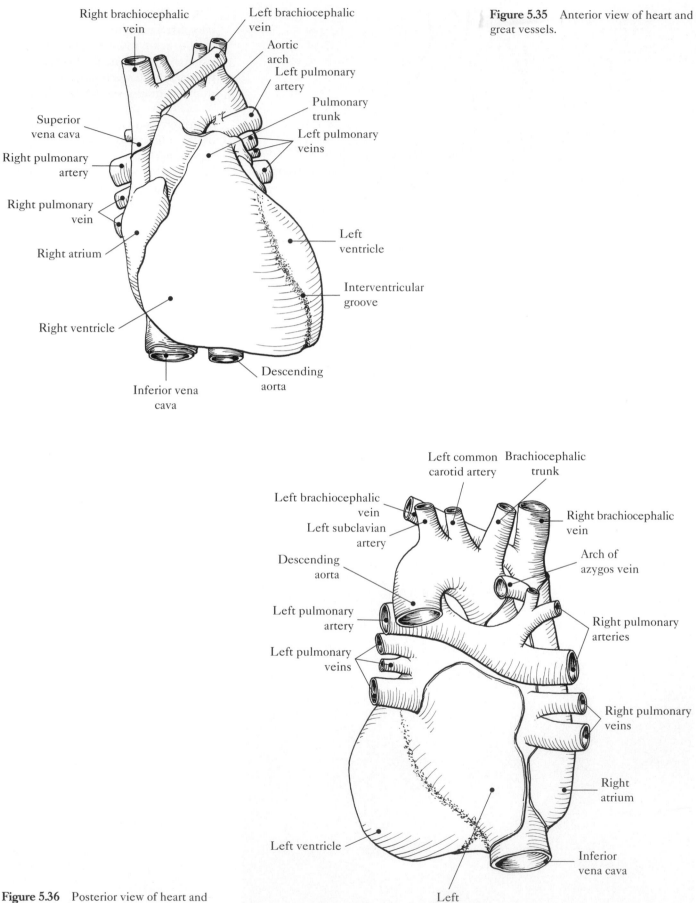

Right brachiocephalic vein

Left brachiocephalic vein

Aortic arch

Left pulmonary artery

Pulmonary trunk

Superior vena cava

Left pulmonary veins

Right pulmonary artery

Right pulmonary vein

Left ventricle

Right atrium

Interventricular groove

Right ventricle

Inferior vena cava

Descending aorta

Figure 5.35   Anterior view of heart and great vessels.

Left common carotid artery

Brachiocephalic trunk

Left brachiocephalic vein

Left subclavian artery

Right brachiocephalic vein

Descending aorta

Arch of azygos vein

Left pulmonary artery

Right pulmonary arteries

Left pulmonary veins

Right pulmonary veins

Right atrium

Left ventricle

Inferior vena cava

Left atrium

Figure 5.36   Posterior view of heart and great vessels.

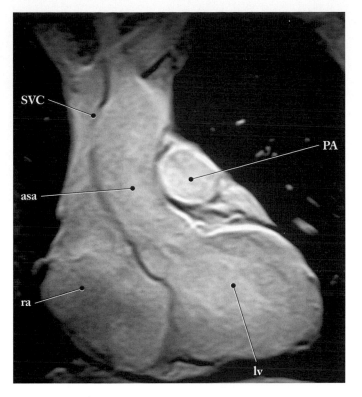

Figure 5.37   Coronal MR scan of chest with aortic arch. (Courtesy GE Medical Systems, Milwaukee, Wisc.)   (R2.B)

Key.   a aorta; **asa** ascending aorta; **ca** carina; **lv** left ventricle; **PA** pulmonary arteries; **PV** pulmonary veins; **ra** right atrium; **SVC** superior vena cava.

Figure 5.38   Coronal MR scan of chest with pulmonary arteries. (Courtesy Anne Marie Sawyer, Radiologic Sciences Laboratory, Stanford University School of Medicine, Stanford, Calif.)   (R2.C)

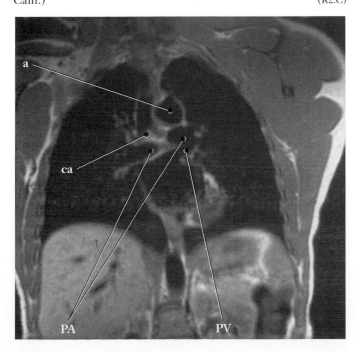

GREAT VESSELS.   Blood travels to and from the heart through the **great vessels**, which include the **aorta, pulmonary trunk,** and **superior** and **inferior venae cavae** (Figures 5.35 through 5.38). The aorta is the largest artery of the body and can be divided into the **ascending aorta, aortic arch,** and **descending aorta.** The ascending aorta begins at the base of the left ventricle and curves superiorly and posteriorly as the aortic arch from which three major vessels branch (Figures 5.39 and 5.40). The descending aorta is the continuation of the aortic arch, lying slightly anterior and to the left of the vertebral column as it descends through the thoracic and abdominal cavities (Figures 5.41 and 5.42). The pulmonary trunk arises from the right ventricle adjacent to the ascending aorta (Figures 5.43 and 5.44). It ascends to the level of the aortic arch, where it bifurcates into the **right** and **left pulmonary arteries.** The right pulmonary artery courses laterally and anterior to the right mainstem bronchus, whereas the left pulmonary artery immediately arches over and descends posterior to the left mainstem bronchus. At the hilum of the lungs, the pulmonary arteries branch out along the divisions of the bronchial tree. Inferior to the pulmonary arteries are four **pulmonary veins,** two extending from each lung to enter the left atrium (Figures 5.45 through 5.48).

Obstruction of a pulmonary artery or one of its branches is known as a *pulmonary embolism.* This condition prevents blood flow to the alveoli and, if left in place for several hours, will result in permanent collapse of the alveoli. It is usually caused by thrombosis in lower extremities.

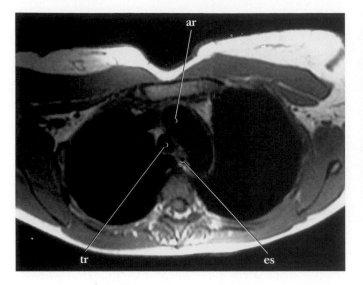

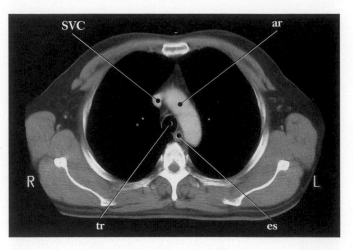

Figure 5.40 Axial CT scan of chest with aortic arch. (R1.E)

Figure 5.39 Axial MR scan of chest with aortic arch. (Courtesy Anne Marie Sawyer, Radiologic Sciences Laboratory, Stanford University School of Medicine, Stanford, Calif.) (R1.E)

Key. **ar** aortic arch; **asa** ascending aorta; **ca** carina; **da** descending aorta; **es** esophagus; **SVC** superior vena cava; **tr** trachea.

Figure 5.41 Axial MR scan of chest with ascending and descending aortae. (Courtesy Anne Marie Sawyer, Radiologic Sciences Laboratory, Stanford University School of Medicine, Stanford, Calif.) (R1.F)

Figure 5.42 Axial CT scan of chest with ascending and descending aortae. (R1.F)

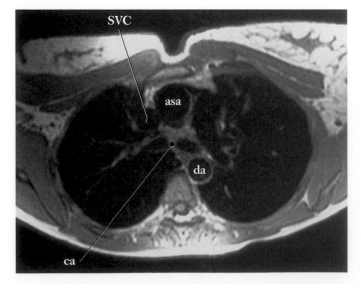

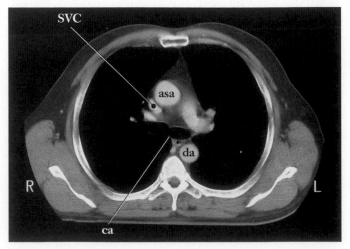

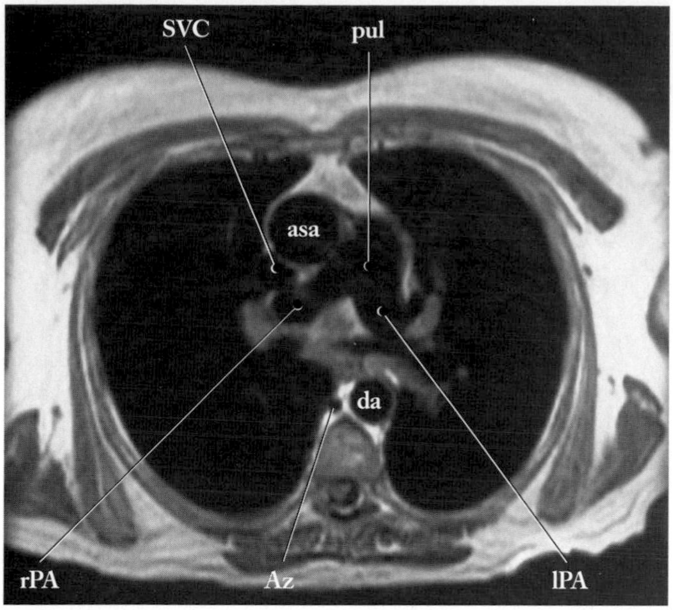

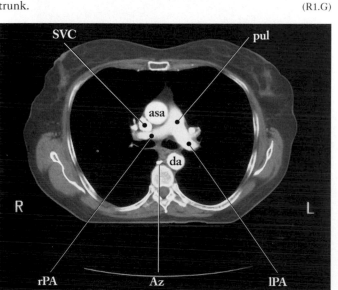

Figure 5.43   Axial MR scan of chest with pulmonary trunk.   (R1.G)

The superior and inferior venae cavae are the largest veins of the body. The superior vena cava is formed by the junction of the brachiocephalic veins and enters the upper portion of the right atrium. The inferior vena cava is formed by the junction of the common iliac veins and enters the lower portion of the right atrium. It ascends the abdominal and thoracic cavities slightly anterior to the vertebral column and to the right of the descending aorta (Figures 5.41 through 5.45).

CIRCULATION OF BLOOD THROUGH THE HEART. Deoxygenated blood is brought to the right atrium from the peripheral tissues by the inferior and superior venae cavae. The right atrium contracts, forcing blood through the tricuspid (right atrioventricular) valve into the right ventricle. The right ventricle pumps blood through the pulmonary semilunar valve to the pulmonary arteries, which enter into the lungs. Oxygenated blood returns to the heart via the pulmonary veins, which enter the left atrium. The left atrium forces blood through the bicuspid (mitral) valve into the left ventricle, where it is then pumped through the aortic semilunar valve to the aorta (see Figure 5.23).

Key. asa ascending aorta; **Az** azygous vein; **da** descending aorta; **lPA** left pulmonary artery; **pul** pulmonary trunk; **rPA** right pulmonary artery; **SVC** superior vena cava.

Figure 5.44   Axial CT scan of chest with pulmonary trunk.   (R1.G)

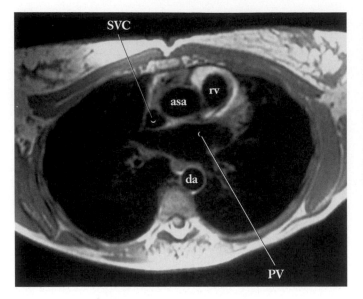

Figure 5.45 Axial MR scan of chest with pulmonary veins. (Courtesy Anne Marie Sawyer, Radiologic Sciences Laboratory, Stanford University School of Medicine, Stanford, Calif.)   (R1.I)

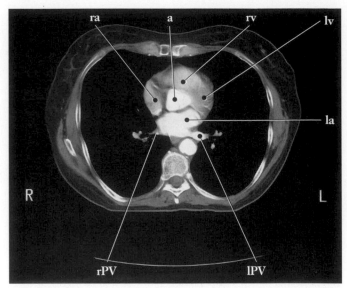

Figure 5.46 Axial CT scan of chest with pulmonary veins.   (R1.I)

Key. **a** aorta; **ab** aortic bulb; **ar** aortic arch; **asa** ascending aorta; **da** descending aorta; **IVC** inferior vena cava; **la** left atrium; **lPV** left pulmonary vein; **lv** left ventricle; **mbr** mainstem bronchi; **ra** right atrium; **rPA** right pulmonary artery; **rPV** right pulmonary vein; **rv** right ventricle; **SVC** superior vena cava; **tr** trachea.

Figure 5.47 Sagittal MR scan of left mediastinum. (Courtesy Anne Marie Sawyer, Radiologic Sciences Laboratory, Stanford University School of Medicine, Stanford, Calif.)   (R2.E)

Figure 5.48 Sagittal MR scan of right mediastinum. (Courtesy Anne Marie Sawyer, Radiologic Sciences Laboratory, Stanford University School of Medicine, Stanford, Calif.)   (R2.I)

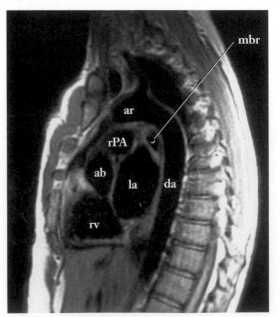

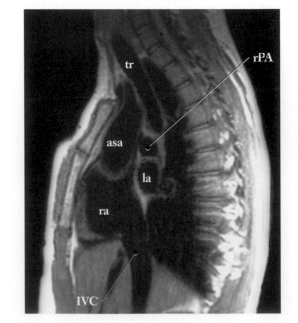

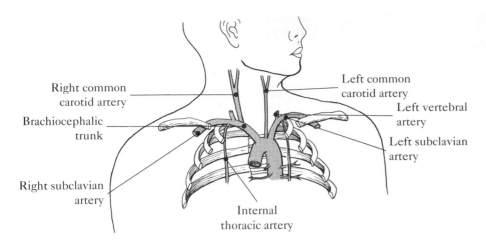

Figure 5.49   Branches of the aortic arch.

Key. brT brachiocephalic trunk; **lCCA** left common carotid artery; **lSA** left subclavian artery; **lVA** left vertebral artery; **rCCA** right common carotid artery; **rSA** left subclavian artery; **rVA** right vertebral artery.

Figure 5.50   MRA of aortic arch. (Courtesy GE Medical Systems, Milwaukee, Wisc.)

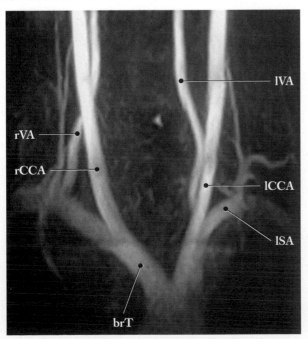

BRANCHES OF THE AORTIC ARCH

The three main branches of the aortic arch are the brachiocephalic trunk, left common carotid artery, and left subclavian artery (Figures 5.49 through 5.51). The **brachiocephalic (innominate) trunk** is the first major vessel to branch from the aortic arch. It passes upward and to the right of the trachea before dividing, behind the right sternoclavicular joint, into the **right common carotid** and **right subclavian arteries** (Figures 5.50 and 5.51). The right common carotid artery ascends the neck lateral to the trachea. The right subclavian artery curves posterior to the clavicle into the axillary region, where it becomes the axillary artery. The **left common carotid artery** is the second vessel to branch from the aortic arch. It arises just behind the left sternoclavicular joint and ascends into the neck along the left side of the trachea. The **left subclavian artery** arises from the aortic arch posterior to the left common carotid artery and arches laterally in a manner similar to that of the right subclavian artery. The common carotid arteries supply blood to the head and neck, whereas the subclavian arteries supply blood to the upper extremities (Figures 5.52 and 5.53).

Key.   ar aortic arch; **brT** brachiocephalic trunk; **lCCA** left common carotid artery; **lSA** left subclavian artery; **rCCA** right common carotid artery; **rSA** right subclavian artery.

Figure 5.51   CTA of aortic arch. (Courtesy Picker International, Cleveland, Ohio.)

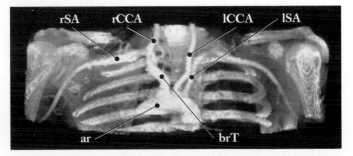

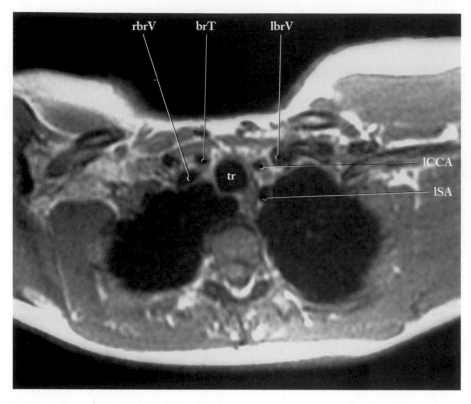

Figure 5.52   Axial MR scan of chest with aortic arch branches and superior vena cava tributaries. (Courtesy Anne Marie Sawyer, Radiologic Sciences Laboratory, Stanford University School of Medicine, Stanford, Calif.)   (R1.C)

Key. brT brachiocephalic trunk; **es** esophagus; **lbrV** left brachiocephalic vein; **lCCA** left common carotid artery; **lSA** left subclavian artery; **rbrA** right brachiocephalic artery; **rbrV** right brachiocephalic vein; **tr** trachea.

Figure 5.53   Axial CT scan of chest with aortic arch branches and superior vena cava tributaries.
                                                                    (R1.C)

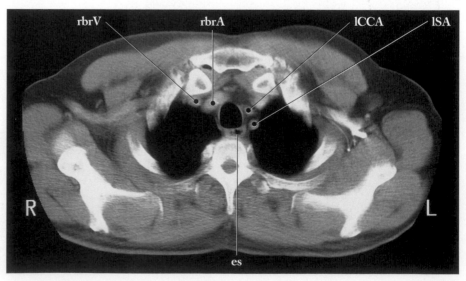

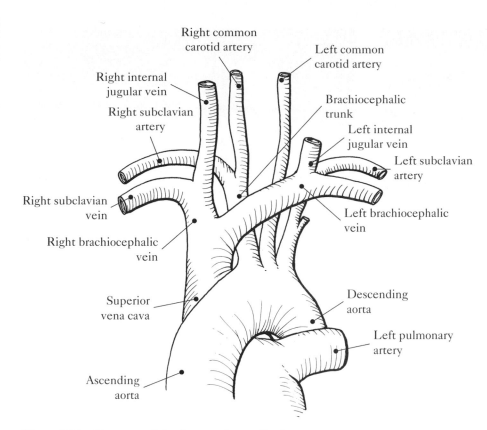

Figure 5.54   Great vessels in the superior mediastinum.

TRIBUTARIES OF THE SUPERIOR VENA CAVA

The superior vena cava receives blood from the head and neck via the **internal** and **external jugular veins** and from the upper extremities via the subclavian veins (Figures 5.54 through 5.56). The subclavian veins arise from the axillary veins and course posterior to the clavicles. The subclavian veins receive blood from the external jugular veins before uniting with the internal jugular veins behind the sternoclavicular joints, where they continue as the **brachiocephalic veins.** The left brachiocephalic vein courses across the midline, anterior to the branches of the aorta, to unite with the right brachiocephalic vein just posterior to the sternum (Figures 5.57 and 5.58). The union of the two brachiocephalic veins forms the superior vena cava, which empties into the right atrium of the heart.

TRACHEA AND ESOPHAGUS

Throughout their course in the mediastinum, the trachea runs anterior to the esophagus. In cross section, the trachea appears as a round, air-filled structure to the point at which it bifurcates at the carina. The **esophagus** appears as an oval-shaped structure that descends through the diaphragm to enter the stomach at the gastroesophageal junction (Figures 5.57 through 5.59).

Key.   EJV external jugular vein; **IJV** internal jugular vein; **lCCA** left common carotid artery; **rCCA** right common carotid artery; **rJV** right jugular vein; **VA** vertebral artery.

Figure 5.55   Axial MR scan of neck with jugular veins.   (R1.D)

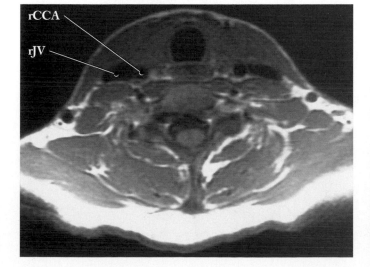

Figure 5.56   Axial CT scan of neck with jugular veins.   (R1.A)

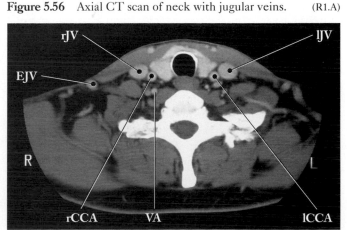

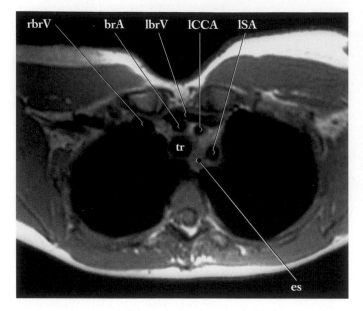

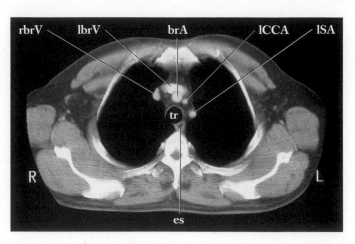

Figure 5.58   Axial CT scan of chest with aortic arch branches and brachiocephalic veins.   (R1.C)

Figure 5.57   Axial MR scan of chest with aortic arch branches and brachiocephalic veins. (Courtesy Anne Marie Sawyer, Radiologic Sciences Laboratory, Stanford University School of Medicine, Stanford, Calif.)   (R1.C)

Key. **brA** brachiocephalic artery; **es** esophagus; **lbrV** left brachiocephalic vein; **lCCA** left common carotid artery; **lSA** left subclavian artery; **rbrV** right brachiocephalic vein; **tr** trachea.

LYMPH NODES

Lymph nodes in the mediastinum are generally clustered around the great vessels, esophagus, bronchi, and carina. Lymph vessels and nodes are difficult to visualize in cross section unless they are enlarged as a result of an abnormality (Figure 5.59).

THORACIC DUCT

The **thoracic duct** is the main vessel of the lymph system, draining most of the lymph of the body. It passes from the abdominal cavity into the thorax through the aortic hiatus of the diaphragm. It ascends the thorax, lying between the azygos vein and the descending aorta. At the level of the clavicle, the thoracic duct empties into the subclavian vein (Figure 5.60).

Figure 5.59   Anterior view of esophagus and trachea.

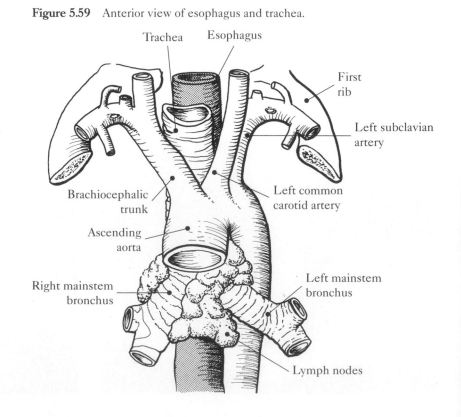

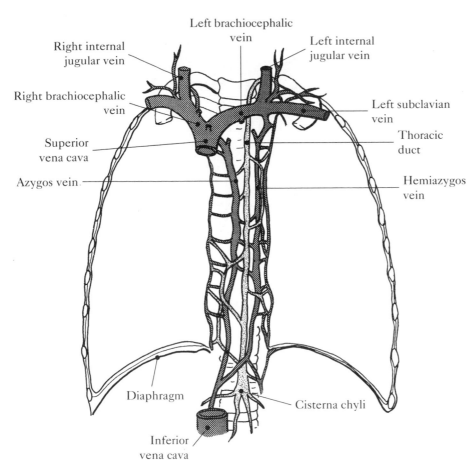

Right internal
jugular vein

Left brachiocephalic
vein

Left internal
jugular vein

Right brachiocephalic
vein

Left subclavian
vein

Superior
vena cava

Thoracic
duct

Azygos vein

Hemiazygos
vein

Diaphragm

Cisterna chyli

Inferior
vena cava

Figure 5.60   Thoracic duct and azygos venous system.

AZYGOS VENOUS SYSTEM

The **azygos venous system,** which provides collateral circulation between the inferior and superior venae cavae, can be divided into the **azygos** and **hemiazygos veins** (Figure 5.60). Together, they drain blood from most of the posterior thoracic wall and from the bronchi, pericardium, and esophagus. The azygos vein ascends along the right side of the vertebral column, whereas the hemiazygos vein ascends along the left side. The hemiazygos vein crosses to the right behind the aorta to join the azygos vein at approximately T7-T9. The azygos vein then arches over the hilum of the right lung to empty into the posterior superior vena cava (Figures 5.61 and 5.62).

Key.   **Az** azygos vein; **da** descending aorta; **es** esophagus; **hemi** hemiazygos vein.

Figure 5.61   Axial MR scan of chest with azygos and hemiazygos veins.   (R1.M)

Figure 5.62   Axial CT scan of chest with azygos and hemiazygos veins.   (R1.G)

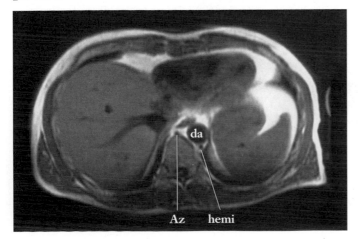

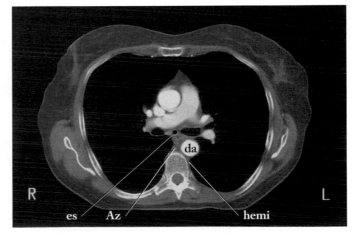

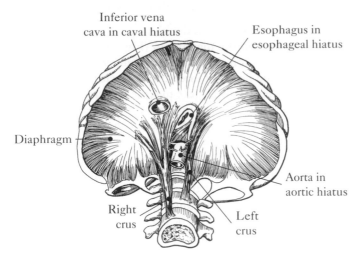

Figure 5.67 Inferior view of diaphragm.

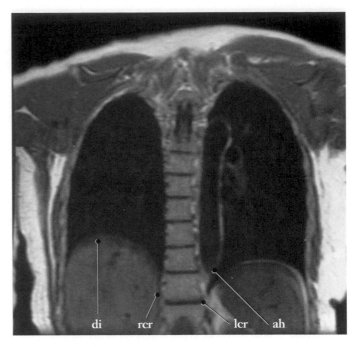

Figure 5.68 Coronal MR scan of chest with diaphragm.   (R2.D)

Key.   ah aortic hiatus; **da** descending aorta; **di** diaphragm; **in** intercostals; **IVC** inferior vena cava; **lcr** left crus; **rcr** right crus.

Figure 5.69 Axial MR scan of lumbar region with crura.   (R1.N)

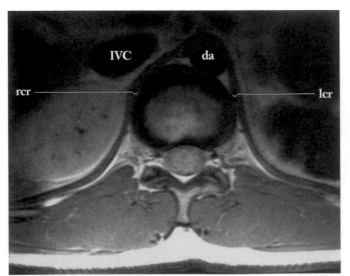

Figure 5.70 Axial CT scan of chest with crura.   (R1.M)

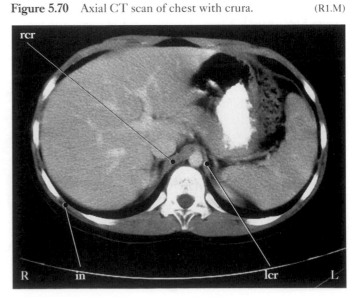

Breast

Subcutaneous, Mammary, and Retromammary Layers

The female **breast,** or **mammary gland,** lies within the subcutaneous tissue overlying the pectoralis major muscle.

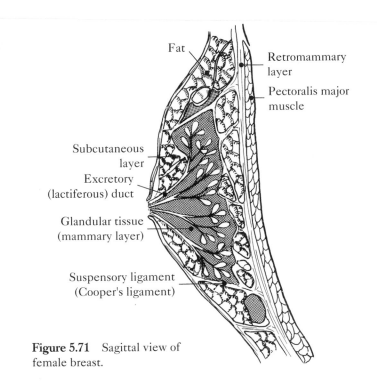

Figure 5.71 Sagittal view of female breast.

Typically, the breast extends from the sternum to the axilla and from the second rib to the seventh rib. The breast consists of three layers of tissue: **subcutaneous layer, mammary layer,** and **retromammary layer** (Figures 5.71 and 5.72). The subcutaneous layer contains the skin and all of the subcutaneous fat. The mammary layer consists of glandular tissue, excretory (lactiferous) ducts, and connective tissues. The **glandular tissue** consists of 15 to 20 lobes arranged radially around a centrally located nipple. The glandular lobes are embedded in connective tissue and fat, which give the breast its size and shape. **Excretory (lactiferous) ducts** extend from each lobe to the nipple, where they terminate as small openings. Cords of connective tissue coursing throughout the mammary layer, from the dermis to the thoracic fascia, are known as the suspensory ligaments of the breast or **Cooper's ligaments.** These ligaments provide support for the breasts. The retromammary layer contains muscle, deep connective tissue, and retromammary fat (Figures 5.72 and 5.73).

Axillary lymph nodes drain the lymphatics from the breast, arm, and integument of the back. They are frequently clustered around the axillary vessels, the lower border of the pectoralis major muscle, and the lower margin of the posterior wall.

Answer to Figure 5.1

Pulmonary trunk and right ventricle.

Key. gl glandular; **mam** mammary layer; **n** nipple; **pec** pectoralis major muscle; **ret** retromammary layer; **subq** subcutaneous layer.

Figure 5.72 Sagittal MR scan of female breast. (Courtesy GE Medical Systems, Milwaukee, Wisc.)

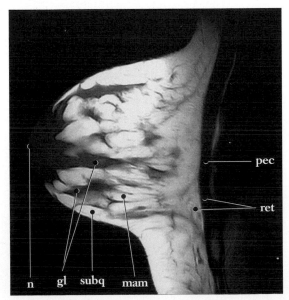

Figure 5.73 Axial MR scan of female breast. (Courtesy GE Medical Systems, Milwaukee, Wisc.)

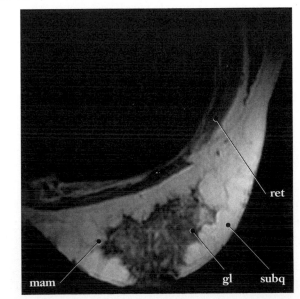

Chapter 6

1

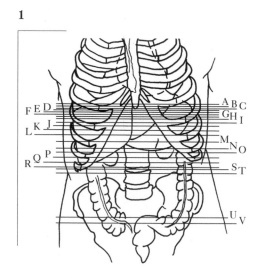

2

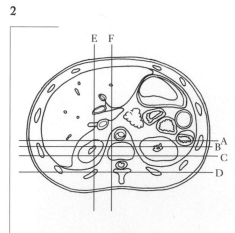

Reference illustrations

Abdomen

A man's liver is his carburetor.

Anonymous

In Figure 6.1, which structures are abnormal? (Answer on p. 201.)

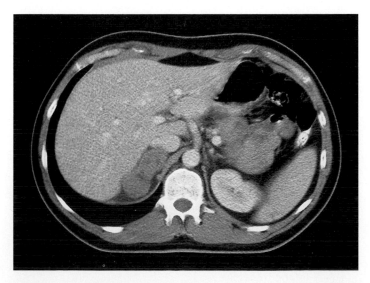

Figure 6.1 Axial CT scan of abdomen.

The abdominal cavity houses many critical structures that have a large array of functions. It is for this reason that cross-section imaging of the abdomen is so essential in visualizing these various organs and body systems. This chapter demonstrates cross-section anatomy of the following structures:

Abdominal Cavity
peritoneum
peritoneal spaces
retroperitoneum
retroperitoneal spaces

Liver
portal hepatic system
vasculature of the liver

Gallbladder and Biliary System

Pancreas

Spleen

Adrenal Glands

Urinary System

Stomach

Intestines

Abdominal Aorta and Branches
unpaired branches
paired branches

Inferior Vena Cava and Tributaries
lumbar veins
gonadal veins
renal veins
hepatic veins

Abdominal Muscles

ABDOMINAL CAVITY

The **abdominal cavity** is the region located between the diaphragm and sacral promontory (Figure 6.2). The abdominal and pelvic cavities are commonly divided into four quadrants or nine distinct regions. Contents of the abdominal cavity include the liver, gallbladder and biliary system, pancreas, spleen, adrenal glands, kidneys, ureters, stomach, intestines, and vascular structures.

PERITONEUM

The walls of the abdominal cavity are lined by a thin serous membrane called the **peritoneum.** This membrane is divided into the **parietal layer,** which lines the abdominal walls, and the **visceral layer,** which covers the organs (Figures 6.3 through 6.5). The peritoneum forms a cavity that encloses the following organs of the abdomen: liver (except for the bare area), gallbladder, spleen, stomach, ovaries, and majority of intestines. Numerous folds of peritoneum extend between the organs, serving to hold them in position and at the same time enclose the vessels and nerves proceeding to each part. The peritoneal folds that connect certain parts of the intestine with the abdominal wall are termed **mesentery.** Other folds of peritoneum that relate specifically to the stomach are the **greater** and **lesser omentum** (Figure 6.6). The greater omentum drapes over the greater curvature of the stomach, whereas the lesser omentum attaches the duodenum and lesser curvature of the stomach to the liver.

Inflammation of the peritoneal cavity is termed *peritonitis*. Acute peritonitis is most commonly caused by the leaking of infection through a perforation in the bowel.

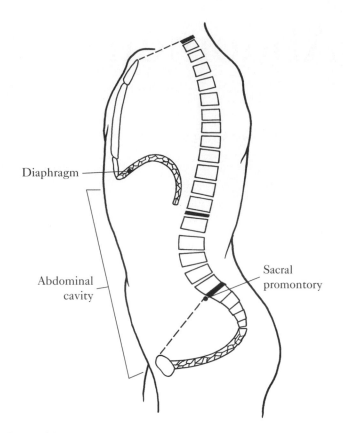

Figure 6.2   Sagittal view of the abdominal cavity.

Figure 6.3   Axial view of peritoneum.

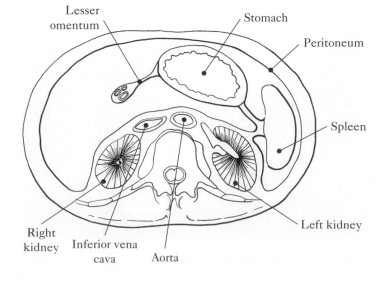

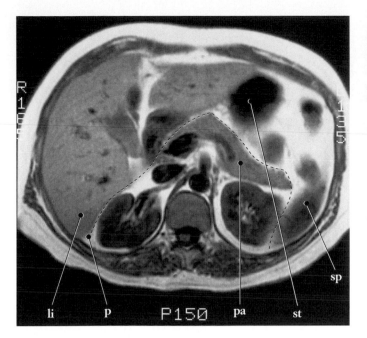

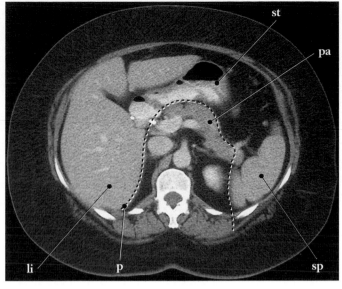

Figure 6.4   Axial MR scan of peritoneal and retroperitoneal structures (separated by dotted line). (Courtesy Luann Culbreth, Baylor University Medical Center, Dallas, Tex.)   (R1.H)

Key.   **li** liver; **p** peritoneum; **pa** pancreas; **sp** spleen; **st** stomach.

Figure 6.5   Axial CT scan of peritoneal and retroperitoneal structures (separated by dotted line).   (R1.H)

Key.   **li** liver; **p** peritoneum; **pa** pancreas; **sp** spleen; **st** stomach.

Figure 6.6   Sagittal view of peritoneal structures.

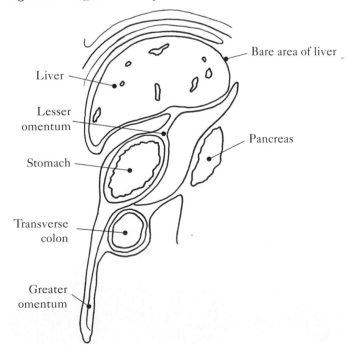

PERITONEAL SPACES

The peritoneal cavity contains potential spaces resulting from the folds of peritoneum that extend from the viscera to the abdominal wall. These spaces can be divided into the **supracolic** and **infracolic compartments** (Figure 6.7).

The supracolic compartment is located above the transverse colon and contains the **right** and **left subphrenic spaces** and the **right** and **left subhepatic spaces.** The subphrenic spaces are located between the diaphragm and the anterior portion of the liver. They are divided into right and left compartments by the **falciform ligament** (Figures 6.8 and 6.9). The subhepatic spaces are located posterior and inferior between the liver and the abdominal viscera. The right subhepatic space, located between the liver and kidney, contains **Morison's pouch,** which is the deepest point of the abdominal cavity in a supine patient and a common site for the collection of fluid (Figures 6.10 and 6.11).

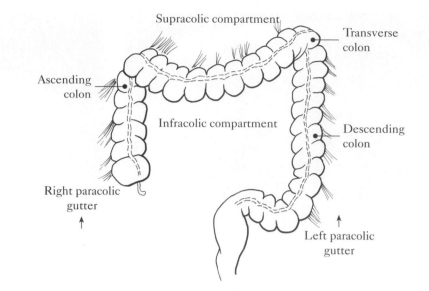

Figure 6.7   Supracolic and infracolic compartments.

Key.   bare bare area of liver; **Lsphr** left subphrenic compartment; **Rsphr** right subphrenic compartment.

Figure 6.9   Axial CT scan of abdomen with subphrenic spaces.

(R1.A)

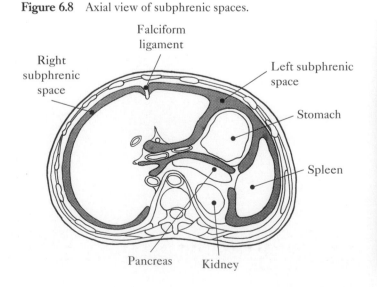

Figure 6.8   Axial view of subphrenic spaces.

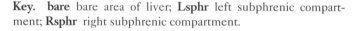

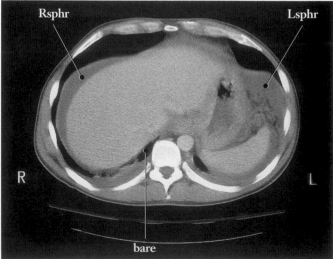

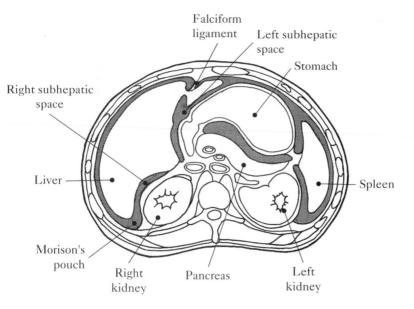

Figure 6.10 Axial view of subhepatic spaces and Morison's pouch.

Below the transverse colon is the infracolic compartment, which consists of the paracolic gutters. The **right** and **left paracolic gutters** are trough-like spaces located lateral to the ascending and descending colon. The deeper right gutter is a common site for free fluid collections (Figure 6.12).

Key. **Mo** Morison's pouch; **Rshep** right subhepatic space; **Rsphr** right subphrenic compartment.

Figure 6.11 Axial CT scan of abdomen with subhepatic spaces and Morison's pouch.   (R1.N)

Key. **asc** ascending colon; **Lpar** left paracolic gutter; **Rpar** right paracolic gutter.

Figure 6.12 Axial CT scan of abdomen with paracolic gutters.   (R1.Q)

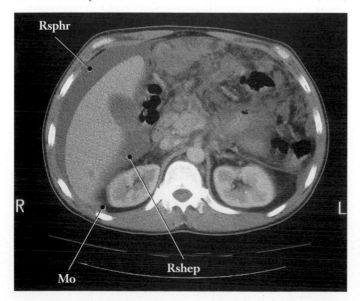

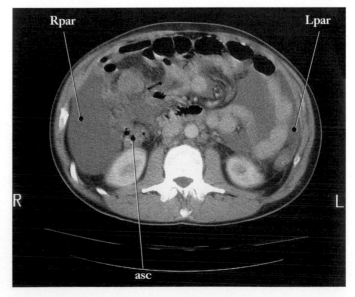

RETROPERITONEUM

Structures located posterior to the peritoneum, yet lined by it anteriorly, are considered to be in the **retroperitoneum** and include the kidneys, ureters, adrenal glands, pancreas, duodenum, aorta, inferior vena cava, bladder, uterus, and prostate gland. In addition, the ascending and descending colon and most of the duodenum are situated in the retroperitoneum (Figures 6.13 through 6.15).

RETROPERITONEAL SPACES

The **anterior pararenal space** is located between the anterior surface of **renal fascia (Gerota's fascia)** and the posterior portion of the peritoneum. It contains the retroperitoneal portions of the ascending and descending colon, the pancreas, and the duodenum. The **posterior pararenal space** is located between the posterior renal fascia and the muscles of the posterior abdominal wall. There are no solid organs located in this space, just fat and vessels (Figures 6.16 and 6.17).

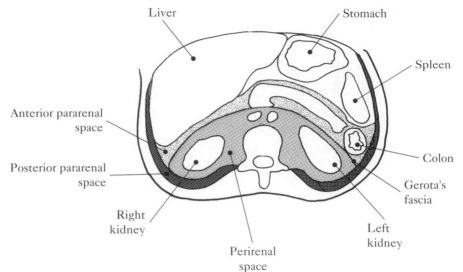

Figure 6.13   Axial view of retroperitoneum.

Key. **ad** adrenal gland; **k** kidney; **pa** pancreas; **retro** retroperitoneum; **sp** spleen; **st** stomach.

Figure 6.14   Axial MR scan of retroperitoneal structures (posterior to dotted line).   (R1.H)

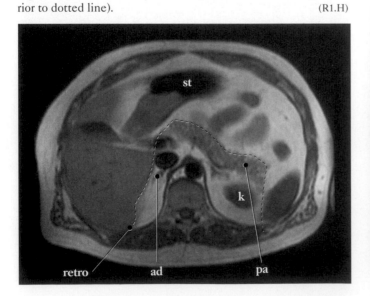

Figure 6.15   Axial CT scan of retroperitoneal structures (posterior to dotted line).   (R1.H)

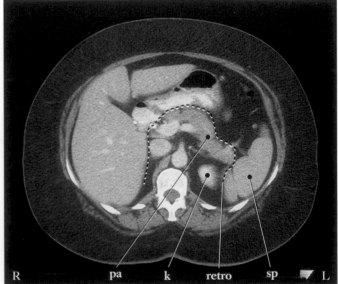

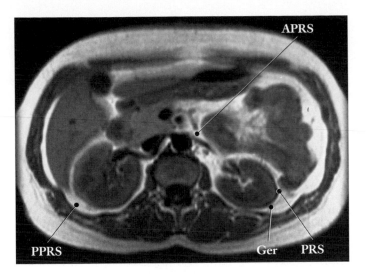

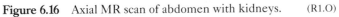

Figure 6.16   Axial MR scan of abdomen with kidneys.   (R1.O)

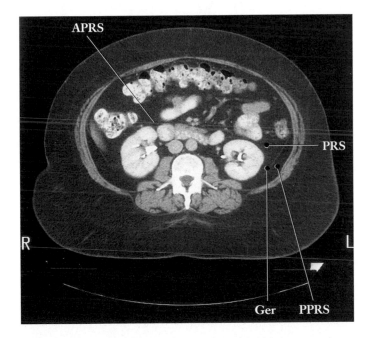

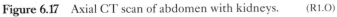

Figure 6.17   Axial CT scan of abdomen with kidneys.   (R1.O)

Key. APRS anterior pararenal space; **Ger** Gerota's fascia; **PPRS** posterior pararenal space; **PRS** perirenal space.

The **perirenal space** is the area located directly around the kidney and is completely enclosed by renal fascia (Figure 6.13). This space contains the kidneys, adrenal glands, lymph nodes, blood vessels, and perirenal fat. The perirenal fat separates the adrenal glands from the kidneys and provides cushioning for the kidney.

Table 6.1   Peritoneal and retroperitoneal spaces

SPACE	LOCATION
PERITONEAL SPACES	
SUPRACOLIC COMPARTMENT	Above transverse colon
Subphrenic space	Between diaphragm and anterior liver
Right	Right and left spaces divided by
Left	falciform ligament
Subhepatic space	Posterior and inferior to liver
Right	Between right lobe of liver and kidney; contains Morison's pouch
Left	Between left lobe of liver and kidney; includes lesser omentum
INFRACOLIC COMPARTMENT	Below transverse colon
Paracolic gutters	
Right	Between ascending colon and right abdominal wall
Left	Between descending colon and left abdominal wall
RETROPERITONEAL SPACES	
PARARENAL SPACES	
Anterior	Between renal (Gerota's) fascia and posterior surface of peritoneum
Posterior	Between renal (Gerota's) fascia and muscles of posterior abdominal wall
PERIRENAL SPACE	
Right	Around kidney and adrenal
Left	glands; completely enclosed by renal (Gerota's) fascia

LIVER

The **liver** is the largest organ of the abdomen, occupying a major portion of the right upper quadrant. The liver functions as the primary center for metabolism, and it also supports multiple body systems. The liver can be divided into lobes according to surface anatomy or into segments according to the vascular supply (Figures 6.18 and 6.19).

The four lobes commonly used for reference are the **left, right, caudate,** and **quadrate.** The left lobe is the most anterior of the liver lobes, extending across the midline. It is separated from the right lobe by the **main lobar fissure,** an imaginary line drawn through the gallbladder fossa and the middle hepatic vein to the inferior vena cava (Figure 6.19). The upper surface of the right lobe, the largest of the four lobes, lies close to the right lateral abdominal wall directly

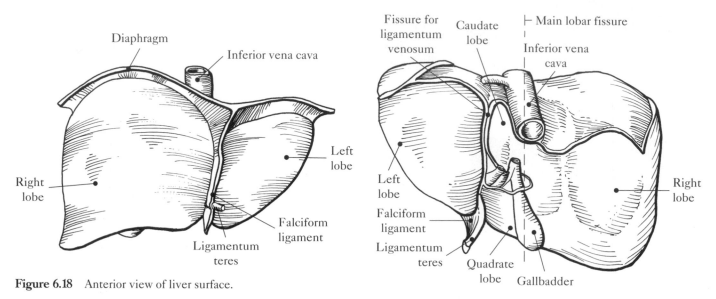

Figure 6.18   Anterior view of liver surface.

Figure 6.19   Posterior view of liver surface.

Key.   cau caudate lobe of liver; **fal** falciform ligament; **LL** left lobe of liver; **RL** right lobe of liver; **ven** ligamentum venosum.

Figure 6.20   Axial MR scan of abdomen with lobes of liver.

(R1.C)

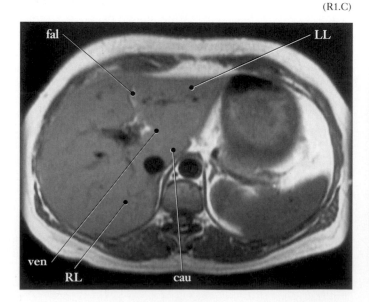

Figure 6.21   Axial CT scan of abdomen with lobes of liver.

(R1.C)

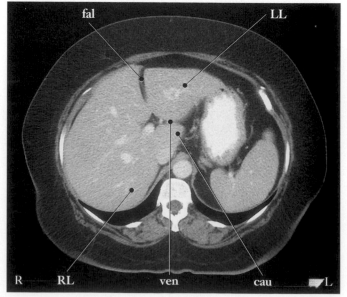

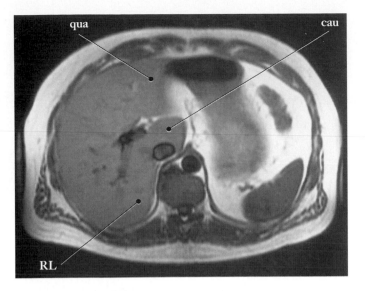

Figure 6.22   Axial MR scan of liver with quadrate lobe.   (R1.D)

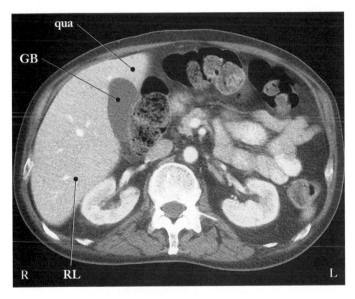

Figure 6.23   Axial CT scan of liver with quadrate lobe.   (R1.G)

Key.   cau caudate lobe of liver; **GB** gallbladder; **qua** quadrate lobe of liver; **RL** right lobe of liver.

under the diaphragm. The inferior and posterior surface of the right lobe is bordered by the porta hepatis, gallbladder, and inferior vena cava (Figures 6.18 and 6.19). The smallest lobe is the caudate lobe, which is located on the inferior and posterior liver surface, sandwiched between the inferior vena cava and the **ligamentum venosum** (Figures 6.19 to 6.21). The quadrate lobe is located on the anteroinferior surface of the left lobe between the gallbladder and the **ligamentum teres** (Figures 6.19, 6.22 and 6.23). The round, cord-like, ligamentum teres is a remnant of the fetal umbilical vein and runs along the free edge of the falciform ligament. The falciform ligament provides the structural support that attaches the upper surfaces of the liver to the diaphragm and upper abdominal wall. The hilum of the liver, the **porta hepatis**, is located on the inferomedial border of the liver. It is the central location for vessels to enter and exit the liver.

Current practice favors dividing the liver into eight segments, according to the vascular supply, which can aid in surgical planning. The right and left lobes are demarcated by the middle hepatic vein and gallbladder fossa. The right lobe contains four separate segments, and the left has three segments, with the quadrate lobe comprising the most medial segment. The caudate lobe remains a separate segment (Figure 6.24).

Figure 6.24   Coronal view with segmental anatomy of the liver.

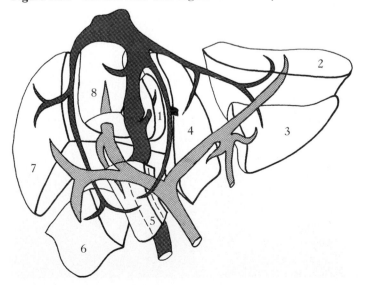

PORTAL HEPATIC SYSTEM

The liver receives nutrient-rich blood from the gastrointestinal tract via the portal hepatic system (Figure 6.25). The major vessel of this system is the **portal vein,** which is formed by the union of the **superior** and **inferior mesenteric veins** and the **splenic vein** (Figures 6.26 through 6.29). The superior mesenteric vein drains the small intestine and ascending and transverse colon. It ascends the abdomen to the right of the superior mesenteric artery and joins the splenic vein near the neck of the pancreas (Figures 6.30 and 6.31). The inferior mesenteric vein drains blood from the descending colon, sigmoid colon, and rectum. For most of its course, it runs anterior to the left psoas muscle to meet the splenic vein just posterior to the body of the pancreas (Figures 6.32 and 6.33). The splenic vein, which drains the spleen and receives blood from the gastric and pancreatic veins, curves along the posterior surface of the pancreas to unite with the superior mesenteric vein to form the portal vein behind the head of the pancreas.

Portal hypertension is caused by obstruction of blood flow in the portal hepatic system. This condition can lead to splenomegaly and ascites.

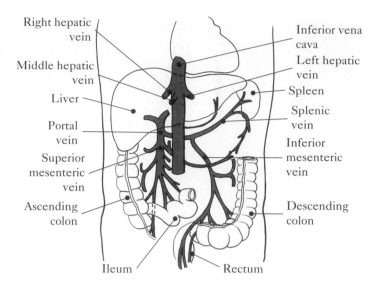

Figure 6.25   Anterior view of portal hepatic system.

Key.   GV gastric vein; **IVC** inferior vena cava; **LL** left lobe of liver; **LV** left ventricle; **PorV** portal vein; **RA** right atrium; **RHV** right hepatic vein; **RL** right lobe of liver; **sp** spleen.

Figure 6.26   MRA with portal vein. (Courtesy GE Medical Systems, Milwaukee, Wisc.)

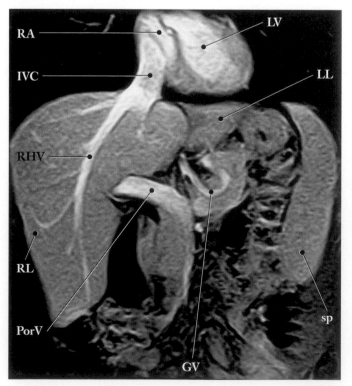

Key.   A aorta; **IVC** inferior vena cava; **li** liver; **PorV** portal vein.

Figure 6.27   Axial CT scan with portal vein.   (R1.G)

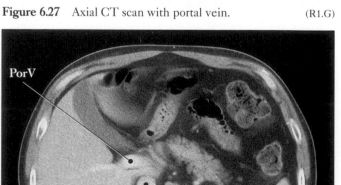

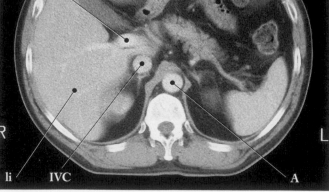

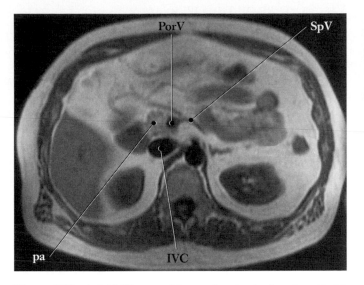

Figure 6.28   Axial MR scan with portal and splenic vein.   (R1.M)

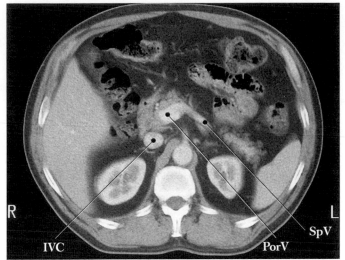

Figure 6.29   Axial CT scan with portal and splenic vein.   (R1.M)

Key.   **A** aorta; **IMV** inferior mesenteric vein; **IVC** inferior vena cava; **pa** head of pancreas; **PorV** portal vein; **SMA** superior mesenteric artery; **SMV** superior mesenteric vein; **SpV** splenic vein.

Figure 6.30   Axial MR scan with superior mesenteric vein.
(R1.N)

Figure 6.31   Axial CT scan with superior mesenteric vein.
(R1.N)

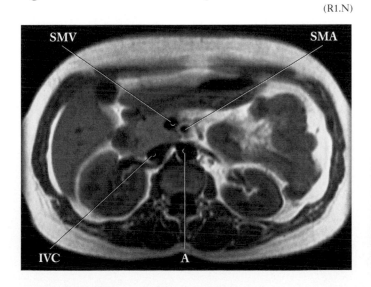

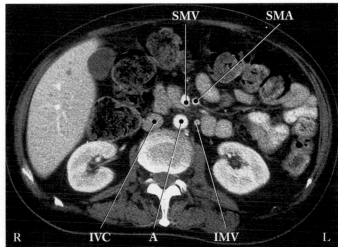

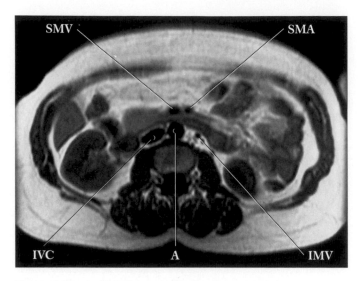

Figure 6.32 Axial MR scan with superior and inferior mesenteric veins. (R1.P)

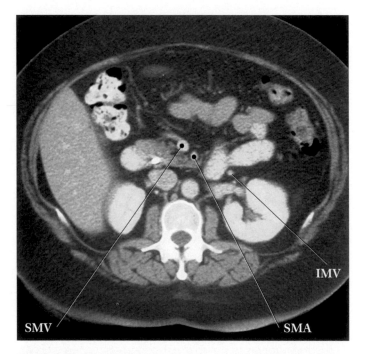

Figure 6.33 Axial CT scan with superior and inferior mesenteric veins. (R1.O)

Key. **A** aorta; **IMV** inferior mesenteric vein; **IVC** inferior vena cava; **SMA** superior mesenteric artery; **SMV** superior mesenteric vein.

VASCULATURE OF THE LIVER

Arterial blood is supplied to the liver via the **common hepatic artery,** which is one of the three branches of the celiac artery (Figure 6.34). The hepatic artery passes into the liver medial to the bile duct and anterior to the portal vein. Before entering the porta hepatis, it divides into the left and right hepatic arteries which continue to branch and supply the lobes of the liver, respectively (Figures 6.35 and 6.36). The venous drainage of the liver is composed of the **right, middle,** and **left hepatic veins,** which drain the corresponding locations of the liver into the inferior vena cava just below the diaphragm (Figures 6.25, 6.26, 6.37 and 6.38).

Figure 6.34 Anterior view of hepatic arteries.

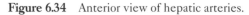
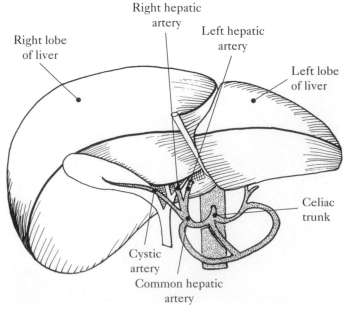

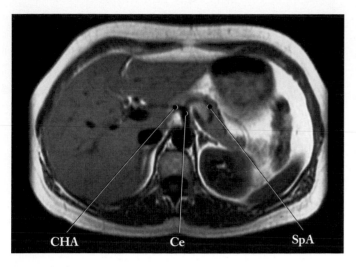

Figure 6.35 Axial MR scan with celiac trunk and hepatic artery.   (R1.I)

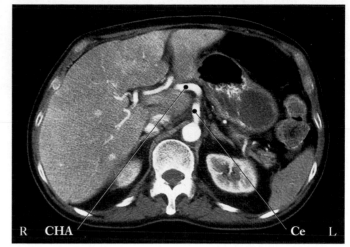

Figure 6.36 Axial CT scan with celiac trunk and hepatic artery.   (R1.I)

Key.   Ce celiac axis; **CHA** common hepatic artery; **SpA** splenic artery.

Key.   di diaphragm; **es** esophagus; **IVC** inferior vena cava; **LHV** left hepatic vein; **MHV** middle hepatic vein; **RHV** right hepatic vein.

Figure 6.37 Axial MR scan with hepatic veins.   (R1.C)

Figure 6.38 Axial CT scan with hepatic veins.   (R1.A)

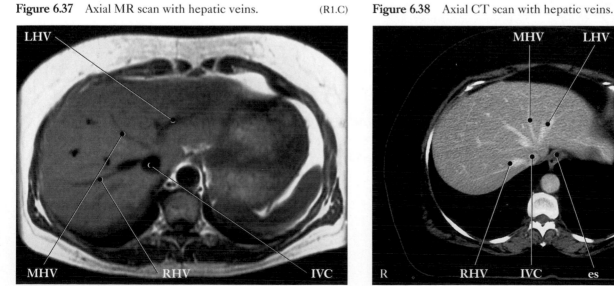

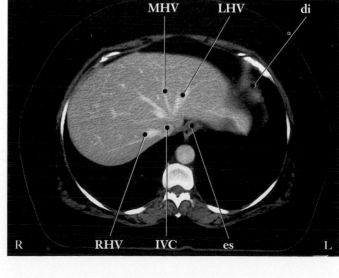

GALLBLADDER AND BILIARY SYSTEM

The pear-shaped **gallbladder** is located in a fossa on the anteroinferior portion of the right lobe of the liver. It acts as a reservoir for bile. The body of the gallbladder tapers into the neck of the gallbladder and then continues as the **cystic duct** (Figure 6.39). Bile enters and leaves the gallbladder by way of the cystic duct.

Bile is produced in the liver and drains into the **right** and **left hepatic ducts.** The right and left hepatic ducts leave the liver through the porta hepatis and unite to form the **common hepatic duct.** The common hepatic duct is joined by the cystic duct of the gallbladder to form the **common bile duct** (Figures 6.39, 6.40, and 6.41). The common bile duct penetrates the duodenal wall in conjunction with the **pancreatic duct (duct of Wirsung)** at the **ampulla of Vater.** The basic function of the biliary system is to store bile and then drain it when needed to aid in digestion.

PANCREAS

The **pancreas** is a long, narrow organ that lies behind the stomach and extends transversely from the duodenum toward the spleen (see Figure 6.39). It can be divided into a head, neck, body, and tail. The head is located in the curve of the duodenum, and the neck lies just anterior to the portal and superior mesenteric veins (Figures 6.42 and 6.43). The body curves laterally from the neck toward the spleen, and the short tail extends to the hilum of the spleen. Arterial blood is supplied to the pancreas by the splenic, superior mesenteric, and hepatic arteries, whereas the splenic vein drains the pancreas. The pancreatic duct (duct of Wirsung) runs the length of the gland beginning in the tail and traversing the body and head, where it meets the common bile duct from the liver and gallbladder to form the ampulla of Vater just before entering the duodenum (Figures 6.44 and 6.45). The pancreas is both an exocrine and an endocrine gland. Exocrine cells secrete pancreatic juice into the small intestine and endocrine cells secrete insulin and glucagon into the bloodstream. The pancreas has a distinct lobulated appearance, making identification easy in cross section.

> Acute pancreatitis can lead to the leakage of powerful digestive enzymes. As the enzymes "digest" the surrounding tissue, pancreatic necrosis results.

Figure 6.39 Anterior view of biliary system.

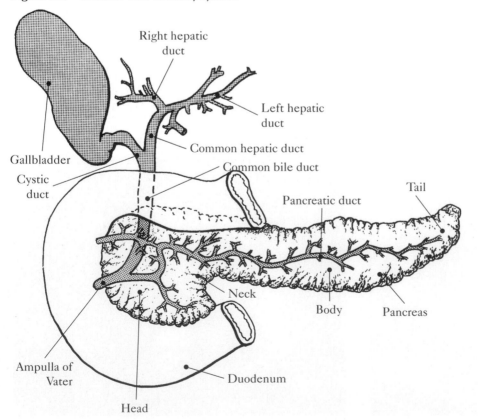

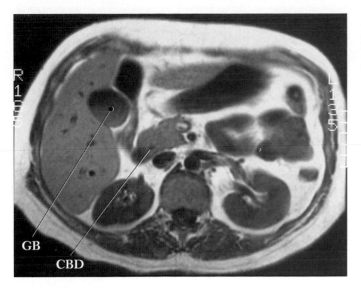

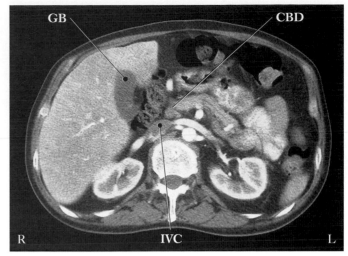

Figure 6.40   Axial MR scan with gallbladder and common bile duct. (Courtesy Luann Culbreth, Baylor University Medical Center, Dallas, Tex.)   (R1.K)

Figure 6.41   Axial CT scan with gallbladder and common bile duct.   (R1.K)

Key.   CBD common bile duct; **duo** duodenum; **GB** gallbladder; **IVC** inferior vena cava; **pa** pancreas; **SMV** superior mesenteric vein; **st** stomach.

Figure 6.42   Axial MR scan with head of pancreas and duodenum.   (R1.L)

Figure 6.43   Axial CT scan with head of pancreas and duodenum.   (R1.J)

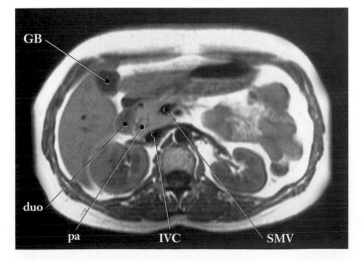

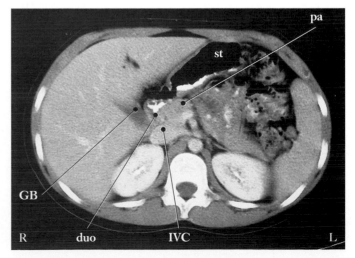

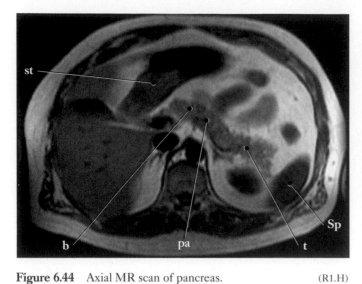

Figure 6.44 Axial MR scan of pancreas. (R1.H)

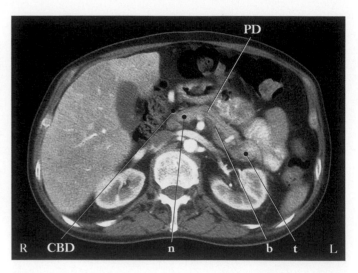

Figure 6.45 Axial CT scan of pancreas and pancreatic duct. (R1.G)

Key. **b** body of pancreas; **CBD** common bile duct; **n** neck of pancreas; **pa** pancreas; **PD** pancreatic duct; **sp** spleen; **st** stomach; **t** tail of pancreas.

Figure 6.46 Anterior view of spleen.

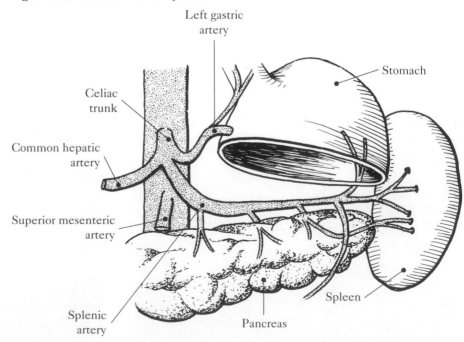

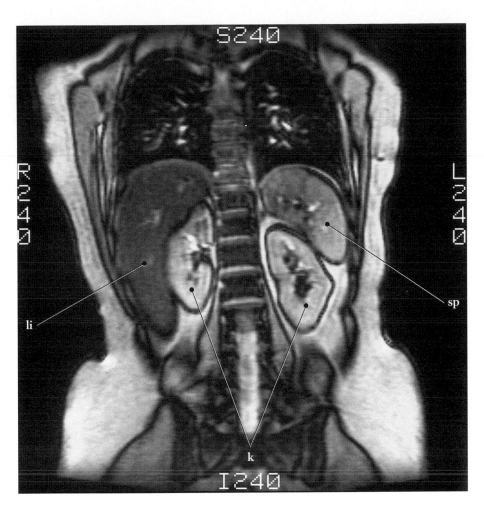

Figure 6.47   Coronal MR scan of spleen. (Courtesy Luann Culbreth, Baylor University Medical Center, Dallas, Tex.)   (R2.C)

SPLEEN

The **spleen** is the largest lymph organ in the body. It is located posterior to the stomach in the left upper quadrant of the abdomen (Figures 6.46 and 6.47). It is protected by the ninth through eleventh ribs. The spleen is in contact with the stomach, left kidney, and diaphragm. The splenic artery and vein enter and exit the spleen at the **hilum** between the gastric and renal depressions (Figures 6.48 and 6.49). The tail of the pancreas is also located at the hilum. The spleen is a highly vascular organ that functions to filter abnormal blood cells from the blood, store iron from red blood cells, and initiate the immune response.

Key.   **hi** hilum; **IVC** inferior vena cava; **k** kidney; **li** liver; **sp** spleen; **SpV** splenic vein; **st** stomach; **t** tail of pancreas.

Figure 6.48   Axial MR scan of spleen.   (R1.E)

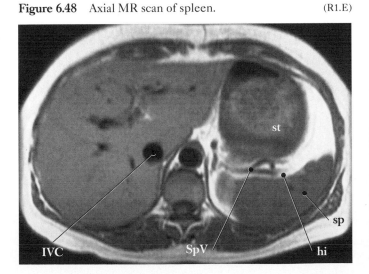

Figure 6.49   Axial CT scan of spleen.   (R1.E)

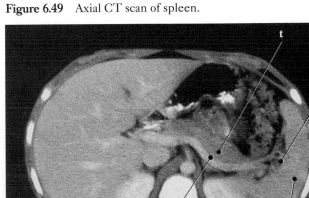

ADRENAL GLANDS

The pyramid-shaped **adrenal (suprarenal) glands** sit on the upper border of each kidney (Figures 6.50 and 6.51). They are separated from the kidney by perirenal fat. The **right adrenal gland** is located in the angle between the superior pole of the kidney and the inferior vena cava. The right gland is generally lower and more medial than the left gland and commonly appears as a **V** on cross section (Figures 6.52 through 6.54). The **left adrenal gland** extends down the medial border of the kidney toward the hilum. It commonly appears as a triangular or **Y**-shaped configuration (Figures 6.55 and 6.56). The posterior surfaces of both the right and left glands border the crus of the diaphragm. The adrenal glands are responsible for the production of steroids and epinephrine.

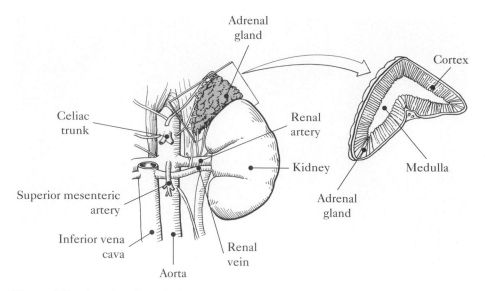

Figure 6.50   Anterior view of adrenal glands.

Key. **cr** crus; **k** kidney; **Lad** left adrenal gland; **li** liver; **Rad;** right adrenal gland.

Figure 6.51   Coronal MR scan with adrenal glands.   (R2.B)

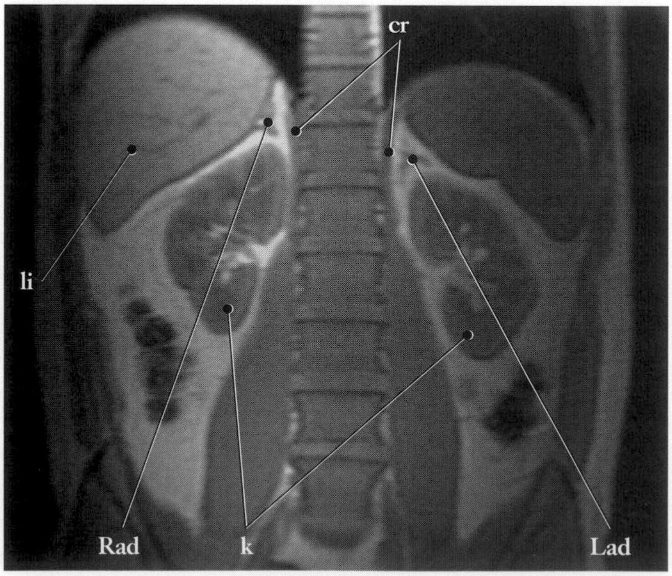

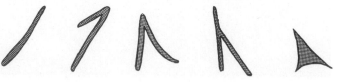

Figure 6.52   Common configurations of adrenal glands.

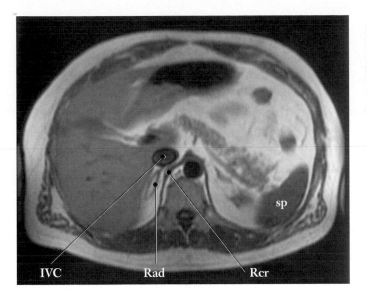

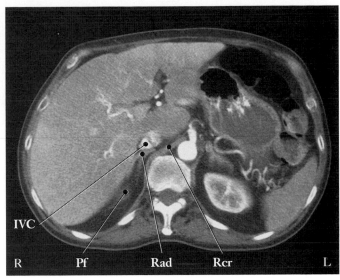

Figure 6.53   Axial MR scan of right adrenal gland.   (R1.H)

Key.   IVC inferior vena cava; **Rad** right adrenal gland; **Rcr** right crus; **sp** spleen.

Figure 6.54   Axial CT scan of right adrenal gland.   (R1.H)

Key.   IVC inferior vena cava; **Pf** perirenal fat; **Rad** right adrenal gland; **Rcr** right crus.

Key.   k kidney; **Lad** left adrenal gland; **Lcr** left crus; **t** tail of pancreas.

Figure 6.55   Axial MR scan of left adrenal gland.   (R1.I)

Key.   Lad left adrenal; **Lcr** left crus; **Pf** perirenal fat.

Figure 6.56   Axial CT scan of left adrenal gland.   (R1.I)

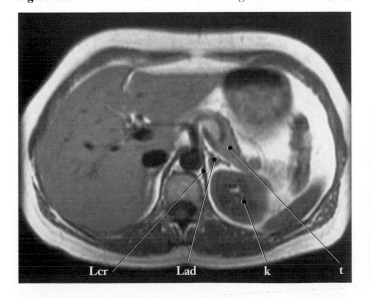

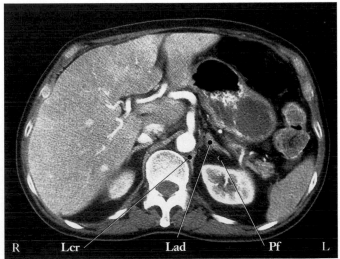

URINARY SYSTEM

The structures of the urinary system include the kidneys, ureters, and bladder (Figure 6.57). The **kidneys** are bean-shaped organs located on each side of the spine between T12 and L4 and are embedded in perirenal fat along the posterior abdominal wall. The left kidney frequently lies slightly higher than the right kidney. Each kidney is composed of an outer cortex and an inner medulla. The **renal cortex** is responsible for filtration of urine, whereas the medulla, consisting of segments called **renal pyramids,** functions as the beginning of the collecting system. Arising from the apices of the pyramids are the cup-shaped **calyces,** which join together to form the **renal pelvis** (Figures 6.58 and 6.59).

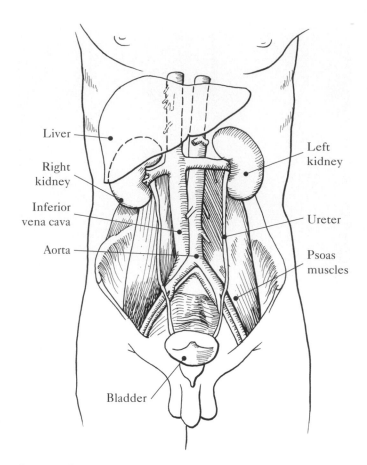

Figure 6.57 Anterior view of urinary system.

Figure 6.58 Coronal view of kidney.

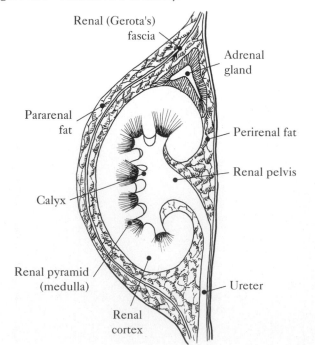

Key. GB gallbladder; **k** kidney; **li** liver; **PorV** portal vein.

Figure 6.59 Sagittal MR scan of kidney. (R2.E)

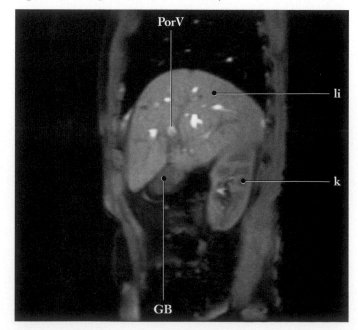

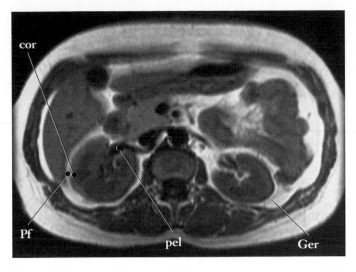

Figure 6.60   Axial MR scan of kidney.   (R1.O)

Key. **cor** renal cortex; **Ger** Gerota's fascia; **pel** renal pelvis; **Pf** perirenal fat.

Surrounding the kidneys and perirenal fat is another protective layer called the renal fascia (Gerota's fascia; Figures 6.60 and 6.61). The renal fascia functions to anchor the kidneys to surrounding structures to prevent bumps and jolts to the body from injuring the kidneys. In addition, the renal fascia acts as a barrier, limiting the spread of infection that may arise from the kidneys. The medial indentation in the kidney is called the hilum; it allows the renal artery and vein and ureters to enter and exit the kidney. The **ureters** are paired muscular tubes that transport urine to the **urinary bladder.** Each ureter originates at the renal pelvis and descends anteriorly and medially to the **psoas muscles** (Figure 6.62). The ureters then enter the posterior wall of the bladder at an oblique angle. The primary function of the urinary system is to filter blood, produce and excrete urine, and help to maintain normal body physiology.

Key. **cal** calyx; **Ger** Gerota's fascia; **pel** renal pelvis; **Pf** perirenal fat.

Figure 6.61   Axial CT scan of kidney.   (R1.O)

Key. **IVC** inferior vena cava; **Lur** left ureter; **ps** psoas muscles; **Rur** right ureter.

Figure 6.62   Axial CT scan with ureters.   (R1.S)

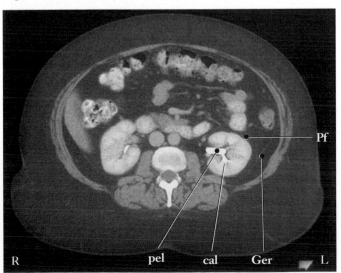

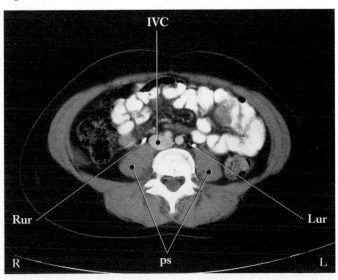

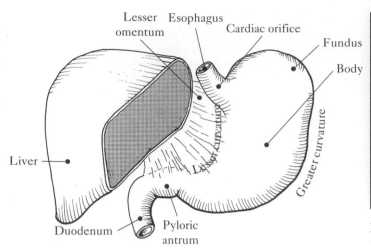

Figure 6.63 Anterior view of stomach.

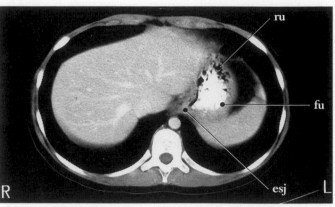

Figure 6.64 Axial CT scan at esophagogastric junction.

(R1.B)

Key. **esj** esophagogastric junction; **fu** fundus of stomach; **ru** rugae.

Key. **air** air; **b** body of stomach; **gcur** greater curvature; **lcur** lesser curvature.

Figure 6.66 Axial CT scan with body of stomach and curvatures.

(R1.G)

Key. **b** body of stomach; **lom** lesser omentum.

Figure 6.65 Axial MR scan with body of stomach and curvatures.

(R1.D)

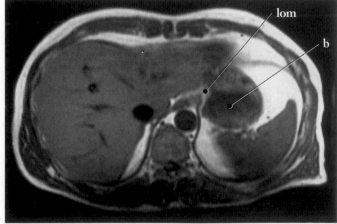

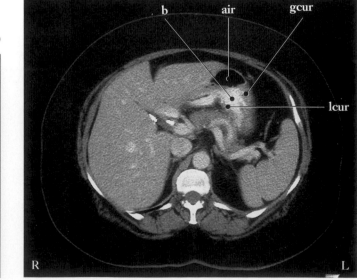

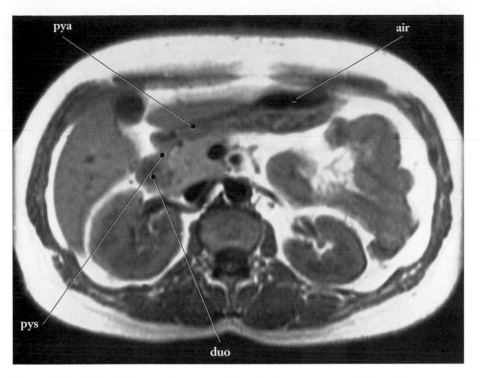

Figure 6.67   Axial MR scan of stomach with pyloric antrum and pyloric sphincter. (R1.N)

Key. air air in stomach; **duo** duodenum; **pya** pyloric antrum; **pys** pyloric sphincter.

STOMACH

The **stomach** is the dilated portion of the digestive system that is responsible for the early stages of digestion (Figure 6.63). It is located under the left dome of the diaphragm, with the superior portion joining the esophagus at the **cardiac orifice,** creating the **esophagogastric junction** (Figure 6.64). The stomach has two borders called the **lesser** and **greater curvatures.** Between the two curvatures is the largest portion of the stomach, termed the **body** (Figures 6.65 and 6.66). On the superior surface of the body is a rounded surface called the **fundus.** The inferior portion (**pyloric antrum**) empties into the duodenum through the **pyloric sphincter** (Figures 6.67 and 6.68). The anterior surface is in contact with the diaphragm, anterior abdominal wall, and left lobe of the liver. Just posterior to the stomach is the gastric portion of the spleen. The stomach commonly extends from the level of T11 to L1. Arterial blood and venous drainage are supplied by branches of the gastric artery and gastric vein, respectively.

Figure 6.68   Axial CT scan of stomach with pyloric antrum and pyloric sphincter.   (R1.H)

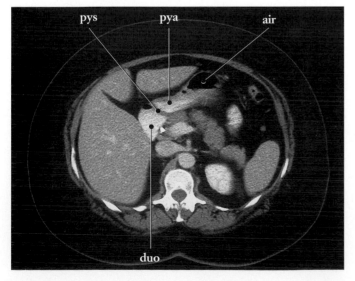

INTESTINES

The **small intestine** consists of loops of bowel averaging 6 to 7 m in length and can be subdivided into the **duodenum, jejunum,** and the **ileum** (Figure 6.69). The proximal portion of the small intestine is the duodenum, which begins at the gastric pylorus and curves around the head of the pancreas, forming the letter C. The duodenum is mostly retroperitoneal, making it less mobile than the rest of the small intestine (Figure 6.70). As the duodenum reenters the peritoneal cavity, it becomes the jejunum. The loops of jejunum occupy the umbilical region of the abdomen and are approximately 2.5 m long. The jejunum then becomes the ileum, which is the longest portion of the small intestine, averaging 3.5 m in length and found in the right lower abdomen (Figure 6.71). The loops of ileum terminate at the **ileocecal valve.**

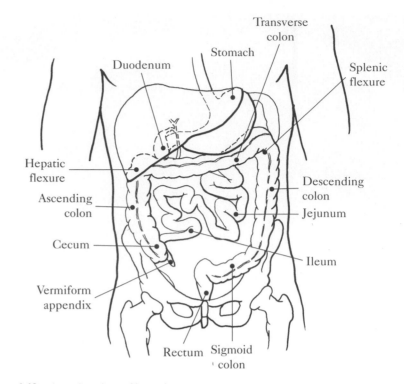

Figure 6.69   Anterior view of intestines.

Key. duo duodenum; **GB** gallbladder; **h** head of pancreas; **IVC** inferior vena cava; **st** stomach.

Figure 6.70   Axial CT scan with duodenum.   (R1.J)

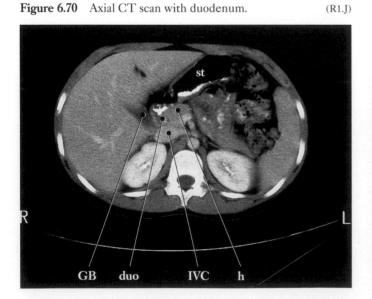

Key. il ileum; **je** jejunum.

Figure 6.71   Axial CT scan with ileum and jejunum.   (R1.S)

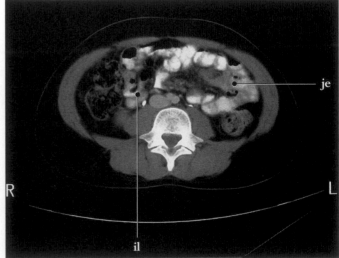

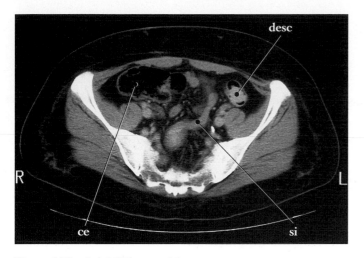

Figure 6.72   Axial CT scan with cecum.   (R1.U)

Key.   ce cecum; **desc** descending colon; **si** sigmoid colon.

The **large intestine** lies inferior to the stomach and liver and almost completely frames the small intestine (Figure 6.69). The large intestine has a diameter larger than the small intestine and starts at the **ileocecal junction,** ending at the anus. The three main divisions of the colon are the **cecum, colon,** and **rectum.** The cecum is a pouchlike section of the proximal portion of the large intestine located at the ileocecal valve (Figure 6.72). The slender **vermiform appendix** attaches to the posteromedial surface of the cecum. The colon is the longest portion of the large intestine and can be subdivided into four distinct portions: **ascending, transverse, descending,** and **sigmoid** (Figure 6.73). The ascending colon commences at the cecum and ascends the right lateral wall of the abdomen to the level of the liver. It then curves sharply to the left, creating the **hepatic flexure.** The hepatic flexure marks the beginning of the transverse colon. The transverse colon travels horizontally across the anterior abdomen toward the spleen, where it bends sharply downward, creating the **splenic flexure** and the beginning of the descending colon. The descending colon continues inferiorly along the left lateral abdominal wall to the **iliac fossa,** where it curves and becomes the S-shaped sigmoid colon posterior to the bladder (Figure 6.74). The sigmoid colon empties into the rectum, which is the terminal portion of the colon. The superior and inferior mesenteric arteries and veins supply and drain blood from the large intestine. The major functions of the large intestine include the reabsorption of water and the storage and elimination of fecal material.

Key.   asc ascending colon; **desc** descending colon; **smb** small bowel; **tra** transverse colon.

Figure 6.73   Axial CT scan with transverse colon.   (R1.O)

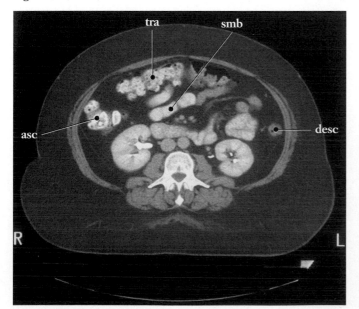

Key.   si sigmoid colon.

Figure 6.74   Axial CT scan with sigmoid colon.   (R1.V)

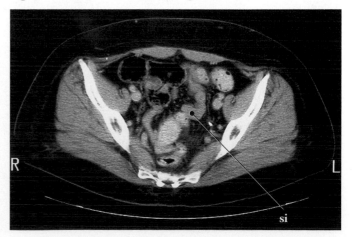

ABDOMINAL AORTA AND BRANCHES

The **abdominal aorta** is a retroperitoneal structure beginning at the aortic hiatus of the diaphragm (Figure 6.75). Typically, it is located just left of midline next to the vertebral bodies and courses midline as it descends the abdominal cavity. At approximately the level of L4, the aorta bifurcates into the **right** and **left common iliac arteries** (Figure 6.76). The major branches of the aorta can be divided into paired and unpaired branches.

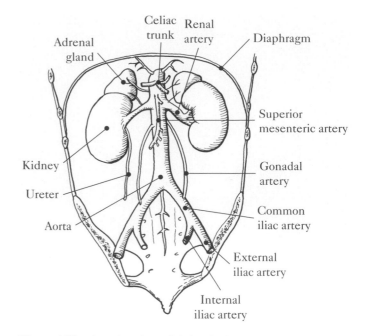

Figure 6.75   Anterior view of abdominal aorta.

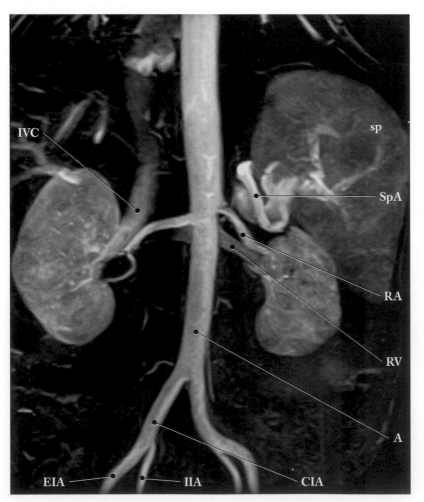

Figure 6.76   MRA of abdominal aorta. (Courtesy GE Medical Systems, Milwaukee, Wisc.)

Key.   **A** aorta; **CIA** common iliac artery; **EIA** external iliac artery; **IIA** internal iliac artery; **IVC** inferior vena cava; **RA** renal artery; **RV** renal vein; **sp** spleen; **SpA** splenic artery.

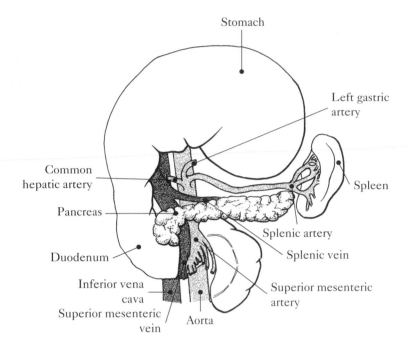

Figure 6.77   Anterior view of celiac trunk.

UNPAIRED BRANCHES

The unpaired branches of the aorta include the celiac trunk (axis), superior mesenteric artery, and inferior mesenteric artery.

CELIAC TRUNK. The **celiac trunk** is the first major branch of the abdominal aorta. It leaves the anterior wall of the aorta just after the aorta passes through the diaphragm. The short celiac trunk divides into three branches: left gastric, common hepatic, and splenic arteries (Figure 6.77). The **left gastric artery** passes to the left to supply the cardiac region of the stomach (Figures 6.78 and 6.79). The **common hepatic artery** crosses to the right and enters the porta hepatis, where it branches into the right and left hepatic arteries. As the common hepatic artery courses toward the liver, it gives off the **right gastric, gastroduodenal,** and **cystic arteries.** The **splenic artery** is the largest branch of the celiac trunk and passes to the left behind the stomach and along the upper border of the pancreas to enter the hilum of the spleen (Figures 6.80 and 6.81). At the point where the splenic artery courses near the border of the pancreas, it gives off numerous **pancreatic branches** that supply the pancreas.

Key.   Ce celiac axis; **GA** left gastric artery; **IVC** inferior vena cava.

Figure 6.78   Axial MR scan with gastric artery.   (R1.D)

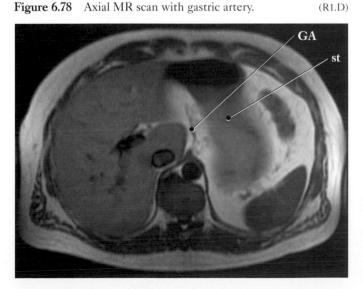

Figure 6.79   Axial CT scan with gastric artery.   (R1.H)

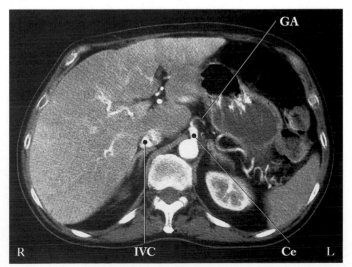

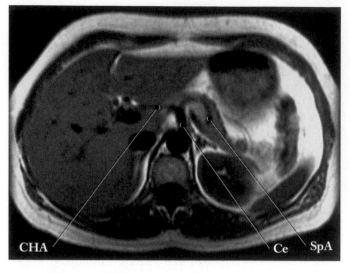

Figure 6.80   Axial MR scan with celiac trunk.   (R1.I)

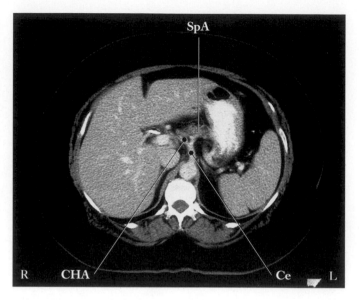

Figure 6.81   Axial CT scan with celiac trunk.   (R1.G)

Key.   **CHA** common hepatic artery; **Ce** celiac axis; **SpA** splenic artery.

Figure 6.82   Anterior view of mesenteric arteries.

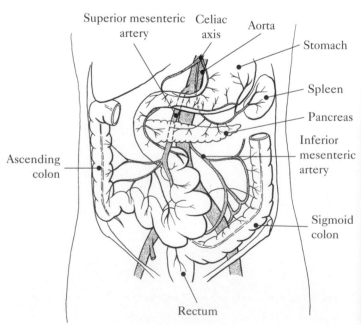

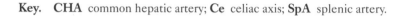

Key.   **IMV** inferior mesenteric vein; **IVC** inferior vena cava; **SMA** superior mesenteric artery; **SMV** superior mesenteric vein.

Figure 6.83   Axial MR scan with superior mesenteric artery.   (R1.O)

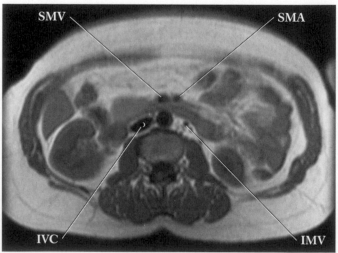

SUPERIOR MESENTERIC ARTERY. The **superior mesenteric artery** is the second vessel to leave the anterior wall of the aorta; it branches off within centimeters of the celiac trunk. It courses anteriorly and inferiorly to branch into several arteries that supply the majority of the small intestine, as well as the ascending and transverse colon (Figures 6.82 through 6.84).

INFERIOR MESENTERIC ARTERY. The **inferior mesenteric artery** leaves the anterior wall of the aorta at approximately the level of L3. It descends for a short distance in front of the aorta and then turns to the left, where it crosses in front of the left psoas muscle. The inferior mesenteric artery branches to supply the distal portion of the transverse colon, descending and sigmoid colon, and rectum (Figures 6.82, 6.85, and 6.86).

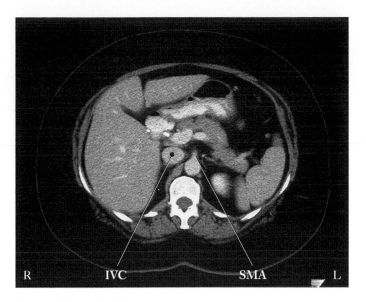

Figure 6.84 Axial CT scan with superior mesenteric artery.   (R1.H)

Key.   **A** aorta; **IMA** inferior mesenteric artery; **IMV** inferior mesenteric vein; **IVC** inferior vena cava; **SMA** superior mesenteric artery; **SMV** superior mesenteric vein.

Figure 6.85 Axial MR scan of inferior mesenteric artery.   (R1.O)

Figure 6.86 Axial CT scan of inferior mesenteric artery.   (R1.O)

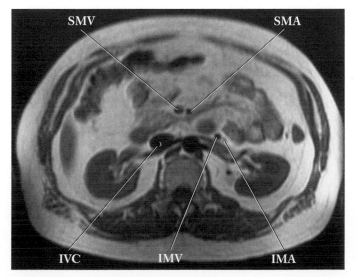

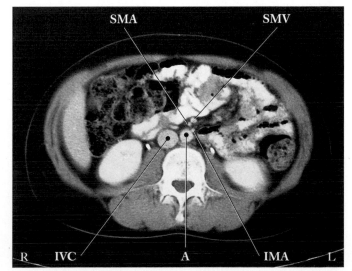

PAIRED BRANCHES

The paired branches of the abdominal aorta include the suprarenal, renal, and gonadal arteries (Figure 6.87).

SUPRARENAL ARTERIES.   The two **suprarenal arteries** exit the lateral walls of the aorta approximately at the level of the superior mesenteric artery. These arteries course laterally and slightly superiorly to supply the adrenal glands (Figure 6.87).

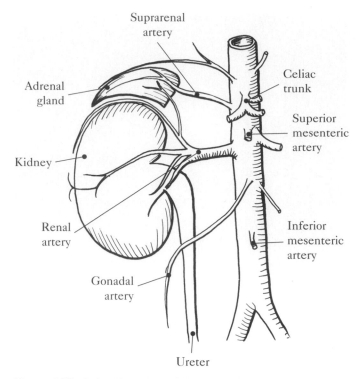

Figure 6.87   Paired branches of the abdominal aorta.

Key.   A aorta; **CIA** common iliac artery; **EIA** external iliac artery; **IIA** internal iliac artery; **IVC** inferior vena cava; **k** kidney; **RA** renal artery; **RV** renal vein; **sp** spleen; **SpA** splenic artery.

Figure 6.88   MRA of renal arteries. (Courtesy GE Medical Systems, Milwaukee, Wisc.)

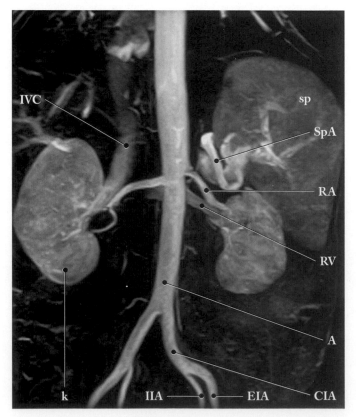

Key.   A aorta; **k** kidney; **RA** renal artery; **ur** ureter.

Figure 6.89   CTA of renal arteries. (Courtesy Picker International, Cleveland, Ohio.)

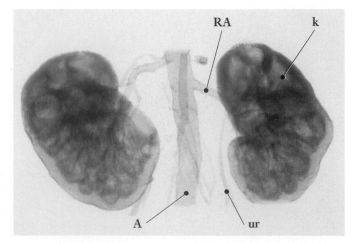

RENAL ARTERIES.   The two large **renal arteries** arise from the lateral walls of the aorta just below the superior mesenteric artery. Each vessel travels horizontally to the hilum of the corresponding kidney (Figures 6.88 and 6.89). Because of the position of the aorta on the left side of the vertebral column, the **right renal artery** is slightly longer than the left renal artery. In addition, the right renal artery passes posterior to the inferior vena cava and right renal vein on its course to the right kidney. Typically, the left kidney is higher than the right kidney, which means the **left renal artery** is generally slightly higher than the right renal artery (Figures 6.90 and 6.91).

> Renal artery stenosis causes renal ischemia and can result in secondary hypertension.

GONADAL ARTERIES.   The **gonadal arteries** originate from the anterior wall of the aorta just inferior to the renal arteries. They descend along the psoas muscles to reach the respective organs. In the male, the gonadal arteries are termed the **testicular arteries,** whereas the gonadal arteries in the female are termed the **ovarian arteries** (see Figure 6.87).

Key.   **A** aorta; **IVC** inferior vena cava; **LRA** left renal artery; **LRV** left renal vein; **RRA** right renal artery.

Figure 6.90   Axial MR scan with renal arteries and veins.   (R1.O)

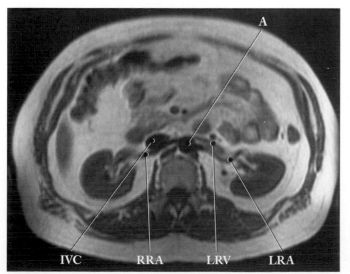

Figure 6.91   Axial CT scan with renal arteries and veins.   (R1.L)

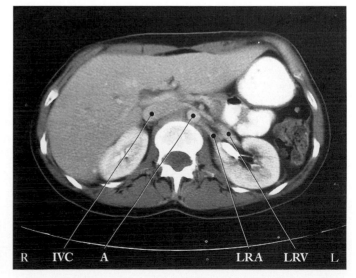

INFERIOR VENA CAVA AND TRIBUTARIES

The **inferior vena cava (IVC)** is the largest vein of the body and is formed by the union of the common iliac veins at approximately the level of L5. The IVC courses superiorly through the retroperitoneum along the anterior aspect of the vertebral column and to the right of the aorta. As it ascends the abdominal cavity, the IVC passes the posterior surface of the liver and pierces the diaphragm at the **caval hiatus** to enter the right atrium of the heart. The IVC receives many tributaries throughout its course in the abdomen, which include the lumbar, right gonadal, renal, and hepatic veins (Figure 6.92).

Figure 6.92   Tributaries of inferior vena cava.

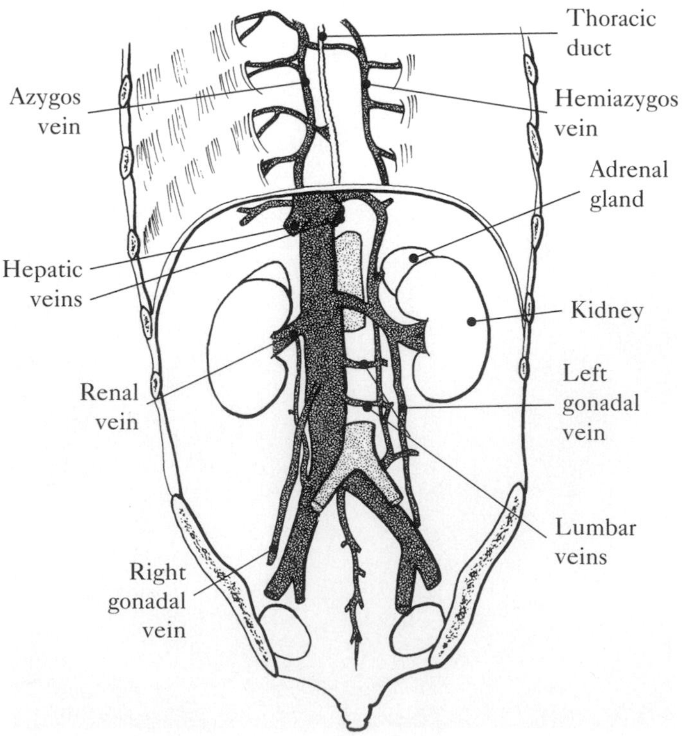

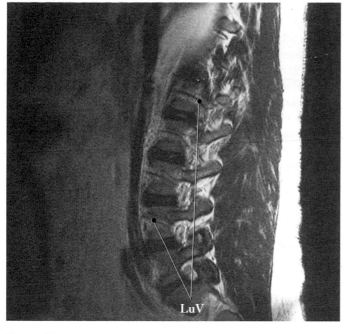

Figure 6.93 Sagittal MR scan with lumbar veins. (R2.F)

Key. **LuV** lumbar veins.

LUMBAR VEINS

The **lumbar veins** consist of four or five pairs of vessels that collect blood from the posterior abdominal wall. These vessels travel horizontally along the transverse processes deep to the psoas muscles (Figure 6.93). The lumbar veins can be found at all lumbar levels, and some continue to empty into the IVC at the level of the renal veins. The arrangement of these veins varies, with some entering the lateral walls of the IVC and others emptying into the azygos venous system. Occasionally, the right lumbar vein continues as the azygos vein and the left lumbar vein continues as the hemiazygos vein.

GONADAL VEINS

The **gonadal veins** ascend the abdomen along the psoas muscle, anterior to the ureters. The **right gonadal vein** enters the anterolateral wall of the IVC just below the opening for the right renal vein, whereas the **left gonadal vein** empties into the left renal vein (Figures 6.92, 6.94, and 6.95).

Key. **lGoA** gonadal artery; **lGoV** gonadal vein; **ur** ureters.

Figure 6.94 Axial MR scan with gonadal veins. (R1.R)

Key. **rGoV** right gonadal vein; **ur** ureters.

Figure 6.95 Axial CT scan with gonadal veins. (R1.R)

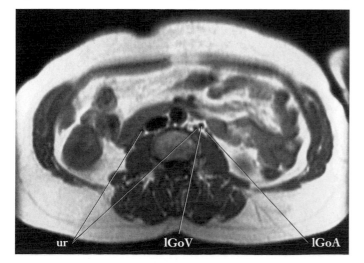

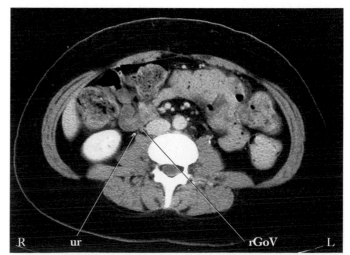

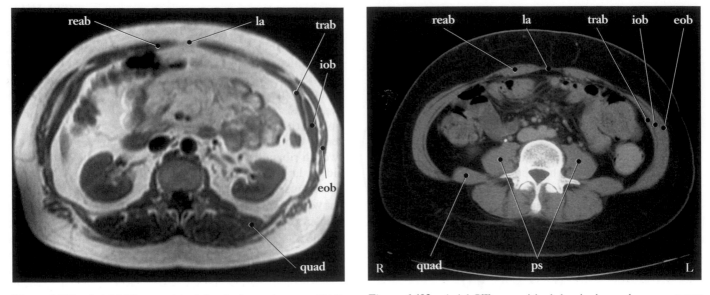

Figure 6.101   Axial MR scan with abdominal muscles.   (R1.S)

Figure 6.102   Axial CT scan with abdominal muscles.   (R1.T)

Key.   eob external oblique; **iob** internal oblique; **la** linea alba; **ps** psoas muscles; **quad** quadratus lumborum; **reab** rectus abdominus; **trab** transverse abdominus.

Table 6.2   Abdominal muscles

MUSCLE	ORIGIN	INSERTION	FUNCTION
Rectus abdominis	Pubic bone near symphysis	Costal cartilage of fifth, sixth, seventh ribs; xiphoid process of sternum	Flex trunk
External oblique	Lower eight ribs	Linea alba and iliac crest	Compress abdominal viscera, flex and rotate spine
Internal oblique	Iliac crest and lumbodorsal fascia	Lower three ribs	Compress abdominal viscera, flex and rotate spine
Transversus abdominis	Lower six ribs, iliac crest, and lumbodorsal fascia	Pubic bone and linea alba	Compress abdominal viscera
Quadratus lumborum	Iliac crest	Twelfth rib and transverse processes of lumbar vertebrae	Flex spine laterally
Psoas	Anterior surfaces and transverse processes of T12-L5	Lesser trochanter of femur	Flex thigh and trunk

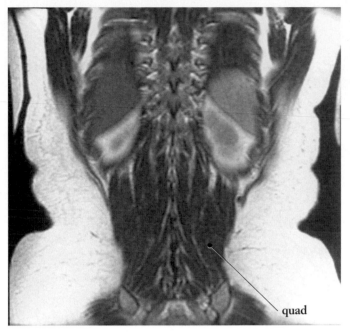

Figure 6.103   Coronal MR scan of quadratus lumborum muscles.   (R2.D)

Key.   quad quadratus lumborum.

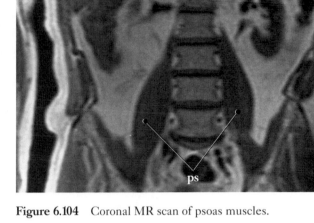

Figure 6.104   Coronal MR scan of psoas muscles.   (R2.A)

Key.   ps psoas muscles.

ANSWER TO FIGURE 6.1

The abnormal structure is the right adrenal gland. The right adrenal mass measures approximately 3 cm in diameter and is associated with an abnormal retrocaval node, measuring approximately 4 × 2.5 cm.

1

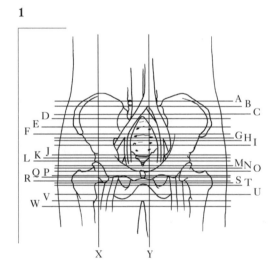

2

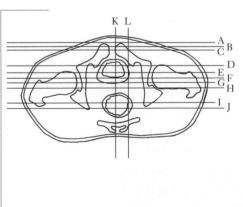

Reference illustrations

Pelvis

The pelvis provides structural support for the body and encloses the male and female reproductive organs. Because of its role as a support mechanism for the body, the pelvis has a large amount of musculoskeletal anatomy, which, together with the differences in male and female anatomy, make this area challenging to learn. This chapter demonstrates cross-section anatomy of the following structures:

Bony Pelvis
sacrum
coccyx
os coxae

Muscles of the Pelvic Region
extrapelvic muscles
pelvic wall muscles
pelvic diaphragm muscles

Pelvic Viscera
urinary bladder
rectum
female reproductive organs
male reproductive organs

Pelvic Vasculature

Lymph Nodes

In Figure 7.1, what portion of the femur is involved in this disease process? (Answer on p. 235.)

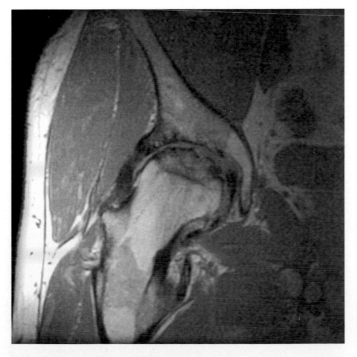

Figure 7.1   Coronal MR scan of hip.

BONY PELVIS

SACRUM, COCCYX, AND OS COXAE

The bony pelvis is formed by the **sacrum, coccyx,** and two **os coxae** (Figures 7.2 and 7.3). The sacrum is a triangular-shaped bone formed by the fusion of five vertebral segments. The first sacral segment has a prominent ridge located on the anterior surface of the body termed the **sacral promontory,** which acts as a bony landmark separating the abdominal cavity from the pelvic cavity. The transverse processes of the five sacral segments combine to form the **lateral mass (ala),** which articulates with the os coxae at the **sacroiliac joints** (Figure 7.4). Articulating with the fifth sacral segment is the coccyx, which consists of three to five small fused bony segments.

The os coxae is made up of three bones: **ilium, pubis,** and **ischium** (Figures 7.5 and 7.6). The ilium, the largest and most superior portion, consists of a **body** and a large winglike projection called the **ala** (Figures 7.7 and 7.8). The concave, anterior surface of the ala is termed the **iliac fossa,** which is separated from the body by the **arcuate line.** This arch-shaped line, located on the anterior surface of the ilium, forms part of the pelvic brim. The superior ridge of the ala is termed the **iliac crest;** it slopes down to give rise to the **superior** and **inferior iliac spines** on both the anterior and posterior surfaces. The body of the ilium creates the upper portion of the **acetabulum,** which is a deep fossa that articulates with the head of the femur (Figures 7.9 and 7.10). The pubis, or pubic bone, forms the lower anterior portion of the acetabulum and consists of a body and a **superior** and **inferior pubic rami** (Figures 7.11 and 7.12). The bodies of the two pubic bones meet at the midline to form the **pubic symphysis.** Located on the upper surface of the superior pubic ramus is a ridge termed the **pectineal line,** which is continuous with the arcuate line of the ilium, forming the **pelvic brim** (Figures 7.13 and 7.14).

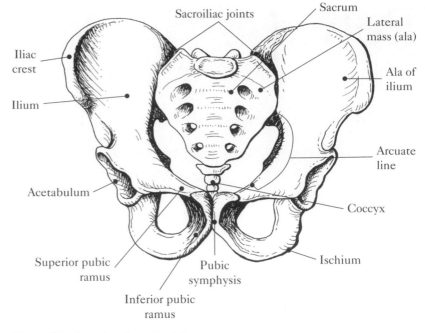

Figure 7.2 Anterior view of pelvis.

Key. **ace** acetabulum; **fn** femoral neck; **gtro** greater trochanter; **ili** iliac fossa; **isch** ischium; **obt** obturator foramen; **pub** pubic symphysis.

Figure 7.3 3D CT scan of anterior view of pelvis.

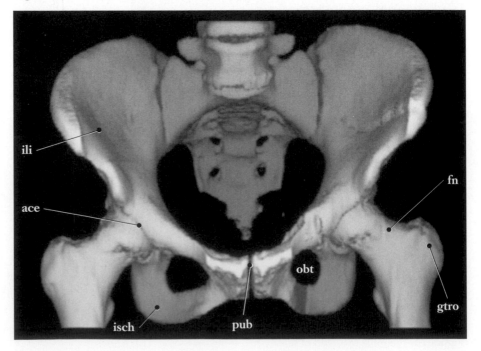

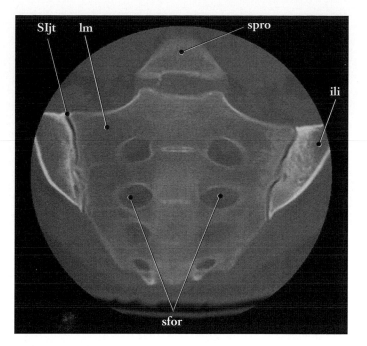

Figure 7.4   Coronal CT scan of sacroiliac joints.

Key.   il ilium; **lm** lateral mass; **sfor** sacral foramina; **SIjt** sacroiliac joint; **spro** sacral promontory.

The superior pubic ramus extends laterally from the body to meet the ilium, whereas the inferior pubic ramus extends inferiorly from the body to meet the ischium at an indistinct point; as a result, the two together are often referred to as the **ischiopubic ramus.** The ischium, the inferior portion of the os coxae, like the pubis is composed of a body and two rami. The **body** of the ischium forms the lower posterior portion of the acetabulum (Figures 7.15 and 7.16). The **superior ischial ramus** extends posteriorly and inferiorly to a roughened, enlarged area termed the **ischial tuberosity** (Figures 7.17 and 7.18). From the ischial tuberosity, the **inferior ischial ramus** extends anteriorly and medially to join the inferior pubic ramus. The **ischial spine** projects from the superior ischial ramus between two prominent notches on the posterior surface of the os coxae. The **greater sciatic notch** extends from the posterior inferior iliac spine to the ischial spine, and the **lesser sciatic notch** extends from the ischial spine to the ischial tuberosity. The two notches are spanned by ligaments, which create a foramina for the passage of nerves and vessels. The union of the pubic rami and ischium surrounds a large opening termed the **obturator foramen,** which is enclosed by the obturator muscles.

Key.   AIIS anterior inferior iliac spine; **ASIS** anterior superior iliac spine; **cr** crest; **cx** coccyx; **gsn** greater sciatic notch; **ispi** ischial spine; **lsn** lesser sciatic notch; **sa** sacrum; **tub** ischial tuberosity.

Figure 7.6   3D CT scan of lateral os coxae.

Figure 7.5   Lateral view of os coxae.

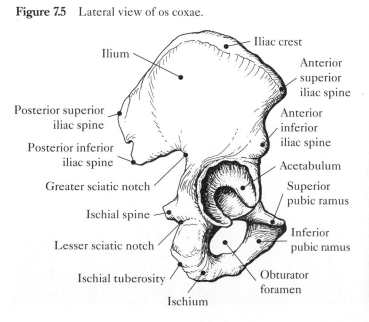

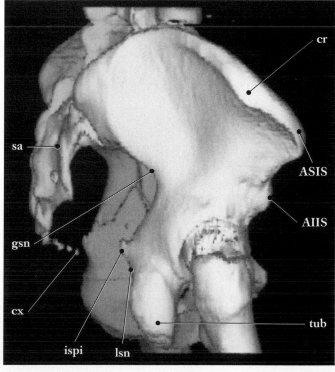

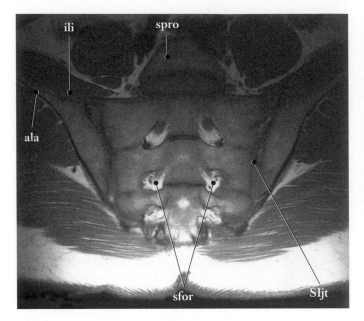

Figure 7.7   Coronal oblique MR scan of sacroiliac joints.

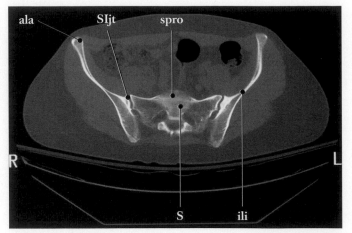

Figure 7.8   Axial CT scan of sacroiliac joints with ala of ilium.   (R1.D)

Key.   **ala** ala of ilium; **ili** iliac fossa; **s** sacrum; **sfor** sacral foramina; **SIjt** sacroiliac joint; **spro** sacral promontory.

Key.   **ace** acetabulum; **b** body of ilium; **cr** crest; **f** femur; **ili** iliac fossa; **isch** ischium.

Figure 7.9   Coronal MR scan of acetabulum.   (R2.F)

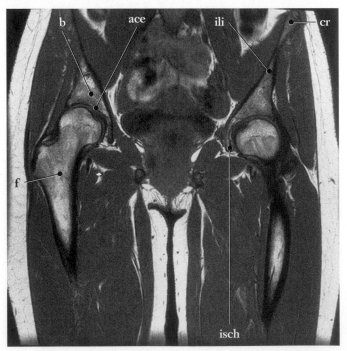

Figure 7.10   Coronal CT reformat of pelvis with acetabulum.
                                                          (R2.G)

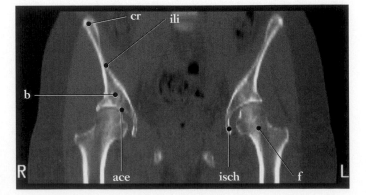

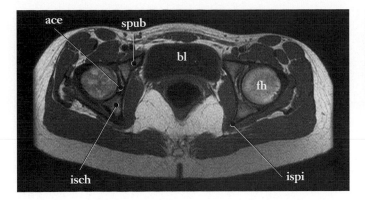

Figure 7.11 Axial MR scan of acetabulum and superior pubic ramus. (R1.P)

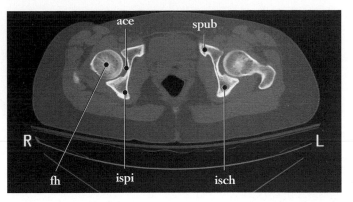

Figure 7.12 Axial CT scan of acetabulum and superior pubic ramus. (R1.Q)

Key. ace acetabulum; **bl** bladder; **fh** femoral head; **isch** ischium; **ispi** ischial spine; **spub** superior pubic ramus.

Key. ace acetabulum; **arc** arcuate line; **brim** pelvic brim; **il** ilium; **pec** pectineal line; **pub** pubic symphysis.

Figure 7.13 Coronal MR scan of pelvis with pelvic brim. (R2.D)

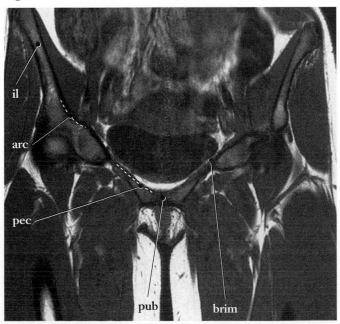

Figure 7.14 Coronal CT scan with pelvic brim. (R2.E)

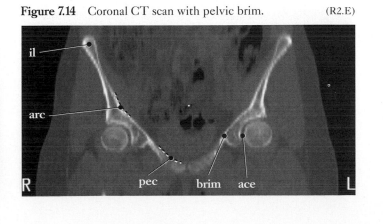

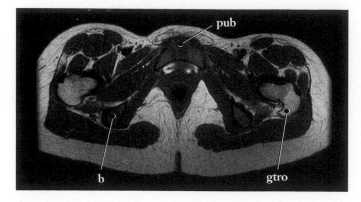

Figure 7.15 Axial MR scan of body of pubic and ischial bones. (R1.S)

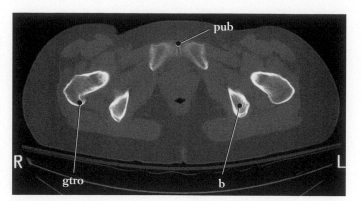

Figure 7.16 Axial CT of body of pubic and ischial bones. (R1.S)

Key. **b** body of ischium; **gtro** greater trochanter; **pub** pubic symphysis.

Key. **ipub** inferior pubic ramus; **pub** pubic symphysis; **tub** ischial tuberosity.

Figure 7.17 Axial MR scan of inferior pubic ramus and ischial tuberosity. (R1.U)

Figure 7.18 Axial CT scan of inferior pubic ramus and ischial tuberosity. (R1.U)

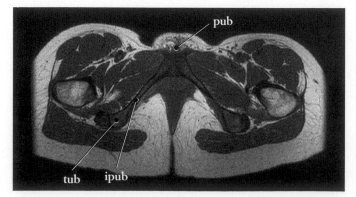

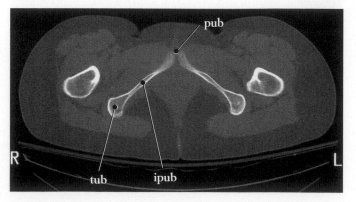

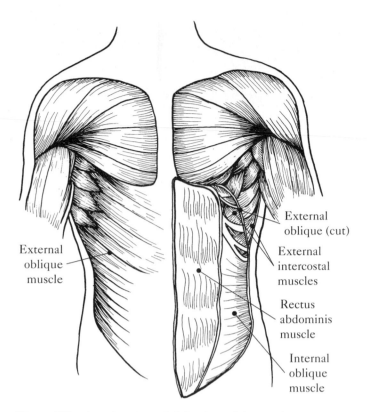

External oblique muscle

External oblique (cut)

External intercostal muscles

Rectus abdominis muscle

Internal oblique muscle

Figure 7.19   Anterior view of abdominopelvic muscles.

MUSCLES OF THE PELVIC REGION

Multiple muscles are visualized in the pelvis. For ease of description, the major pelvic muscles have been divided into functional groups: extrapelvic, pelvic wall, and pelvic diaphragm.

EXTRAPELVIC MUSCLES

Several of the muscles visualized in the pelvis are actually abdominal muscles such as the **rectus abdominis, psoas, and internal and external oblique muscles.** The rectus abdominis muscles, visualized on the anterior surface of the abdomen and pelvis, originate from the symphysis pubis and extend to the xiphoid process and the costal cartilage of the fifth, sixth, and seventh ribs. They function to flex the lumbar vertebrae and support the abdomen. The psoas muscles extend along the lateral surfaces of the lumbar vertebrae and act to flex the thigh or trunk. The external and internal oblique muscles are located on the outer lateral portion of the abdomen and span primarily between the cartilages of the lower ribs to the level of the iliac crest (Figures 7.19 through 7.21).

Key. **ilia** iliacus muscle; **la** linea alba; **ps** psoas muscles; **reab** rectus abdominus.

Figure 7.20   Axial MR scan of pelvis with oblique, psoas, and rectus abdominis muscles.   (R1.C)

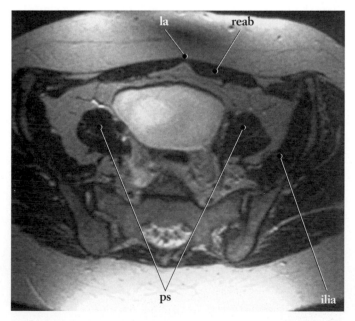

la   reab

ps   ilia

Key. **eob** external oblique muscle; **iob** internal oblique muscle; **ps** psoas muscles; **reab** rectus abdominus.

Figure 7.21   Axial CT scan of pelvis with oblique, psoas, and rectus abdominis muscles.   (R1.A)

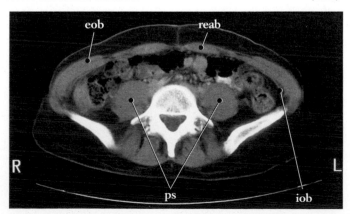

eob   reab

R   L

ps   iob

The oblique muscles work together to flex and rotate the vertebral column and compress the abdominal viscera. An inferior band of fibrous connective tissue from the external oblique muscle folds back on itself to form the **inguinal ligament,** which spans between the anterior superior iliac spine and the pubic tubercle (Figure 7.22).

> Indirect inguinal hernias are protrusions of the intestine at the inguinal ring. They account for approximately 80% of all hernias.

Many of the muscles visualized in the pelvis are considered to be muscles of the hip. The largest of this group are the **gluteus muscles (maximus, medius, minimus),** which function together to abduct, rotate, and extend the thigh (Figure 7.23). The largest and most superficial is the gluteus maximus muscle, which makes up the bulk of the buttocks. The gluteus medius and minimus muscles are smaller in size, respectively, and are deep to the gluteus maximus muscle (Figures 7.24 through 7.26).

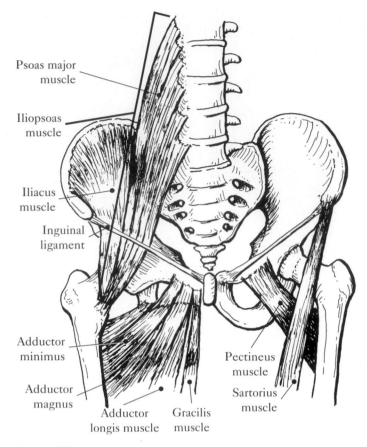

Figure 7.22   Anterior view of iliopsoas muscle.

Figure 7.23   Posterior view of gluteus muscle group.

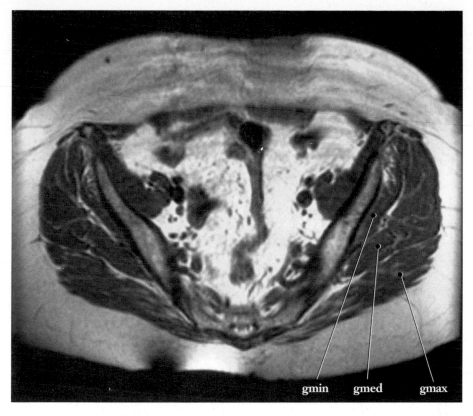

Figure 7.24   Axial MR scan of pelvis with gluteus muscle group.   (R1.H)

Key. ace acetabulum; **gmax** gluteus maximus; **gmed** gluteus medius; **gmin** gluteus minimus.

Figure 7.26   Coronal MR scan of pelvis with gluteus muscle group.   (R2.H)

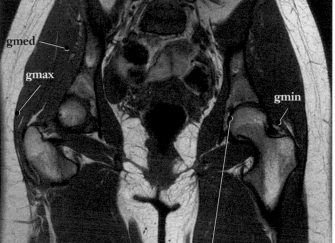

Figure 7.25   Axial CT scan of pelvis with gluteus muscle group.   (R1.J)

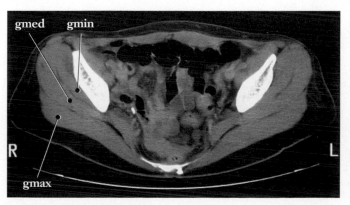

PELVIC WALL MUSCLES

The muscles of the pelvis include the **piriformis, obturator internus** and **externus,** and **iliacus muscles** (Figures 7.27 and 7.28; see also Figure 7.22). The piriformis muscle, which acts to rotate the thigh laterally, originates from the ilium and the sacrum and passes through the greater sciatic notch to insert on the greater trochanter of the femur (Figures 7.29 and 7.30). Also functioning to rotate the thigh laterally is the obturator internus muscle. This fan-shaped muscle extends from the pubic bone and obturator foramen to pass through the lesser sciatic notch and attaches to the greater trochanter of the femur. Inserting on the greater trochanter just below the obturator internus muscle is the obturator externus muscle. This strong muscle originates on the obturator foramen, aiding in adduction and rotation of the thigh. Extending from the iliac crest and sacrum is the triangular-shaped iliacus muscle (Figures 7.31 and 7.32). As the iliacus muscle spans the iliac fossa, it is joined by the psoas muscle to form the **iliopsoas muscle,** which extends to insert on the lesser trochanter of the femur. The iliopsoas muscle is the most important muscle for flexing the leg, which makes walking possible (Figures 7.33 through 7.35).

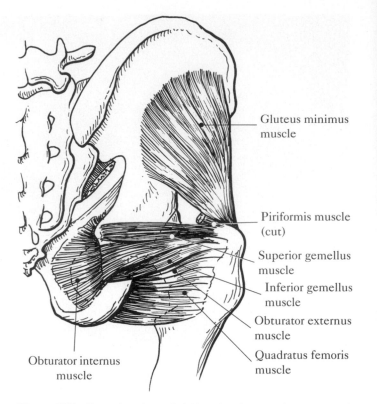

Figure 7.27   Posterior view of piriformis, obturator internus, and obturator externus muscles.

Key.   ilia iliacus; **obe** obturator externus; **obi** obturator internus.

Figure 7.28   Coronal MR scan of pelvis with obturator internus and obturator externus muscles.   (R2.F)

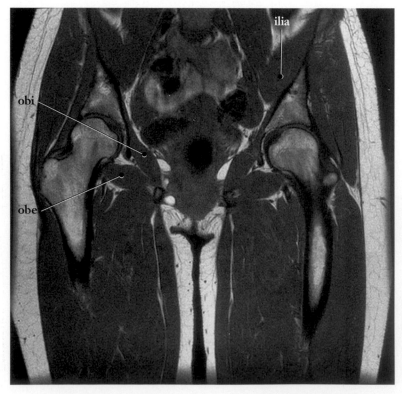

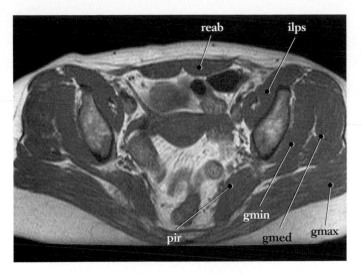

Figure 7.29   Axial MR scan of pelvis with piriformis muscle.

(R1. J)

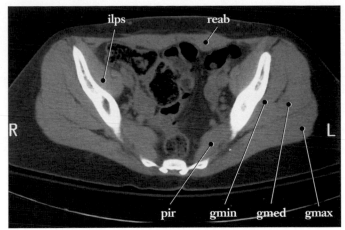

Figure 7.30   Axial CT scan of pelvis with piriformis muscle.

(R1.I)

Key.   gmax gluteus maximus; **gmed** gluteus medius; **gmin** gluteus minimus; **ilia** iliacus; **ilps** iliopsoas; **lym** lymph nodes; **pir** piriformis; **ps** psoas muscle; **reab** rectus abdominus.

Figure 7.31   Axial MR scan of pelvis with iliacus muscle.   (R1.C)

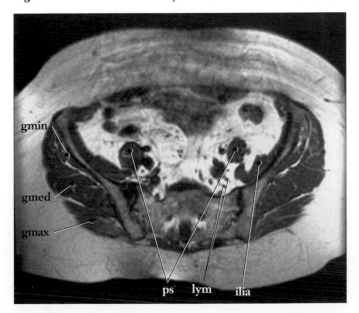

Figure 7.32   Axial CT scan of pelvis with iliacus muscle.   (R1.E)

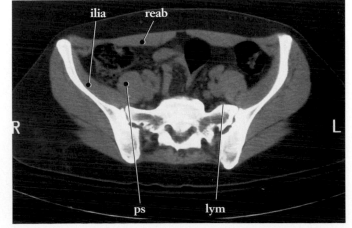

PELVIC DIAPHRAGM MUSCLES

The funnel-shaped **pelvic diaphragm** is a layer of muscles and fascia that forms the greatest majority of the pelvic floor. The primary muscles of the pelvic diaphragm are the **levator ani** and **coccygeus muscles** (Figures 7.36 through 7.39). The two levator ani muscles are the largest and most important muscles of the pelvic floor, originating from the symphysis pubis and ischial spines to form winglike arches that attach to the coccyx (Figures 7.40 and 7.41). The two coccygeus muscles form the posterior portion of the pelvic floor, arising from the ischial spines and fanning out to attach to the lower sacrum and coccyx. Together, the levator ani and coccygeus muscles provide support for the pelvic contents (Figures 7.42 and 7.43).

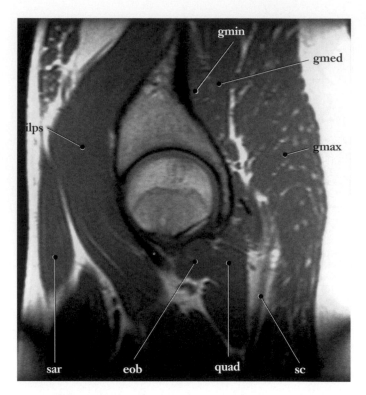

Figure 7.33 Sagittal MR scan of pelvis with iliopsoas muscle.
(R1. X)

Key. **eob** external oblique; **gmax** gluteus maximus; **gmed** gluteus medius; **gmin** gluteus minimus; **ilps** iliopsoas muscle; **quad** quadratus femoris; **sar** sartorius; **sc** sciatic nerve.

Key. **f** femur; **gmax** gluteus maximus; **ilps** iliopsoas; **isch** ischium; **obe** obturator externus; **obi** obturator internus; **pec** pectineus muscle; **pub** pubic symphysis.

Figure 7.34 Axial MR scan of pelvis with iliopsoas muscle.
(R1.P)

Figure 7.35 Axial CT scan of pelvis with iliopsoas muscle.
(R1.S)

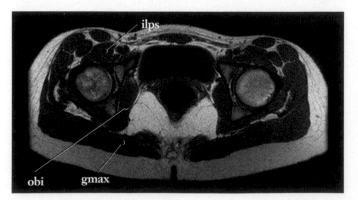

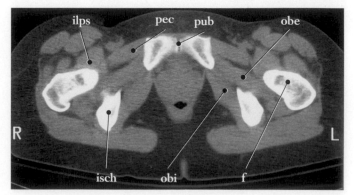

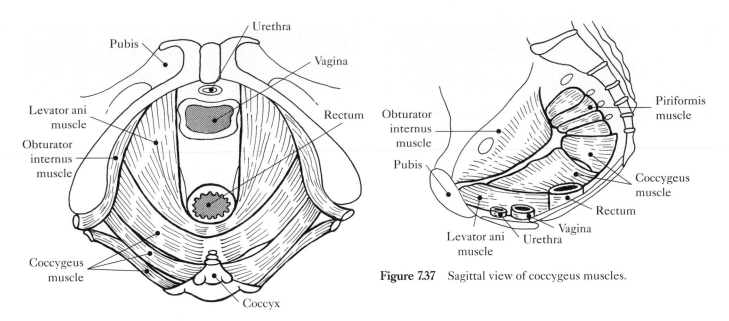

Figure 7.36 Inferior view of pelvic diaphragm muscles.

Figure 7.37 Sagittal view of coccygeus muscles.

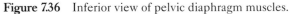

Key. **cerv** cervix; **lev** levator ani; **ut** uterus; **v** vagina.

Figure 7.38 Coronal MR scan of pelvis with pelvic diaphragm muscles.   (R2. J)

Key. **bl** bladder; **lev** levator ani; **pub** pubic symphysis; **reab** rectus abdominus.

Figure 7.39 Sagittal MR scan of pelvis with pelvic diaphragm muscles.   (R2. L)

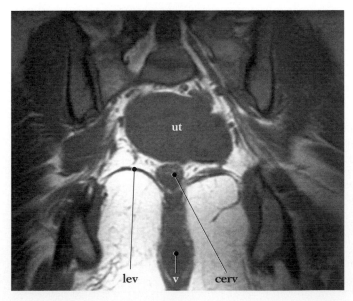

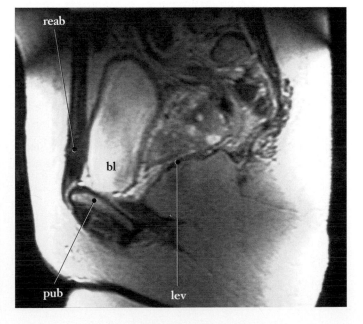

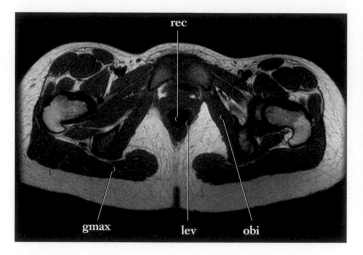

Figure 7.40   Axial MR scan of pelvis with levator ani muscle.
(R1.S)

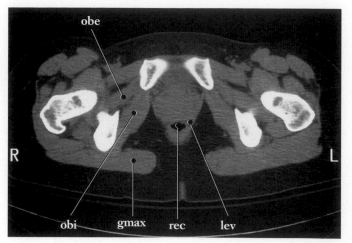

Figure 7.41   Axial CT scan of pelvis with levator ani muscle.
(R1.S)

Key.   gmax gluteus maximus; **lev** levator ani; **obe** obturator externus; **obi** obturator internus; **rec** rectum.

Table 7.1   Muscles of the pelvic wall and diaphragm

Muscle	Origin	Insertion	Function
Piriformis	Ilium and sacrum	Greater trochanter of femur	Laterally rotate and adduct thigh
Obturator internus	Obturator foramen and pubic bone	Greater trochanter of femur (medial surface)	Laterally rotate thigh
Obturator externus	Obturator foramen	Greater trochanter of femur (trochanteric fossa)	Laterally rotate and adduct thigh
Iliacus	Iliac crest and sacrum	Lesser trochanter of femur (tendon fused with that of psoas muscle)	Flex hip
Levator ani	Symphysis pubis and ischial spine	Coccyx	Support pelvic viscera, flex coccyx, elevates and retracts anus
Coccygeus	Ischial spine	Sacrum and coccyx	Assist in support of pelvic floor and flex coccyx

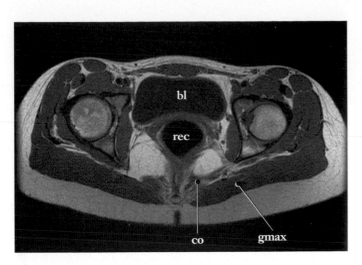

Figure 7.42   Axial MR scan of pelvis with coccygeus muscles.
(R1.P)

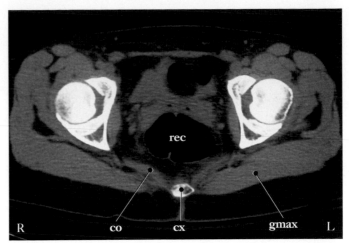

Figure 7.43   Axial CT scan of pelvis with coccygeus muscles.
(R1.P)

Key.   bl bladder; **co** coccygeus; **cx** coccyx; **gmax** gluteus maximus; **rec** rectum.

PELVIC VISCERA

The pelvic cavity contains the urinary bladder, rectum, and internal reproductive organs.

URINARY BLADDER

The **urinary bladder** is a triangular-shaped muscular organ that lies immediately posterior to the symphysis pubis. It functions as a temporary reservoir for the storage of urine. Three openings in the floor of the bladder form a triangular area called the **trigone.** Two of the openings, at the base of the trigone, are created by the ureters (Figure 7.44). The pelvic portions of the ureters run anterior to the internal iliac arteries and enter the posterolateral surface of the bladder at an oblique angle. The third opening is located in the apex of the trigone and is formed by the entrance to the **urethra** (Figures 7.44, 7.45, and 7.46).

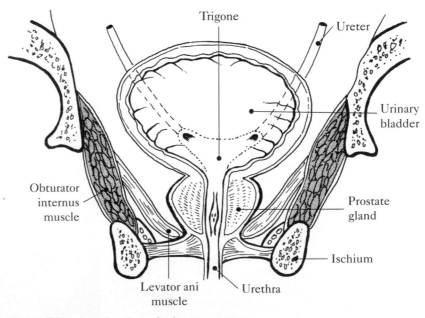

Figure 7.44   Anterior view of urinary system.

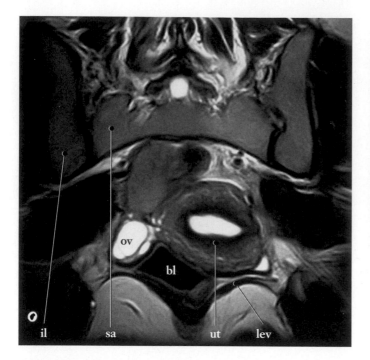

Figure 7.45   Coronal MR scan of female bladder. (Courtesy GE Medical Systems, Milwaukee, Wisc.)   (R2.I)

Key.   bl bladder; **il** ilium; **lev** levator ani; **ov** ovary; **sa** sacrum; **ut** uterus.

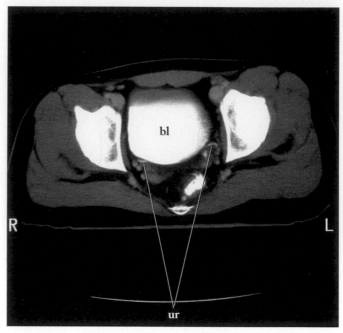

Figure 7.46   Axial CT scan of pelvis with bladder.   (R1.N)

Key.   bl bladder; **ur** ureter.

Key.   bl bladder; **pub** pubic symphysis; **ut** uterus.

Figure 7.48   Sagittal MR scan of pelvis with female bladder.

(R2.K)

Figure 7.47   Lateral view of female bladder.

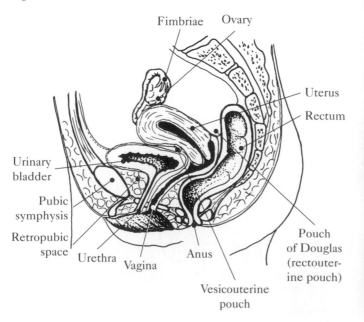

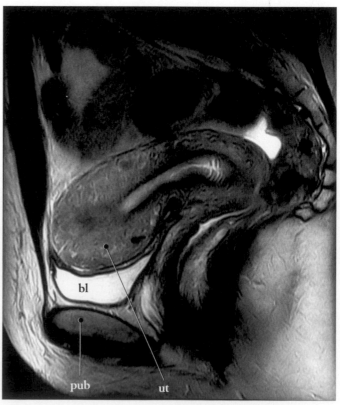

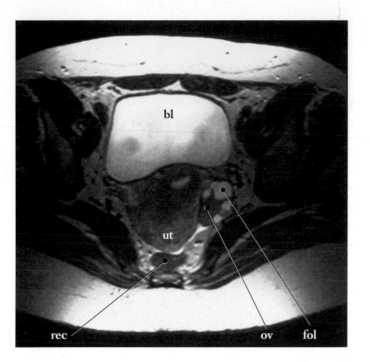

Figure 7.49 Axial MR scan of pelvis with female bladder.   (R1.J)

Key. bl bladder; **fol** follicular cyst; **ov** ovary; **rec** rectum;
ut uterus.

The female urethra is a short muscular tube that drains urine from the bladder. The external urethral opening is located just anterior to the vagina (Figures 7.47 through 7.50). The male urethra is much longer and extends from the inferior portion of the bladder to the tip of the **penis.** It can be subdivided into three regions: **prostatic urethra, membranous urethra,** and **penile urethra** (Figures 7.51 through 7.53). The prostatic urethra passes through the middle of the prostate gland (Figures 7.54 and 7.55). The membranous urethra is the shortest and narrowest portion of the urethra and is the portion that penetrates the external urethral sphincter. The penile urethra is the longest portion, extending from the external urethral sphincter to the tip of the penis.

RECTUM

The **rectum** is the terminal part of the large intestine extending from S3 to the tip of the coccyx. It follows the anteroposterior curve of the sacrum and coccyx and ends by turning inferiorly to become the **anal canal.** The anal canal terminates in the **anus,** which is the opening to the exterior of the body (see Figures 7.47, 7.51, 7.54, and 7.55).

Key. bl bladder; **rec** rectum; **va** vagina.

Figure 7.50 Axial CT scan of pelvis with female bladder.   (R1.O)

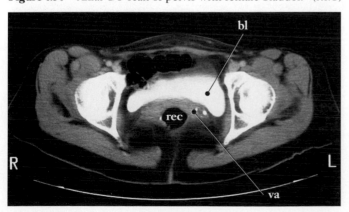

Figure 7.51 Lateral view of male bladder.

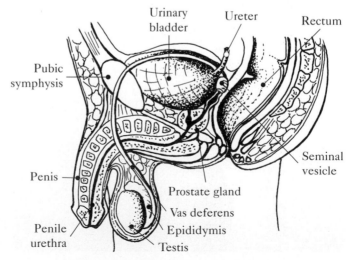

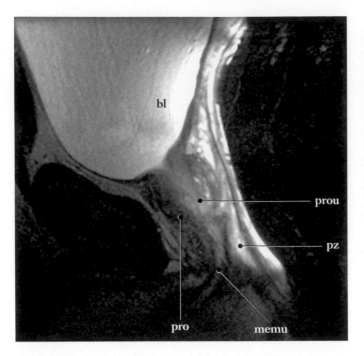

Figure 7.52   Sagittal MR scan of pelvis with male bladder.   (R2.K)

Key. bl bladder; **memu** membranous urethra; **pro** prostate; **prou** prostatic urethra; **pz** peripheral zone.

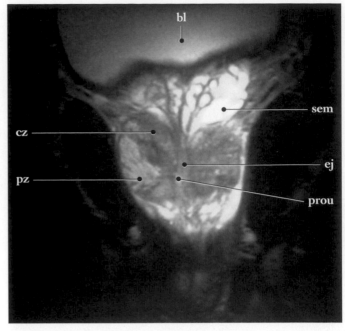

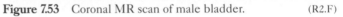

Figure 7.53   Coronal MR scan of male bladder.   (R2.F)

Key. bl bladder; **cz** central zone; **ej** ejaculatory duct; **prou** prostatic urethra; **pz** peripheral zone; **sem** seminal vesicle.

Key. bl bladder; **rec** rectum; **sem** seminal vesicle; **vas** vas deferens.

Figure 7.54   Axial MR scan of pelvis with male bladder.   (R1.O)

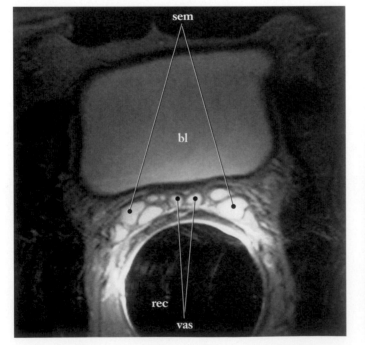

Key. pro prostate gland; **prou** prostatic urethra; **rec** rectum.

Figure 7.55   Axial CT scan of pelvis with male bladder.   (R1.T)

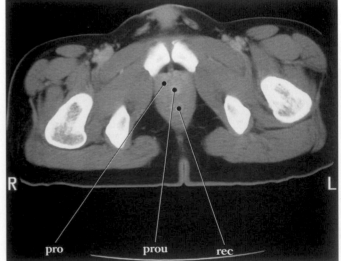

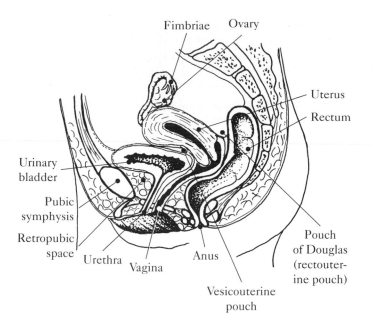

Figure 7.56 illustration labels: Fimbriae, Ovary, Uterus, Rectum, Urinary bladder, Pubic symphysis, Retropubic space, Urethra, Vagina, Anus, Pouch of Douglas (rectouterine pouch), Vesicouterine pouch

Figure 7.56   Sagittal view of female reproductive system.

Key. bl bladder; **cerv** cervix; **myo** myometrium; **pub** pubic symphysis; **rpub** retropubic space; **rute** rectouterine pouch; **ucav** uterine cavity; **ure** urethra; **v** vagina; **ves** vesicouterine pouch.

Figure 7.57   Sagittal MR scan of female reproductive system. (Courtesy GE Medical Systems, Milwaukee, Wisc.)   (R2.K)

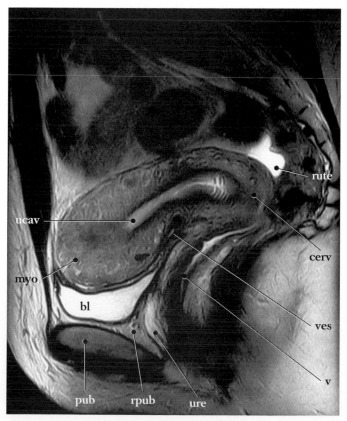

Figure 7.57 MR scan labels: ucav, myo, bl, pub, rpub, ure, rute, cerv, ves, v

FEMALE REPRODUCTIVE ORGANS

The female reproductive system is responsible for producing sex hormones and ova and also functions to protect and support a developing embryo. The principal organs of the female reproductive system are located within the pelvic cavity and include the uterus, ovaries, uterine tubes, and vagina (Figures 7.56 and 7.57).

UTERUS.   The **uterus** is a pear-shaped muscular organ located in the anterior portion of the pelvic cavity between the bladder and the rectum (Figures 7.56 and 7.57). The uterus can be subdivided into two anatomic regions: **body** and **cervix.** The body is the largest division, comprising the upper two thirds of the uterus. The rounded superior portion of the body is called the **fundus,** which is located just superior to the region where the uterine tubes enter the uterus. The narrow, inferior portion of the uterus is called the cervix, which communicates with the vagina via the external orifice (Figure 7.58). There is a bend near the base of the uterus that causes the body of the uterus to project superanteriorly over the bladder. The wall of the uterus is composed of three layers. The **endometrium** is the inner glandular tissue lining the inner wall. The middle muscular layer is the thickest portion of the uterine wall and is called the **myometrium.** The outer layer is a thin serous membrane called the **perimetrium,** which covers the fundus and posterior surface of the uterus. The uterus is the reproductive organ responsible for protecting and nourishing the fetus during development (Figures 7.58, 7.59 and 7.60).

Figure 7.58   Anterior view of uterus.

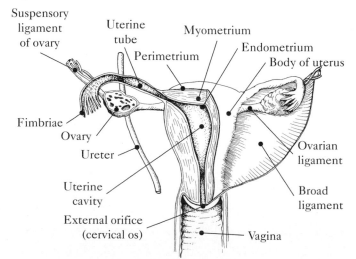

Figure 7.58 illustration labels: Suspensory ligament of ovary, Uterine tube, Myometrium, Perimetrium, Endometrium, Body of uterus, Fimbriae, Ovary, Ureter, Uterine cavity, External orifice (cervical os), Vagina, Ovarian ligament, Broad ligament

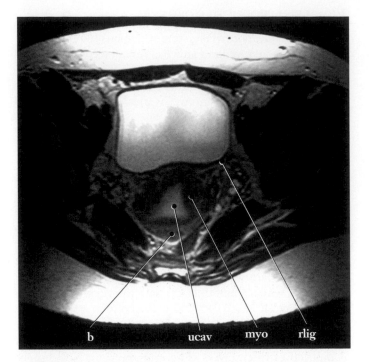

Figure 7.59   Axial MR scan of pelvis with body of uterus.   (R1.H)

Suspensory ligaments of the uterus.   The uterus is stabilized by several pairs of suspensory ligaments (Figure 7.61). The **round ligaments** extend laterally from the body of the uterus to the pelvic wall to prevent posterior movement of the uterus (Figures 7.62 and 7.63). The **uterosacral ligaments** extend from the lateral walls of the cervix to the anterior surface of the sacrum, preventing forward movement of the uterus (Figure 7.64). The **lateral cervical (cardinal) ligaments** extend from the lateral walls of the cervix and vagina to the lateral walls of the pelvis to prevent downward movement of the uterus (Figure 7.65). Additional support is provided by the muscles and fascia of the pelvic floor.

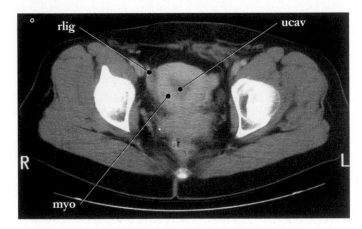

Figure 7.60   Axial CT scan of pelvis with body of uterus.   (R1.N)

Key.   b body of uterus; **myo** myometrium; **rlig** round ligament; **ucav** uterine cavity.

Figure 7.61   Superior view of uterus with ligaments.

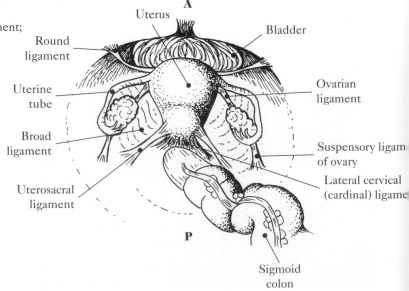

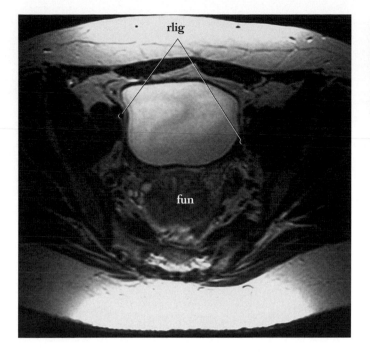

Figure 7.62   Axial MR scan of pelvis with round ligaments.

(R1.F)

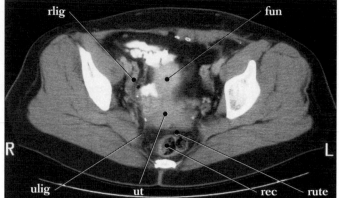

Figure 7.63   Axial CT scan of pelvis with round ligaments.

(R1.L)

Key.   cerv cervix; **clig** cardinal ligament; **fun** fundus of uterus; **rec** rectum; **rlig** round ligament; **rute** retrouterine pouch; **ulig** uterosacral ligament; **ut** uterus; **ves** vesicouterine pouch.

Figure 7.64   Axial MR scan of pelvis with uterosacral ligaments.   (R1.N)

Figure 7.65   Axial MR scan of pelvis with lateral cervical (cardinal) ligaments.   (R1.O)

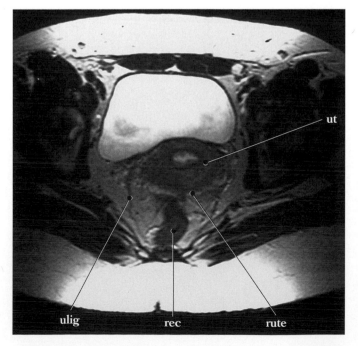

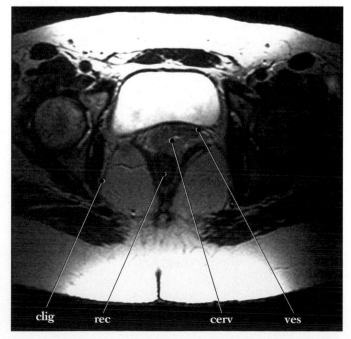

PELVIC SPACES. A peritoneal fold called the **broad ligament** encloses the ovaries, uterine tubes, and uterus (see Figure 7.58). The broad ligament extends from the sides of the uterus to the walls and floor of the pelvis, preventing side-to-side movement of the uterus and dividing the pelvis into anterior and posterior pouches (Figure 7.66). The anterior **vesicouterine pouch** is located between the uterus and the posterior wall of the bladder, whereas the posterior **rectouterine pouch (pouch of Douglas)** lies between the uterus and rectum. Another space in the pelvis is the **retropubic space,** which is located between the pubic bones and the bladder. The pelvic spaces are common areas for the accumulation of fluid within the pelvis (see Figures 7.56, 7.57, 7.63, and 7.64).

OVARIES. The paired **ovaries** are small, almond-shaped organs located on either side of the uterus (see Figures 7.56 and 7.58). They lie in a depression on the lateral walls of the pelvis and are held in place by the **ovarian** and **suspensory ligaments** (Figures 7.67 and 7.68). The cord-like ovarian ligament attaches the ovaries to the lateral surface of the uterus, and the suspensory ligament attaches the ovaries to the pelvic wall. The ovaries are responsible for the production of ova and the secretion of female sex hormones.

A follicular cyst represents the mature oocyte and its surrounding follicular cavity. Fluid increases within the cavity as the oocyte matures.

Key. **b** body of uterus; **myo** myometrium; **ov** ovary; **rlig** round ligament; **ucav** uterine cavity.

Figure 7.67   Axial MR scan of pelvis with ovaries.   (R1.H)

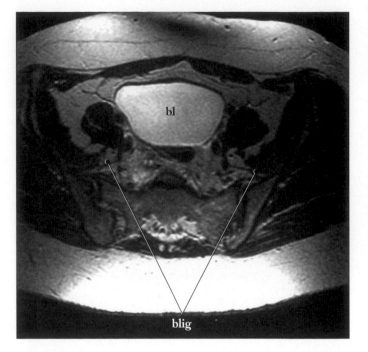

Figure 7.66   Axial MR scan of pelvis with broad ligament. (R1.C)

Key.   **bl** bladder; **blig** broad ligament.

Key.   **ov** ovary; **ut** uterus.

Figure 7.68   Axial CT scan of pelvis with ovaries.   (R1.M)

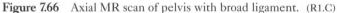

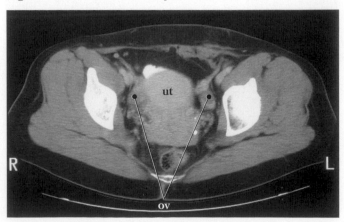

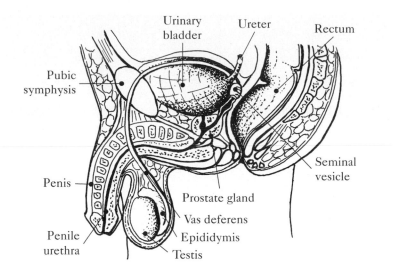

Figure 7.69   Lateral view of male reproductive system.

Key.   bl bladder; **pe** penis; **pro** prostate; **pub** pubic symphysis; **rec** rectum.

Figure 7.70   Sagittal MR scan of male reproductive system.   (R2.K)

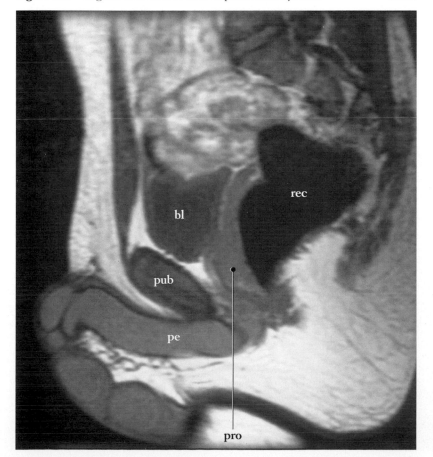

UTERINE TUBES. The **uterine (fallopian) tubes** are slender, muscular tubes extending laterally from the body of the uterus to the peritoneum near the ovaries. They are supported by the broad ligament, and at their distal end expand to form a funnel-shaped **infundibulum.** The infundibulum has numerous fingerlike projections called **fimbriae,** which spread loosely over the surface of the ovaries (see Figures 7.58 and 7.61). During ovulation, the fimbriae trap the ovum and sweep it into the uterine tubes. The proximal portion of the uterine tubes opens into the uterus, and the distal portion opens directly into the peritoneal cavity, immediately superior to the ovaries, thereby providing a direct route for pathogens to enter the pelvic cavity. The uterine tubes provide a method of transport for ova to reach the uterus from the ovaries.

VAGINA.   The **vagina** is a muscular tube extending anteroinferiorly from the cervix of the uterus to the external vaginal orifice. The vagina is located between the bladder and the rectum and functions as a receptacle for sperm and as the lower portion of the birth canal (see Figures 7.50, 7.57, and 7.58).

MALE REPRODUCTIVE ORGANS

The principal structures of the male reproductive system are the testis, epididymis, vas deferens, ejaculatory duct, seminal vesicle, prostate gland, bulbourethral gland, and penis. All these structures, except the testes and penis, are located within the pelvic cavity (Figures 7.69 and 7.70).

TESTES AND EPIDIDYMIS. The paired **testes** are suspended in fleshy, pouchlike scrotal sacs. Each testis produces sperm and male sex hormones. Sperm are transmitted from the testis to the **epididymis,** a tightly coiled, tubular structure, located on the superoposterior surface of each testis. The sperm are stored in the epididymis as they undergo the final stages of maturation (Figures 7.71 and 7.72).

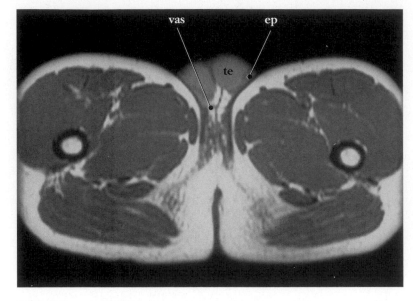

Figure 7.71   Axial MR scan of pelvis with testes.   (R1.W)

Key.   **ep** epididymis; **te** testes; **vas** vas deferens.

Key.   **ep** epididymis; **te** testes.

Figure 7.72   Axial CT scan of pelvis with testes.   (R1.W)

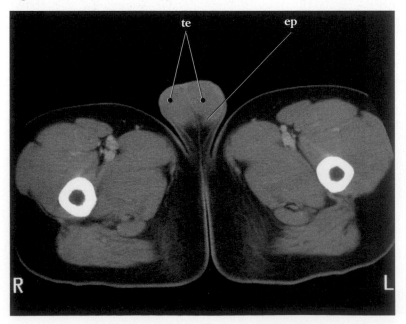

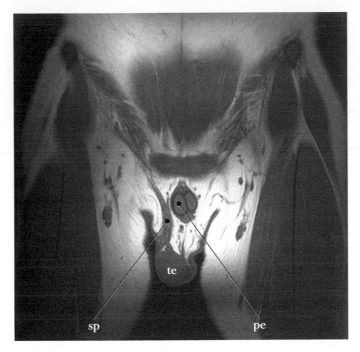

Figure 7.73   Coronal MR scan of pelvis with spermatic cord.

(R2.B)

VAS DEFERENS (DUCTUS) AND EJACULATORY DUCT.

As a continuation of the epididymis, the **vas deferens** is a long muscular tube that broadens near its proximal end and joins with the duct of the seminal vesicle to form the **ejaculatory duct,** which empties into the prostatic urethra (see Figure 7.69). Each vas deferens, along with a testicular artery and vein, is surrounded by the tough connective tissue and muscle of the paired **spermatic cords.** The spermatic cords begin at the inguinal ring and exit through the inguinal ligament to descend into the scrotum (Figures 7.73 through 7.75).

SEMINAL VESICLES.

The **seminal vesicles** are paired accessory glands consisting of coiled tubes that form two pouches, lateral to the vas deferens, on the posterior inferior surface of the bladder. They lie superior to the prostate gland and secrete seminal fluid that mixes with sperm prior to ejaculation (Figures 7.74 and 7.75).

Key. **bl** bladder; **pe** penis; **rec** rectum; **sem** seminal vesicle; **sp** spermatic cord; **te** testes; **vas** vas deferens.

Figure 7.74   Axial MR scan of pelvis with seminal vesicles.

(R1.O)

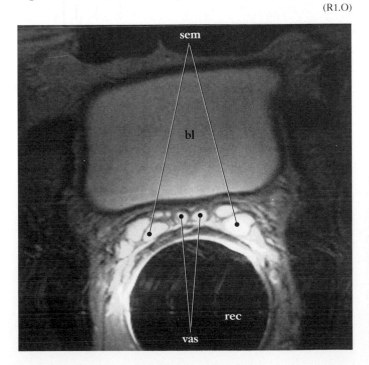

Figure 7.75   Axial CT scan of pelvis with seminal vesicles.

(R1.O)

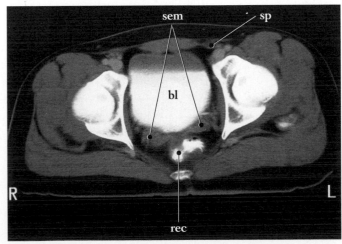

PROSTATE GLAND.   The **prostate gland** is the largest accessory gland of the male reproductive system. It secretes a thin, slightly alkaline fluid that forms a portion of the seminal fluid. The prostate gland surrounds the neck of the bladder, and the urethra courses through the anterior portion of the gland (Figures 7.76 and 7.77). The prostate gland is located inferior to the seminal vesicles between the bladder and rectum. The ejaculatory ducts, which are extensions of the seminal vesicles, descend inferiorly through the posterior portion of the prostate gland to open into the prostatic urethra. In sectional imaging, the prostate gland is divided into zonal anatomy. The three main regions are the **central zone, peripheral zone,** and **transition zone.** The central zone, surrounding the urethra, and the outer peripheral zone are the largest and most easily identified (Figures 7.77 through 7.80).

> Cancer of the prostate gland is the second most common type of cancer in men, occurring with increasing frequency over the age of 55 years.

Key.   bl bladder; **cz** central zone; **ej** ejaculatory duct; **prou** prostatic urethra; **pz** peripheral zone; **sem** seminal vesicle.

Figure 7.76   Coronal view of prostate gland.

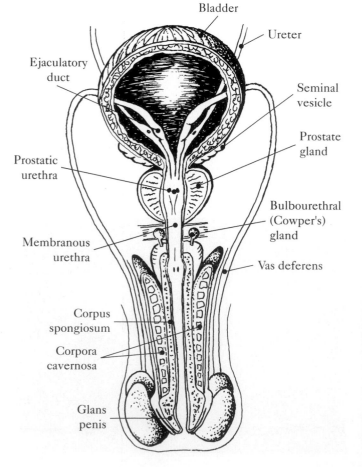

Figure 7.77   Coronal MR scan of prostate gland. (Courtesy GE Medical Systems, Milwaukee, Wisc.)   (R2.F)

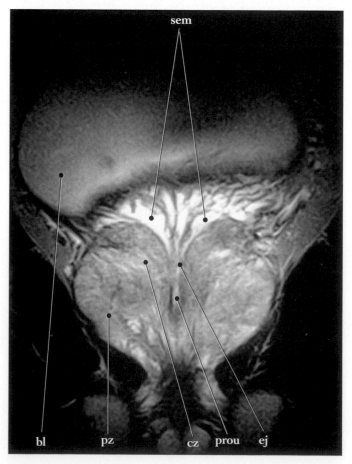

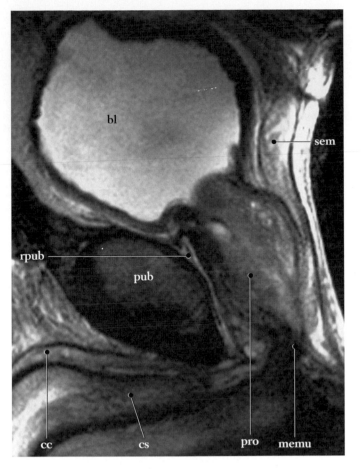

Figure 7.78 Sagittal MR scan of prostate gland. (Courtesy GE Medical Systems, Milwaukee, Wisc.)   (R2.K)

Key. bl bladder; **cc** corpora cavernosum; **cs** corpus spongiosum; **memu** membranous urethra; **pro** prostate gland; **pub** pubic symphysis; **rpub** retropubic space; **sem** seminal vesicle.

BULBOURETHRAL GLANDS. The two small, **bulbourethral glands** (Cowper's glands) lie posterolateral to the membranous urethra. These glands secrete an alkaline fluid into the membranous urethra that forms a portion of the seminal fluid (Figure 7.76).

PENIS. The **penis,** the external reproductive organ, is attached to the pubic arch via suspensory ligaments. Three cylindrical masses of erectile tissue comprise the penis: two **corpora cavernosa** and the **corpus spongiosum.** The two corpora cavernosa form the upper surface, whereas the corpus spongiosum forms the undersurface and contains the greater part of the urethra. The end of the cylindrical masses forms the glans penis (Figures 7.82 through 7.84).

Key. cz central zone; **pz** peripheral zone; **rec** rectum.

Figure 7.79 Axial MR scan of prostate gland and zones. (Courtesy GE Medical Systems, Milwaukee, Wisc.)   (R1.R)

Key. pro prostate gland; **prou** prostatic urethra; **sp** spermatic cord; **sus** suspensory ligament of penis; **rec** rectum.

Figure 7.80 Axial CT scan of prostate gland.   (R1.R)

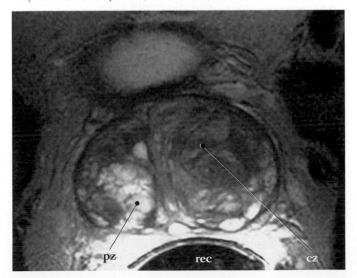

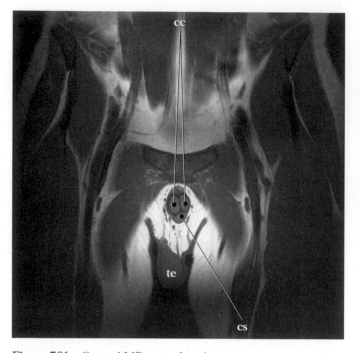

Figure 7.81   Coronal MR scan of penis.   (R2.C)

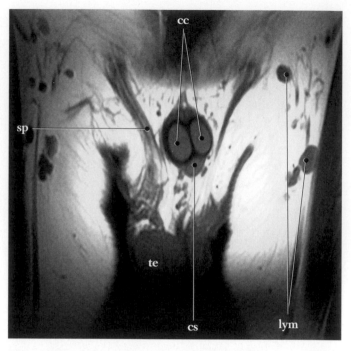

Figure 7.82   Coronal MR scan of spermatic cord.   (R2.A)

Key. **cc** corpora cavernosum; **cs** corpus spongiosum; **lym** lymph nodes; **sp** spermatic cord; **te** testes.

Key. **bulb** bulb of penis; **cc** corpora cavernosum; **gl** glans of penis; **ipub** inferior pubic ramus; **rec** rectum.

Figure 7.83   Axial MR scan of pelvis with penis.   (R1.V)

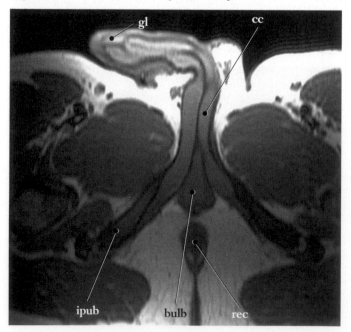

Key. **a** anus; **cc** corpora cavernosum; **cs** corpus spongiosum; **sp** spermatic cord.

Figure 7.84   Axial CT scan of pelvis with penis.   (R1.V)

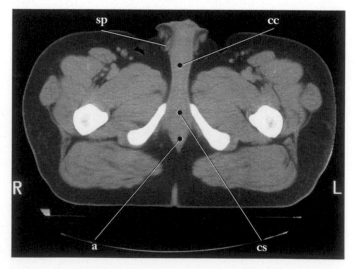

Pelvic Vasculature

The **descending aorta** bifurcates at the level of the fourth lumbar vertebra into the right and left **common iliac arteries** (Figures 7.85 through 7.89). Each common iliac artery bifurcates at the upper margin of the sacroiliac joint into the **internal** and **external iliac arteries** (Figures 7.90 and 7.91). The smaller internal iliac artery extends posteromedially into the pelvis just medial to the external iliac vein, where its numerous branches continue to supply most of the pelvic viscera. The larger external iliac artery, supplying the leg, descends along the medial border of the psoas muscle to become the **femoral artery** at approximately the level of the anterior superior iliac spine (Figures 7.92 and 7.93).

Key.   A aorta; **CIA** common iliac artery; **EIA** external iliac artery; **FA** femoral artery; **IIA** internal iliac artery; **PFA** profunda femoris artery.

Figure 7.86   MRA of the bifurcation of the abdominal aorta. (Courtesy GE Medical Systems, Milwaukee, Wisc.)

Figure 7.85   Anterior view of inferior vena cava and abdominal aorta.

Inferior vena cava

Aorta

Left common iliac artery

Left common iliac vein

Right external iliac artery

Right external iliac vein

Internal iliac artery

Femoral artery

Femoral vein

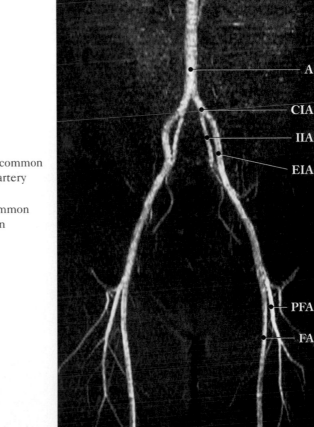

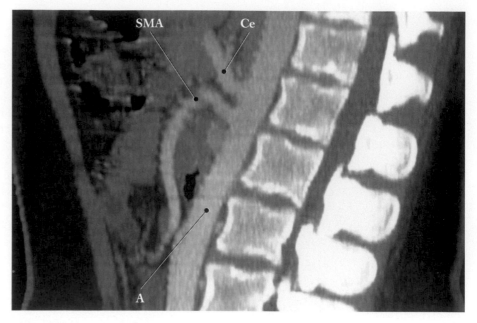

Figure 7.87   Sagittal CT reformat with abdominal aorta.   (R1.Y)

Key.   **A** aorta; **Ce** celiac axis; **SMA** superior mesenteric artery.

Key.   **CIA** right and left common iliac artery; **CIV** right and left common iliac vein;
IVC inferior vena cava; **ps** psoas muscles.

Figure 7.88   Axial MR scan of pelvis with aortic bifurcation.

(R1.A)

Figure 7.89   Axial CT scan of pelvis with aortic bifurcation.

(R1.A)

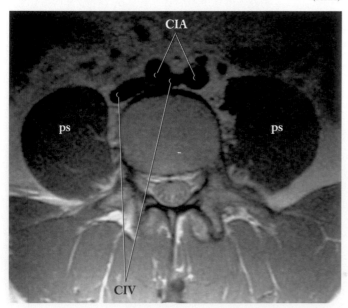

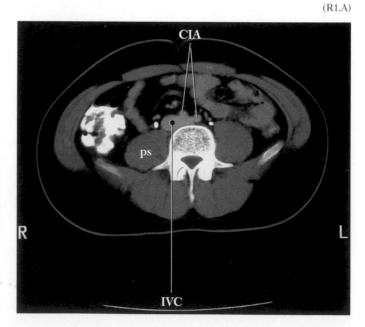

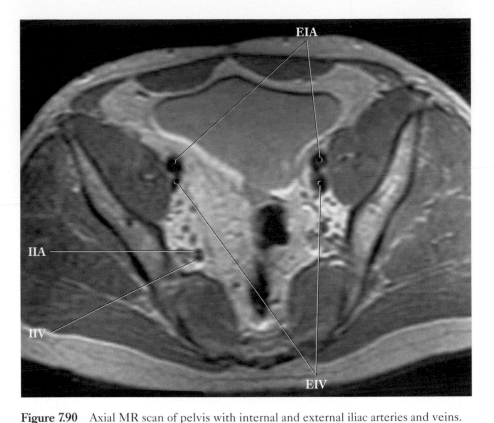

Figure 7.90   Axial MR scan of pelvis with internal and external iliac arteries and veins.

(R1.F)

The **common iliac vein** arises posterior to the common iliac artery from the junction of the **internal** and **external iliac veins** (Figures 7.94 and 7.95). The internal iliac vein ascends the pelvis medial to the internal iliac artery as it returns blood from the pelvic viscera. The external iliac veins, extensions of the femoral veins, return blood from the legs (Figures 7.92 and 7.93). Typically, both external iliac veins course medial to their respective external iliac artery and then change to a posterior position as they ascend to join the common iliac vein at approximately the level of the sacroiliac joint (Figures 7.90 and 7.91).

The **inferior vena cava** is formed at the level of L5, just a little to the right of the midline, by the union of the common iliac veins. From this level, it continues to ascend the abdomen to the right of the abdominal aorta (see Figures 7.88, 7.89, 7.94, and 7.95).

Key.   **EIA** external iliac artery; **EIV** external iliac vein; **IIA** internal iliac artery; **IIV** internal iliac vein.

Figure 7.91   Axial CT scan of pelvis with internal and external iliac arteries and veins.

(R1.D)

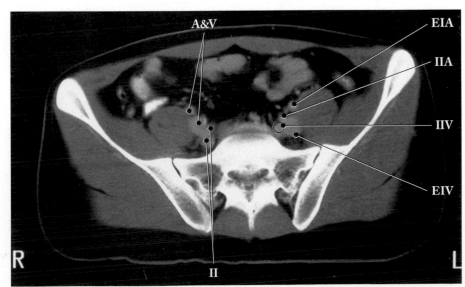

LYMPH NODES

Lymph nodes in the pelvic region are clustered around the iliac arteries, obturator internus muscle, sacrum, and inguinal ligament (see Figures 7.31, 7.32, 7.92, and 7.93).

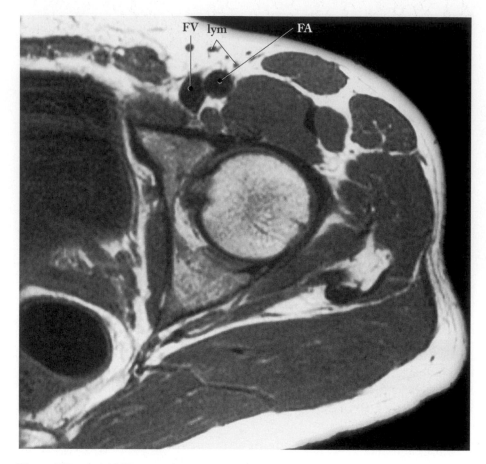

Figure 7.92 Axial MR scan of pelvis with femoral artery and vein.   (R1.P)

Key. **FA** femoral artery; **FV** femoral vein; **lym** lymph nodes.

Figure 7.93 Axial CT scan of pelvis with femoral artery and vein.   (R1.Q)

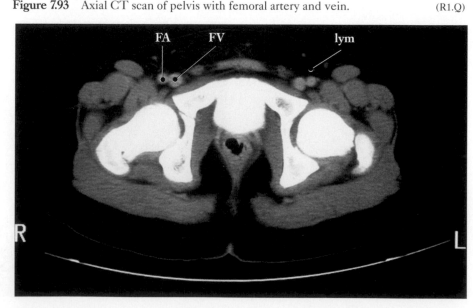

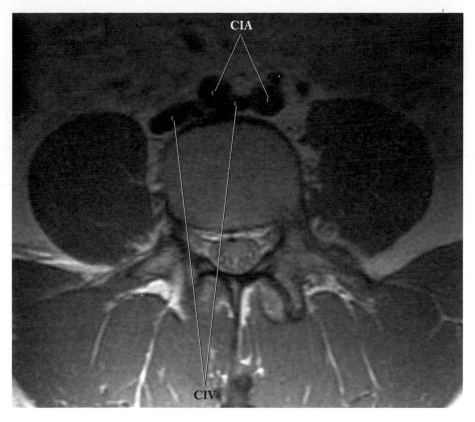

Figure 7.94   Axial MR scan of pelvis with bifurcation of inferior vena cava.   (R1.A)

Answer to Figure 7.1

A zone of avascular necrosis (AVN) involves two thirds of the weight-bearing surface of the femoral head. AVN is the death of bone caused by an interruption of arterial supply or intraosseous or extraosseous venous insufficiency. AVN has numerous causes, which include anemia, steroids, pancreatitis, trauma, and various idiopathic causes.

Key.   CIA right and left common iliac artery; **CIV** right and left common iliac vein.

Figure 7.95   Axial CT scan of pelvis with bifurcation of inferior vena cava.   (R1.B)

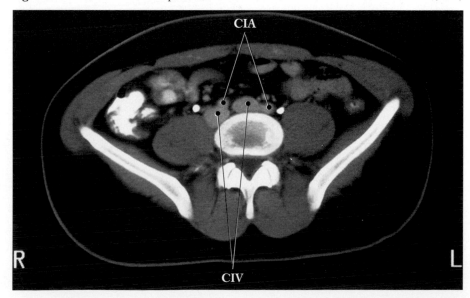

Chapter 8

1

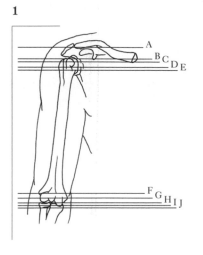

2

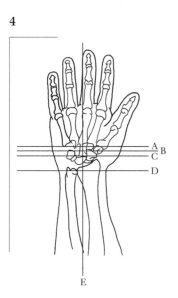

4

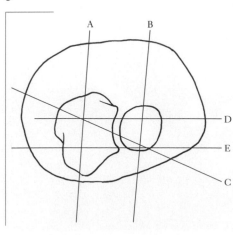

3

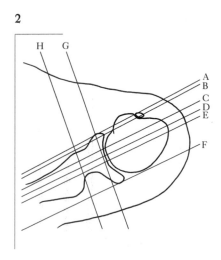

5

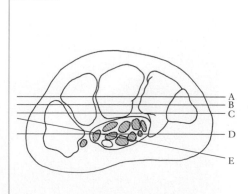

Reference illustrations

Upper Extremity Joints

It is sometimes on one's weakest limbs that one must lean in order to keep going.

Jean Rostand
Substance of Man

The intricate anatomy of the musculoskeletal system can make identification of the joint anatomy challenging. A basic knowledge of the anatomy and kinesiology of these areas increases the ability to identify pathology or injury that may occur.

Shoulder
bony anatomy
muscles and tendons
labrum and ligaments
subacromial-subdeltoid bursa

Elbow
bony anatomy
ligaments
muscles and tendons
neurovasculature

Wrist
bony anatomy
carpal tunnel
tendons
triangular fibrocartilage complex and ligaments
neurovasculature

In Figure 8.1 (an MR postarthrogram image), what structure is abnormal? (Answer on p. 261.)

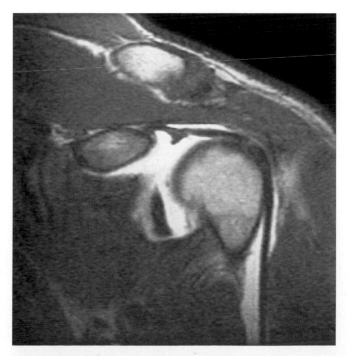

Figure 8.1   Coronal oblique MR scan of shoulder.

SHOULDER

The shoulder joint is a shallow ball-and-socket joint and is considered the most mobile joint of the body.

BONY ANATOMY

The bony anatomy that comprises the shoulder girdle is the **clavicle, scapula, and humerus** (Figures 8.2 and 8.3). Located anteriorly is the long, slender clavicle that extends transversely from the sternum to the acromion of the scapula, creating the **acromioclavicular joint.** The scapula is a triangular-shaped, flat bone that forms the posterior portion of the shoulder girdle. Four projections of the scapula provide attachment sites for the muscles and ligaments contributing to the shoulder girdle. These include the **scapular spine, acromion, coracoid process,** and **glenoid** process (Figures 8.4 through 8.6). The scapular spine arises from the upper third of the posterior surface of the scapula and extends obliquely to give rise to a flattened process termed the acromion. Located on the anterolateral surface of the scapula is a beaklike process termed the coracoid process, which arises just medial to the glenoid. The glenoid process, the largest of the projections, forms the lateral angle of the scapula and ends in a depression called the **glenoid fossa** (Figures 8.7 and 8.8). The shallow articular surface of the glenoid fossa joins with the relatively large articular surface of the humeral head to create a freely moving joint (Figures 8.9 and 8.10). Two tubercles of the humeral head, separated by the **bicipital (intertubercular) groove,** provide attachment sites for tendons and ligaments. The **lesser tubercle** is located on the anterior surface of the humeral head, whereas the **greater tubercle** is located on the lateral surface of the humeral head (Figures 8.2, 8.8 and 8.10).

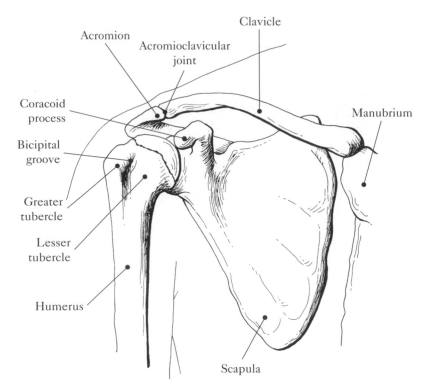

Figure 8.2   Anterior view of shoulder girdle.

Key.   ac acromion process; **cor** coracoid process; **gl** glenoid process; **h** humerus.

Figure 8.3   3D CT scan of shoulder girdle. (Courtesy Picker International, Cleveland, Ohio.)

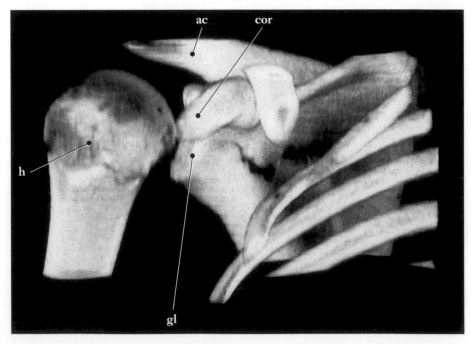

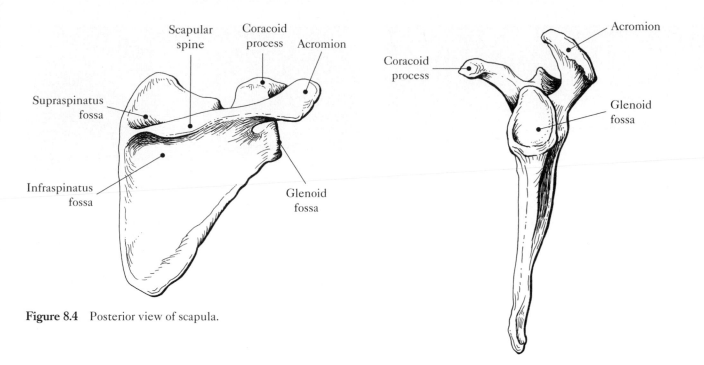

Figure 8.4   Posterior view of scapula.

Figure 8.5   Lateral view of scapula.

Key. **ac** acromion process; **cl** clavicle; **cor** coracoid process; **de** deltoid; **gl** glenoid; **inf** infraspinatus; **sc** scapula; **sub** subscapularis; **sup** supraspinatus; **tm** teres minor.

Figure 8.6   Sagittal oblique MR scan of shoulder.   (R2.G)

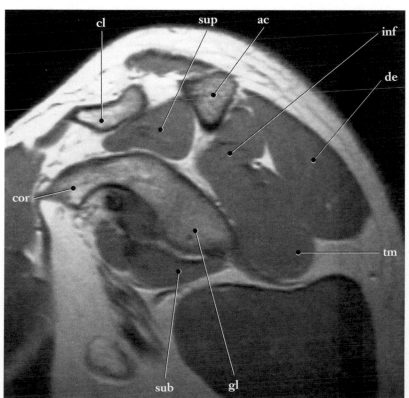

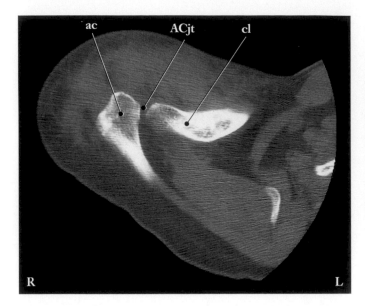

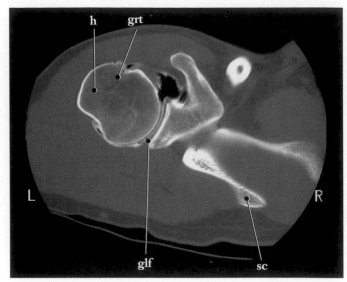

Figure 8.7   Axial CT scan of shoulder with acromioclavicular joint.   (R1.A)

Figure 8.8   Axial CT scan of shoulder, midjoint.   (R1.C)

Key.   **ac** acromion;   **ACjt** acromioclavicular joint;   **cl** clavicle;   **cor** coracoid process; **glf** glenoid fossa;   **grt** greater tubercle;   **h** humerus;   **hh** humeral head;   **sc** scapula.

Figure 8.9   Coronal oblique MR scan of acromioclavicular joint.   (R2.B)

Figure 8.10   Coronal oblique MR scan, midjoint.   (R2.D)

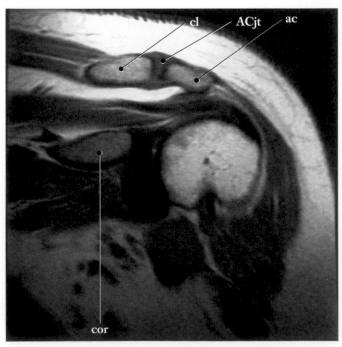

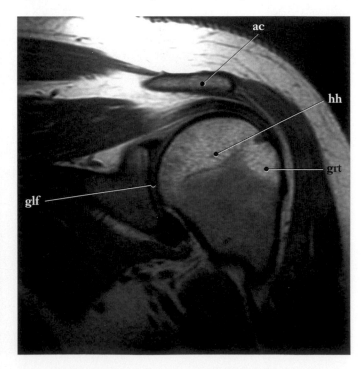

MUSCLES AND TENDONS

Numerous muscles and their tendons provide stability for the shoulder joint and movement of the upper arm. These include the **deltoid, supraspinatus, infraspinatus, teres minor,** and **subscapularis muscles** (Figures 8.11 through 8.14).

The large deltoid muscle originates on the clavicle and acromion and blankets the shoulder joint as it extends to insert on the deltoid tuberosity of the humerus. The primary function of this large muscle is to abduct the arm. The four remaining muscles closely surround the shoulder joint and comprise the **rotator cuff** (Figure 8.15). The supraspinatus, infraspinatus, and teres minor muscles are located on the posterior aspect of the scapula, and their tendons insert on the greater tubercle of the humerus (Figures 8.16 through 8.18). The most frequently injured tendon of the rotator cuff is the **supraspinatus tendon** because it extends under the acromioclavicular joint and continues over the humeral head. The subscapularis muscle is the only muscle of the rotator cuff located on the anterior surface of the scapula; its tendon inserts on the lesser tubercle of the humerus. The rotator cuff provides dynamic stability to the shoulder joint and allows for abduction and rotation of the humerus. Additional support is provided by the **biceps tendon;** it courses through the bicipital groove to insert on the glenoid labrum (Figure 8.19).

> The majority of rotator cuff lesions are a result of chronic impingement of the supraspinatus tendon against the acromial arch. The most susceptible area is approximately 1 cm from the insertion site of the supraspinatus tendon. This location is commonly referred to as the *critical zone.*

Table 8.1 Muscles of the rotator cuff

MUSCLE	ORIGIN	INSERTION	FUNCTION
Supraspinatus	Supraspinous fossa of scapula	Greater tubercle of humerus	Abduct arm
Infraspinatus	Infraspinous fossa of scapula	Greater tubercle of humerus	Rotate arm outward
Teres minor	Axillary border of scapula	Greater tubercle of humerus	Rotate arm outward
Subscapularis	Subscapular fossa of scapula	Lesser tubercle of humerus	Rotate arm medially

Figure 8.11 Anterior view of shoulder muscles.

Figure 8.12 Posterior view of shoulder muscles.

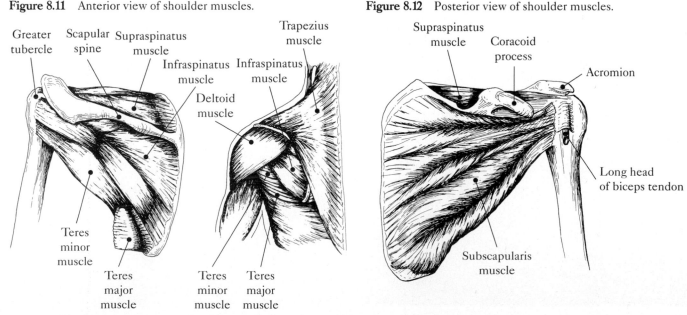

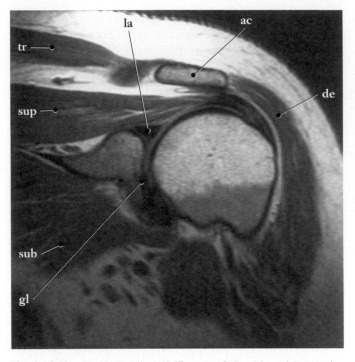

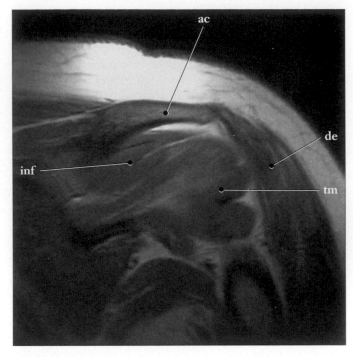

Figure 8.13   Coronal oblique MR scan of shoulder with anterior shoulder muscles.   (R2.C)

Figure 8.14   Coronal oblique MR scan of shoulder with posterior shoulder muscles.   (R2.F)

Key.   ac acromion process; **cl** clavicle; **cor** coracoid process; **de** deltoid; **gl** glenoid; **inf** infraspinatus; **la** labrum; **sub** subscapularis; **sup** supraspinatus; **tm** teres minor; **tr** trapezius.

Figure 8.15   Sagittal oblique MR scan of shoulder with rotator cuff muscles.   (R2.G)

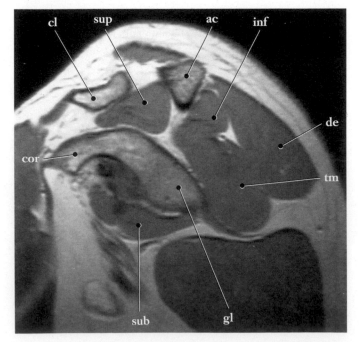

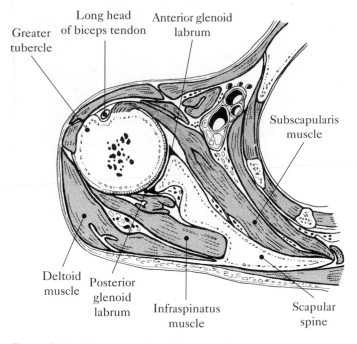

Figure 8.16   Axial view of shoulder muscles.

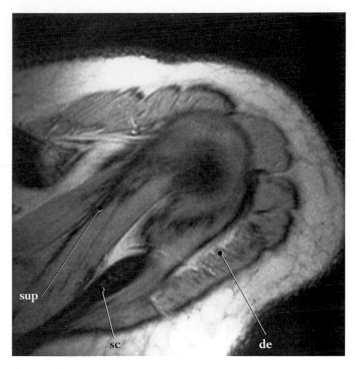

Figure 8.17   Axial MR scan of shoulder with supraspinatus muscle and tendon.   (R1.B)

Key. **bi** biceps tendon; **de** deltoid; **ghl** glenohumeral ligament; **glf** glenoid fossa; **grt** greater tubercle; **inf** infraspinatus; **la** labrum; **sc** scapular spine; **sub** subscapularis; **sup** supraspinatus.

Figure 8.18   Axial MR scan with shoulder muscles, mid-joint.   (R1.C)

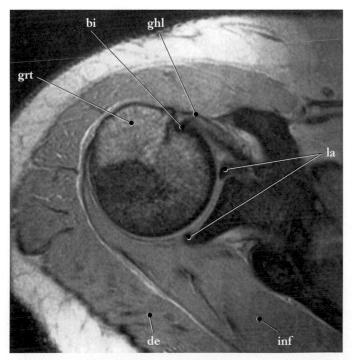

Figure 8.19   Axial CT scan with shoulder muscles.   (R1.C)

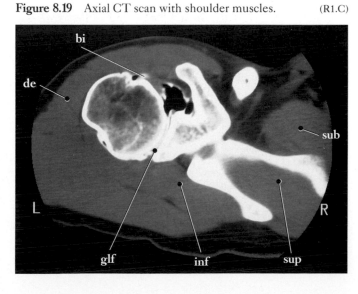

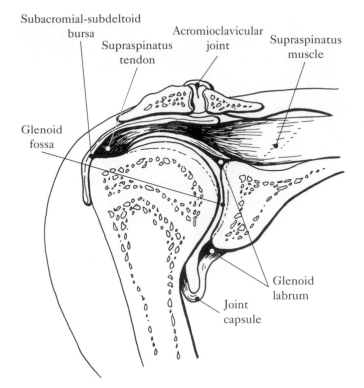

Figure 8.20 showing labels: Subacromial-subdeltoid bursa; Supraspinatus tendon; Acromioclavicular joint; Supraspinatus muscle; Glenoid fossa; Glenoid labrum; Joint capsule.

Figure 8.20 Coronal cross section of shoulder with glenoid labrum.

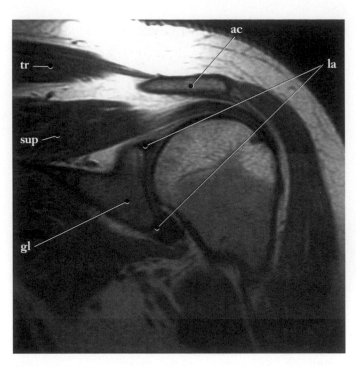

Figure 8.21 Coronal oblique MR scan of shoulder with glenoid labrum. (R2.D)

Key. **ac** acromion process; **gl** glenoid; **la** labrum; **sup** supraspinatus; **tr** trapezius.

Key. **ACjt** acromioclavicular joint; **bi** biceps tendon; **cal** coracoacromial ligament; **cl** clavicle; **cor** coracoid process.

Figure 8.23 Coronal oblique MR scan of shoulder with coracoacromial ligament. (R2.A)

Figure 8.22 Anterior view of shoulder ligaments.

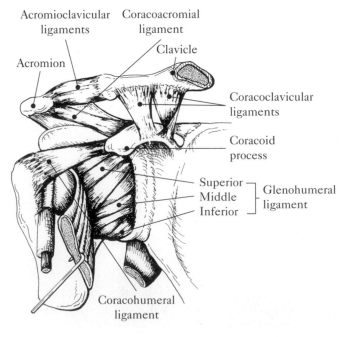

Figure 8.22 showing labels: Acromioclavicular ligaments; Coracoacromial ligament; Acromion; Clavicle; Coracoclavicular ligaments; Coracoid process; Superior / Middle / Inferior Glenohumeral ligament; Coracohumeral ligament.

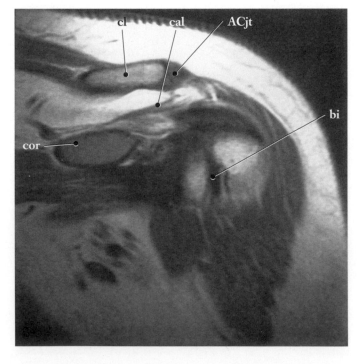

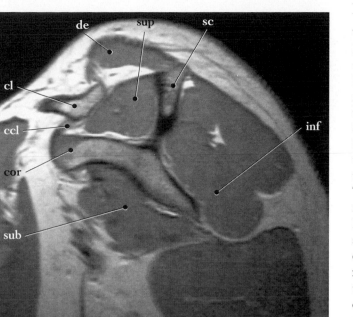

Figure 8.24 Sagittal oblique MR scan of shoulder with coraco-clavicular ligament. (R2.H)

Key. **ccl** coracoclavicular ligament; **cl** clavicle; **cor** coracoid process; **de** deltoid; **inf** infraspinatus; **sc** scapular spine; **sub** subscapularis; **sup** supraspinatus.

LABRUM AND LIGAMENTS

The edge of the glenoid fossa is surrounded by a fibrocartilaginous ring termed the **glenoid labrum,** which deepens the articular surface (Figures 8.20 and 8.21). Three fibrous bands, the **glenohumeral ligaments,** contribute to the formation of the glenoid labrum and extend anteriorly from the lesser tubercle to the glenoid labrum (Figures 8.18 and 8.22). Another structure contributing to the glenoid labrum is the long head of the biceps tendon, which courses through the bicipital groove of the humerus to blend with the superior aspect of the glenoid labrum (Figure 8.23). The **coracoacromial ligament** is another important ligament located on the anterior portion of the shoulder. As this ligament joins the coracoid process and acromion, it forms a strong bridge that protects the humeral head and rotator cuff tendons from direct trauma. The **coracoclavicular ligament** helps to maintain the position of the clavicle, in relation to the acromion, by spanning the distance between the clavicle and coracoid process of the scapula (Figures 8.23 through 8.26).

Figure 8.25 Axial MR scan of shoulder with glenohumeral ligaments. (R1.C)

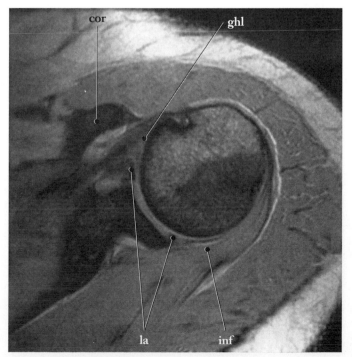

Key. **bi** biceps tendon; **cor** coracoid process; **ghl** glenohumeral ligament; **gl** glenoid; **inf** infraspinatus; **la** labrum.

Figure 8.26 Axial CT scan of shoulder with glenohumeral ligaments and glenoid labrum. (R1.D)

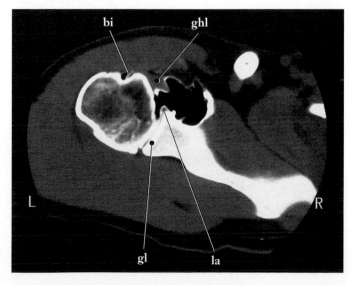

SUBACROMIAL-SUBDELTOID BURSA

The tendons and ligaments of the shoulder joint are cushioned by bursae. The **subacromial-subdeltoid bursa** is the main bursa of the shoulder and the largest bursa within the body (Figure 8.27). Beginning at the coracoid process, the bursa extends laterally just inferior to the acromion and continues beneath the deltoid muscle to the greater tubercle of the humerus (Figures 8.28 and 8.29).

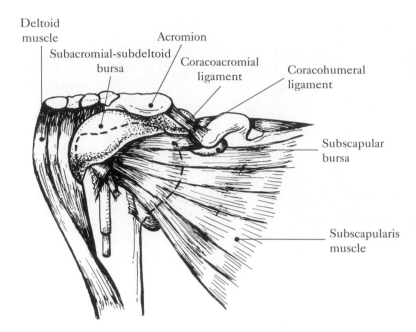

Figure 8.27   Anterior view of shoulder with subacromial-subdeltoid bursa.

Key. ac acromion process; **de** deltoid; **SASD** subacromial-subdeltoid bursa; **sup** supraspinatus tendon.

Figure 8.28   Coronal oblique MR scan of shoulder with subacromial-subdeltoid bursa.   (R2.E)

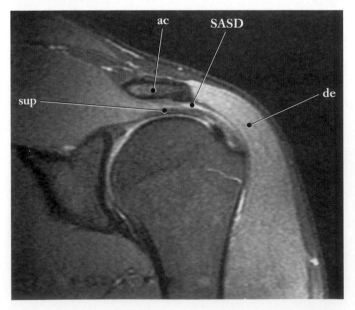

Key.   gl glenoid; **SASD** subacromial-subdeltoid bursa.

Figure 8.29   Axial CT scan of shoulder with subacromial-subdeltoid bursa.   (R1.E)

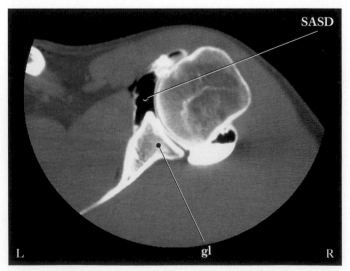

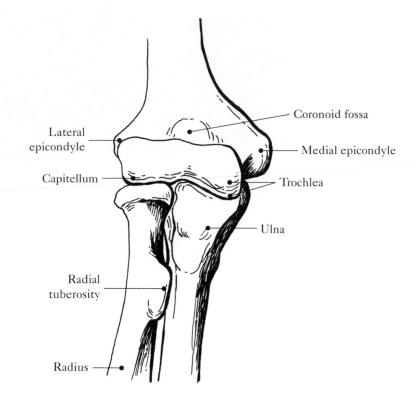

Lateral epicondyle
Coronoid fossa
Capitellum
Medial epicondyle
Trochlea
Ulna
Radial tuberosity
Radius

Figure 8.30   Anterior view of elbow joint.

Figure 8.31   Lateral view of elbow joint.

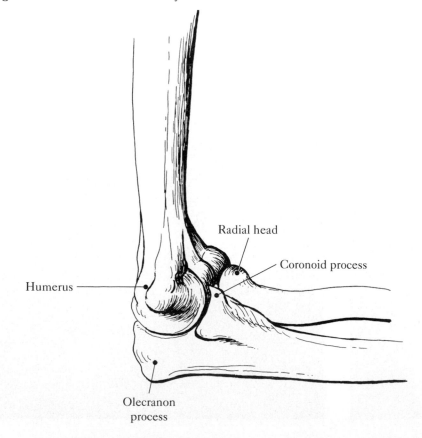

Radial head
Coronoid process
Humerus
Olecranon process

ELBOW

The elbow is a complex hinge-pivot joint created by the articulations of the **humerus, radius,** and **ulna** (Figures 8.30 and 8.31). The radius and ulna are the bones of the forearm, with the radius located on the lateral side. The **radioulnar** and **radiohumeral articulations** create the pivot joint that aids in supination and pronation of the elbow. The radiohumeral and **ulnohumeral articulations** form the hinge joint that allows for flexion and extension.

Bony anatomy

The distal portion of the humerus has two distinct prominences termed the **medial** and **lateral condyles**, with associated **epicondyles**, that provide attachment sites for tendons and ligaments (Figure 8.32). Two depressions located on the distal humerus are the anterior **coronoid fossa** and the deep posterior **olecranon fossa**. These depressions accommodate the **coronoid** and **olecranon processes** of the proximal ulna (Figure 8.33). The **capitellum** and **trochlea** are two articular surfaces of the distal humerus. The capitellum articulates with the **radial head,** whereas the trochlea articulates with the proximal ulna at the **trochlear notch.** The flattened radial head also articulates with the ulna at the **radial notch.** The radial head is cylindrical, which allows for smooth pivotal motions on pronation and supination of the forearm. Just distal to the radial head, on the medial side of the radius, is a roughened process termed the **radial tuberosity,** which is a site for tendon insertion (Figure 8.34).

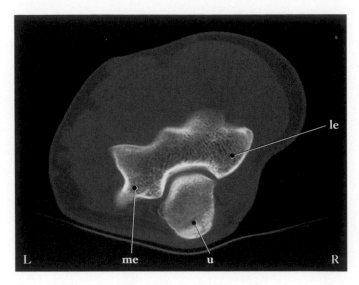

Figure 8.32   Axial CT scan of elbow joint.   (R1.G)

Key. **cap** capitellum; **corn** coronoid process; **h** humerus; **le** lateral epicondyle; **me** medial epicondyle; **of** olecranon fossa; **ol** olecranon; **r** radius; **rh** radial head; **rn** radial notch; **rt** radial tuberosity; **tro** trochlea; **u** ulna.

Figure 8.34   Coronal oblique MR scan of elbow with humerus, radius, and ulna.   (R3.E)

Figure 8.33   Sagittal CT reformat of elbow joint.   (R3.C)

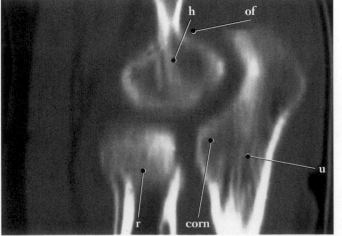

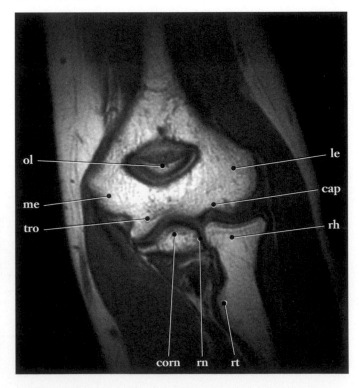

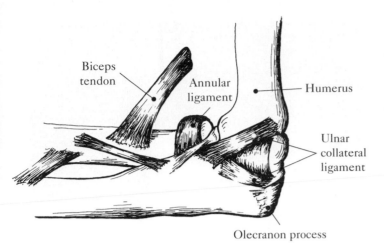

Figure 8.35   Medial view of elbow with ligaments.

LIGAMENTS

The stability of the elbow joint primarily depends on the collateral ligaments. The **ulnar collateral ligament,** reinforcing the medial side, originates on the medial epicondyle of the humerus, and inserts on the coronoid and olecranon processes (Figure 8.35). Reinforcing the lateral side is the **radial collateral ligament,** which arises from the lateral epicondyle of the humerus and attaches on the annular ligament (Figures 8.36 and 8.37). The **annular ligament** forms a partial ring around the radial head to bind it to the radial notch of the ulna (Figures 8.38 and 8.39).

Key. **h** humerus; **lcol** lateral collateral ligament; **mcol** medial collateral ligament; **rh** radial head.

Figure 8.37   Coronal MR scan of elbow with collateral ligaments.
(R3.D)

Figure 8.36   Lateral view of elbow with ligaments.

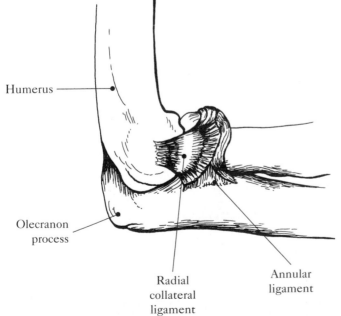

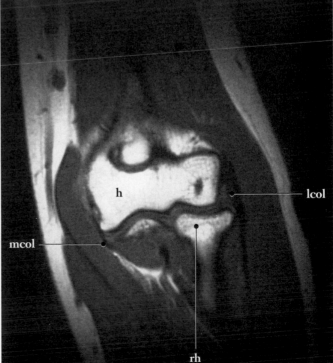

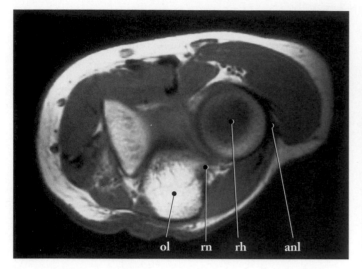

Figure 8.38 Axial MR scan of elbow with annular ligament. (R1.I)

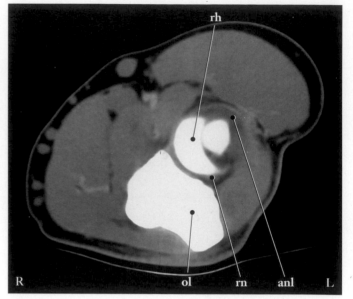

Figure 8.39 Axial CT scan of elbow with annular ligament. (R1.J)

Key. **anl** annular ligament; **ol** olecranon process; **rh** radial head; **rn** radial notch.

Figure 8.40 Anterior surface of elbow with musculature.

Figure 8.41 Posterior surface of elbow with musculature.

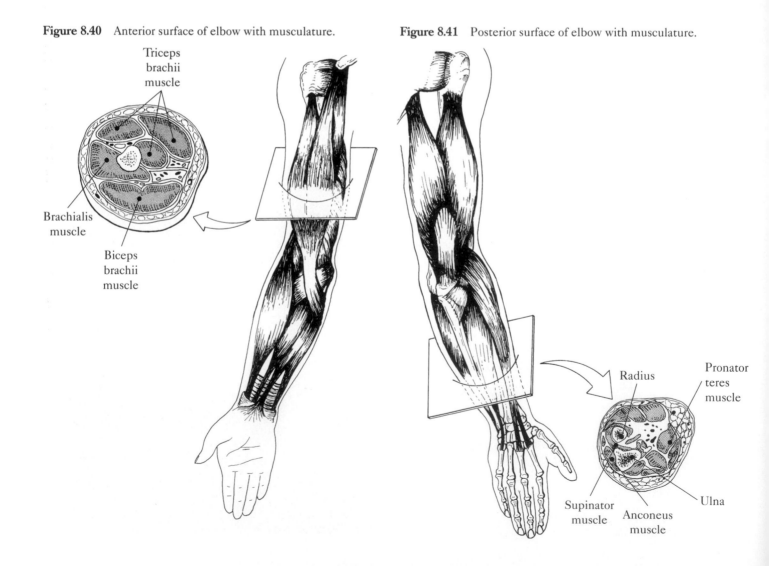

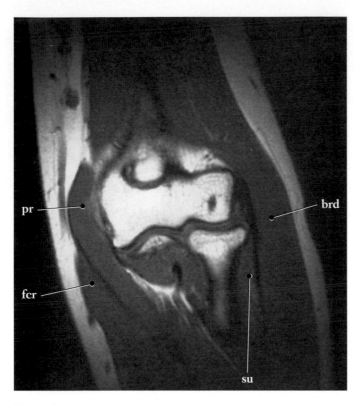

Figure 8.42 Coronal MR scan of elbow with musculature.   (R3.D)

MUSCLES AND TENDONS

Numerous muscles and tendons originate and insert at the elbow. The muscles can be divided into four muscle groups according to their location (Figures 8.40 through 8.44).

Key. **bi** biceps; **br** brachialis; **brd** brachioradialis; **cap** capitellum; **corn** coronoid process; **fcr** flexor carpi radialis; **ol** olecranon; **pr** pronator teres; **rh** radial head; **su** supinator; **tr** triceps; **tro** trochlea.

Figure 8.43 Sagittal MR scan of elbow with lateral muscle group.   (R3.B)

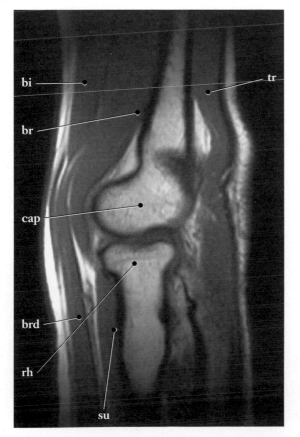

Figure 8.44 Sagittal MR scan of elbow with medial muscle group.   (R3.A)

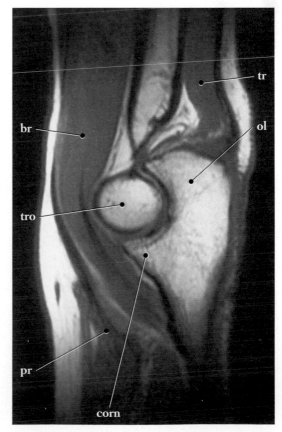

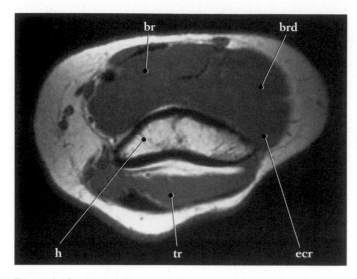

Figure 8.45   Axial MR scan of elbow with anterior muscle groups.   (R1.F)

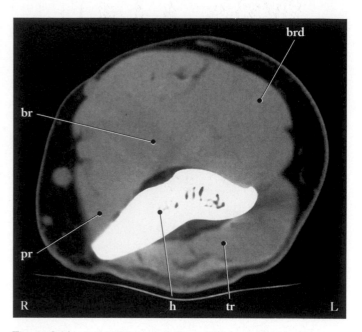

Figure 8.46   Axial CT scan of elbow with anterior muscle groups.   (R1.F)

Key. **an** anconeus; **br** brachialis; **brd** brachioradialis; **ecr** extensor carpi radialis; **h** humerus; **le** lateral epicondyle; **me** medial epicondyle; **pr** pronator teres; **tr** triceps; **u** ulna.

Figure 8.48   Axial CT scan of elbow with posterior muscle groups.   (R1.H)

Figure 8.47   Axial MR scan of elbow with posterior muscle groups.   (R1.G)

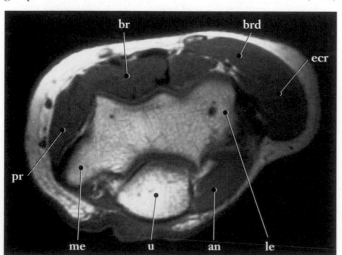

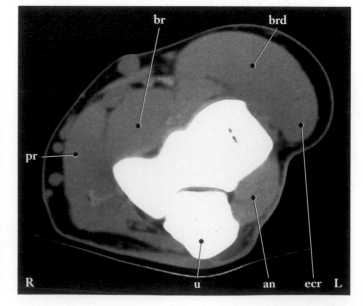

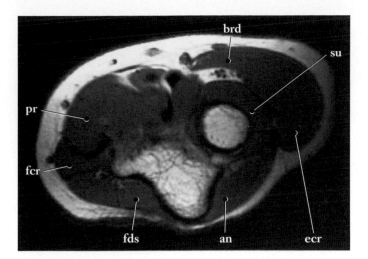

Figure 8.49   Axial MR scan of elbow with lateral and medial muscle groups.   (R1.J)

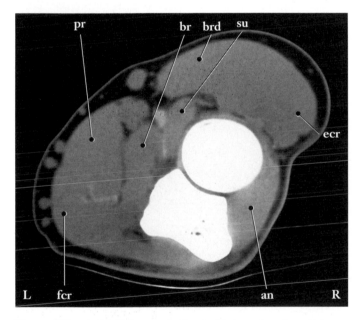

Figure 8.50   Axial CT scan of elbow with lateral and medial muscle groups.   (R1.J)

Key. **an** anconeus; **br** brachialis; **brd** brachioradialis; **ecr** extensor carpi radialis; **fcr** flexor carpi radialis; **fds** flexor digitorum superficialis; **pr** pronator teres; **su** supinator.

ANTERIOR GROUP.   The anterior muscle group consists of the **biceps brachii** and **brachialis muscles** (Figures 8.43, 8.45 and 8.46). The biceps brachii muscle originates from two separate tendons: the short head originates from the coracoid process of the scapula and the long head originates at the superior glenoid labrum. The biceps brachii muscle inserts on the radial tuberosity and flexes and supinates the forearm. The brachialis muscle originates from the anterior surface of the distal humerus and inserts on a roughened area of the proximal and anterior surface of the ulna termed the ulnar tuberosity. The brachialis muscle also flexes the forearm.

POSTERIOR GROUP.   The **triceps brachii** and **anconeus muscles** form the posterior muscle group. The triceps brachii muscle acts as the main extensor of the forearm. It originates from three separate sites about the shoulder joint and inserts on the olecranon process of the ulna. The small, triangular anconeus muscle works to pronate the ulna. It originates on the lateral epicondyle and crosses obliquely to insert on the lateral margin of the olecranon process (Figures 8.45 through 8.48).

LATERAL GROUP.   The lateral group includes the **brachioradialis muscle, extensor muscles** of the fingers and wrist, and **supinator muscle** (Figures 8.43, 8.49 and 8.50). The brachioradialis muscle is the most superficial of the lateral muscle group. This large muscle originates at the lateral epicondyle and inserts on the styloid process of the radius to function as a flexor of the forearm. Posterior and deep to the brachioradialis muscle are the extensor muscles, which include several individual muscles but at the level of the elbow have the appearance of a single structure. The extensor muscles primarily originate at the lateral epicondyle of the humerus and insert at various locations of the hand. The deepest of the lateral muscle group is the supinator muscle, which also originates at the lateral epicondyle of the humerus and inserts just distal to the radial tuberosity.

MEDIAL GROUP.   The **pronator teres** and **flexor muscles** of the fingers and wrist form the medial muscle group of the elbow (Figures 8.44, 8.49 and 8.50). The pronator teres muscle is the most superficial muscle of the medial muscle group. It originates from the medial epicondyle of the humerus and courses obliquely to insert on the lateral surface of the midradius (Figure 8.42). The flexor muscles originate from the medial epicondyle of the humerus and insert on various places about the hand. The flexor muscles, just as the extensor muscles in the lateral group, are visualized as a singular structure in the elbow and appear separate in the forearm.

NEUROVASCULATURE

The major neurovascular structures of the elbow include the **brachial, radial,** and **ulnar arteries; basilic, cephalic,** and **median cubital veins;** and **ulnar nerve** (Figures 8.51 and 8.52). The brachial artery is an extension of the axillary artery, which descends along the anterior aspect of the arm. In its distal segment it courses medial to the biceps brachii muscle and bifurcates into the radial and ulnar arteries at the cubital fossa on the anterior surface of the elbow. The basilic and cephalic veins are tributaries of the axillary vein, with the basilic vein coursing on the medial side of the arm and the cephalic vein coursing on the lateral side. Creating an anastomosis between these two veins is the median cubital vein, which is a common site for venipuncture.

Located between the medial epicondyle of the humerus and the olecranon process is the ulnar nerve (Figures 8.53 through and 8.56).

> Because of its superficial location, the ulnar nerve is the most frequently injured nerve of the body.

Figure 8.52   Anterior view of veins in elbow region.

Figure 8.51   Anterior view of elbow with neurovasculature.

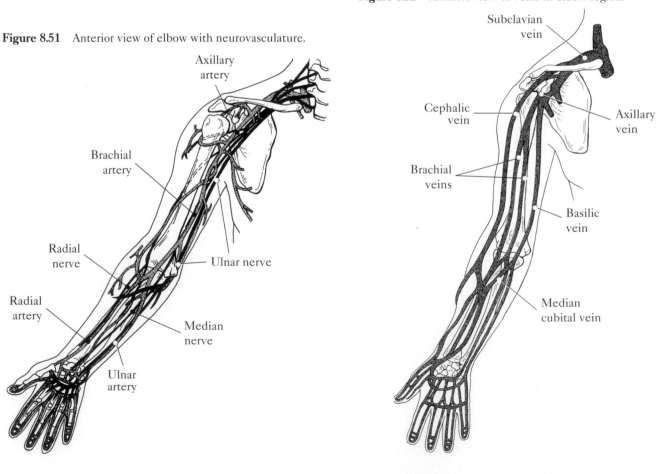

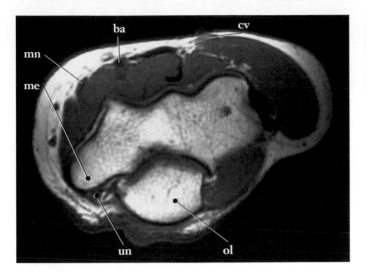

Figure 8.53   Axial MR scan of elbow with ulnar nerve.   (R1.G)

Key. ba brachial artery; **cv** cephalic vein; **me** medial epicondyle; **mn** median nerve; **ol** olecranon process; **un** ulnar nerve.

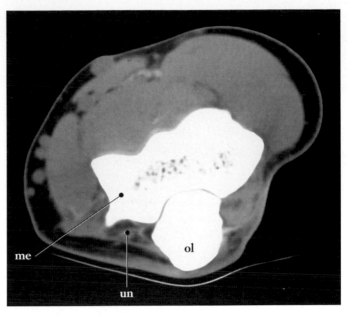

Figure 8.54   Axial CT scan of elbow with ulnar nerve.   (R1.G)

Key. me medial epicondyle; **ol** olecranon process; **un** ulnar nerve.

Key. an anconeus; **br** brachialis; **brd** brachioradialis; **cv** cephalic vein; **ecr** extensor carpi radialis; **fcr** flexor carpi radialis; **pr** pronator teres; **ra** radial artery; **su** supinator.

Figure 8.56   Axial CT scan of elbow with neurovasculature of elbow.   (R1.J)

Key. ba brachial artery; **cv** cephalic vein; **mn** median nerve; **ra** radial artery; **rn** radial nerve; **un** ulnar nerve.

Figure 8.55   Axial MR scan of elbow with neurovasculature of elbow.   (R1.J)

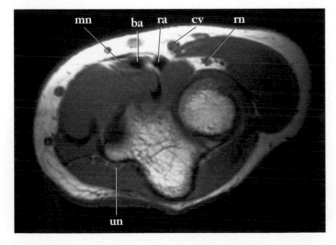

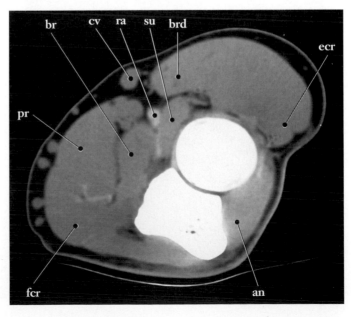

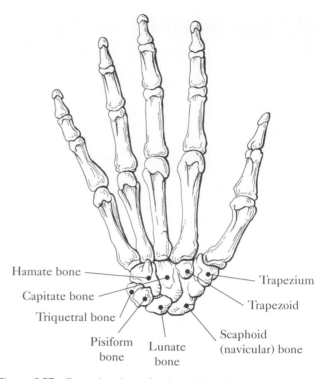

Figure 8.57   Posterior view of wrist and hand.

Key.   **c** capitate; **h** hamate; **l** lunate; **r** radius; **s** scaphoid; **t** triquetrum; **u** ulna.

Figure 8.58   Coronal CT reformat of wrist.   (R5.A)

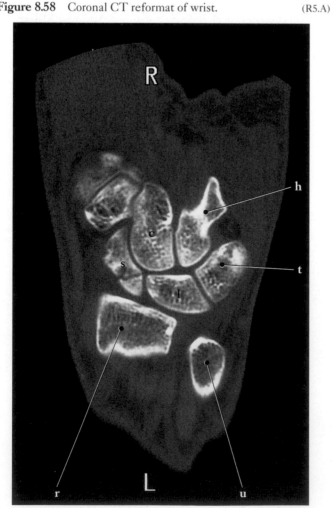

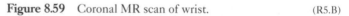

Key.   **c** capitate; **h** hamate; **l** lunate; **r** radius; **s** scaphoid; **t** triquetrum; **u** ulna.

Figure 8.59   Coronal MR scan of wrist.   (R5.B)

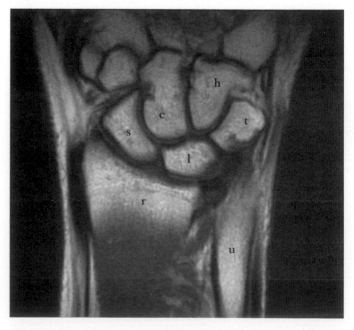

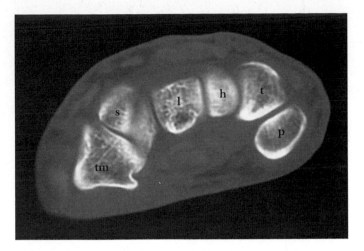

Figure 8.60   Axial CT scan of wrist with proximal row of carpal bones.   (R4.C)

Key.   **h** hamate; **l** lunate; **p** pisiform; **s** scaphoid; **t** triquetrum; **tm** trapezium.

WRIST

The complex anatomy of the wrist provides for a multitude of movements unmatched by any other joint of the body.

BONY ANATOMY

The bony anatomy of the wrist consists of the distal radius and ulna and eight **carpal bones** (Figures 8.57 through 8.59). Both the distal radius and ulna have a conical-shaped styloid process that acts as an attachment site. The **radial styloid process** is located on the lateral surface of the radius, whereas the **ulnar styloid process** is located on the posteromedial side of the ulna. The carpal bones are arranged in proximal and distal rows. Located in the proximal row of carpal bones are the **scaphoid (navicular), lunate, triquetral,** and **pisiform bones** (Figure 8.60). The distal row consists of the **trapezium, trapezoid, capitate,** and **hamate bones** (Figure 8.61).

Key.   **c** capitate; **h** hamate; **td** trapezoid; **1st me** metacarpal.

Figure 8.61   Axial CT scan of wrist with distal row of carpal bones.   (R4.A)

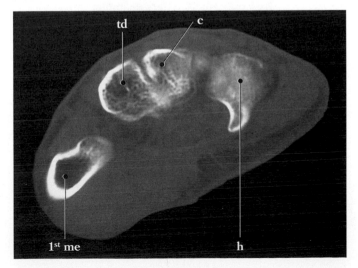

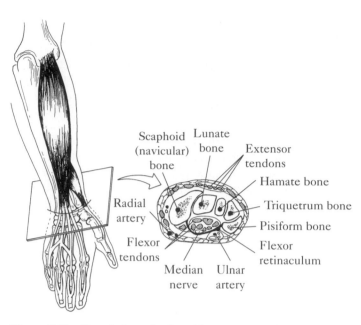

Figure 8.62   Dorsal view of wrist with extensor tendons.

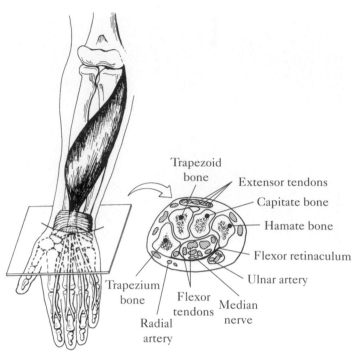

Figure 8.63   Palmar view of wrist with superficial flexor tendons and flexor retinaculum.

Key.   1st me first metacarpal; **fl** flexors; **p** pisiform; **s** scaphoid; **tm** trapezium.

Figure 8.64   Coronal MR scan of wrist with flexor tendons.   (R5.D)

Key.   c capitate; **ex** extensor tendons; **fl** flexors; **l** lunate; **r** radius.

Figure 8.65   Sagittal MR scan of wrist with flexor and extensor tendons.   (R4.E)

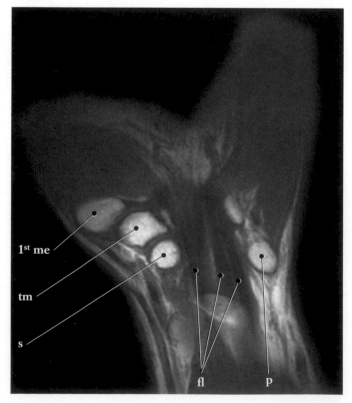

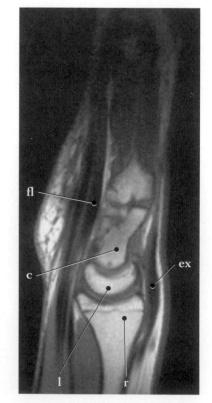

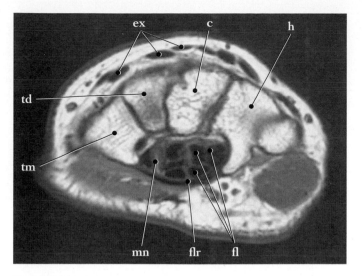

Figure 8.66   Axial MR scan of wrist with flexor and extensor tendons and median nerve.

(R4.B)

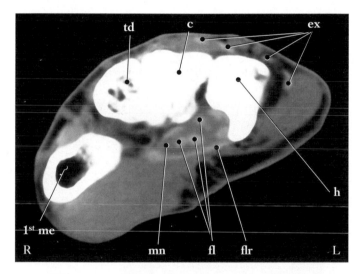

Figure 8.67   Axial CT scan of wrist with flexor and extensor tendons and median nerve.

(R4.A)

Key. **c** capitate; **ex** extensor tendons; **fl** flexor tendons; **flr** flexor retinaculum; **h** hamate; **mn** median nerve; **td** trapezoid; **tm** trapezium; **1st** first metacarpal.

CARPAL TUNNEL

The **carpal tunnel** is created by the concave arrangement of the carpal bones. A ligamentous structure known as the **flexor retinaculum** inserts medially on the pisiform bone and hook of the hamate bone and spans across the wrist to insert laterally on the scaphoid bone and trapezium bone (Figures 8.62 through 8.65). This anatomical arrangement creates an enclosure across the carpal tunnel for the passage of tendons and the **median nerve** (Figures 8.66 and 8.67).

Compression of the median nerve as it passes through the carpal tunnel is called *carpal tunnel syndrome.* Symptoms include pain and numbness of the fingers supplied by the median nerve.

TENDONS

The numerous muscles of the forearm become tendinous just before the wrist joint. The many tendons located in the wrist can be divided into palmar and dorsal tendon groups (Figure 8.62 and 8.63). The **palmar tendon group** collectively flexes the fingers and wrist. As this group courses through the carpal tunnel, the tendons appear to be arranged in two discrete rows (see Figures 8.64 and 8.65). The tendons of the **dorsal tendon group,** spanning the superficial surface of the wrist, are considered the extensors of the fingers and wrist (Figures 8.66 and 8.67).

TRIANGULAR FIBROCARTILAGE COMPLEX AND LIGAMENTS

The **triangular fibrocartilage complex,** also known as the articular disk, is the major stabilizing element of the distal radioulnar joint. This fan-shaped band of fibrous tissue originates on the medial surface of the distal radius and traverses horizontally to insert on the ulnar styloid process (Figure 8.68 through 8.71).

Numerous ligaments provide additional stability to the wrist. The radial and ulnar collateral ligaments support the lateral and medial sides of the wrist, respectively. The many articulations between the carpal bones are supported by the intercarpal ligaments (Figures 8.69 through 8.72).

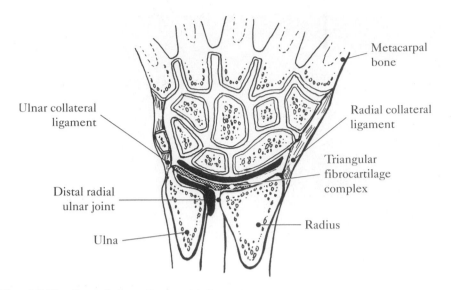

Figure 8.68   Coronal view of wrist with ligaments.

Key.   **r** radius; **TFCC** triangular fibrocartilage complex; **u** ulna.

Figure 8.70   Coronal CT scan of wrist with triangular fibrocartilage complex.   (R5.E)

Key.   **l** lunate; **r** radius; **s** scaphoid; **t** triquetrum; **TFCC** triangular fibrocartilage complex; **u** ulna.

Figure 8.69   Coronal MR scan of wrist with triangular fibrocartilage complex.   (R5.C)

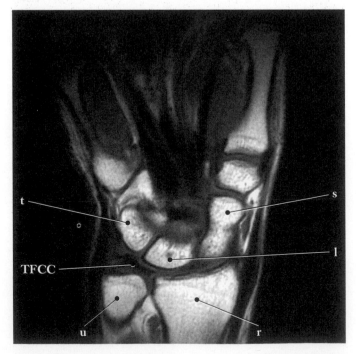

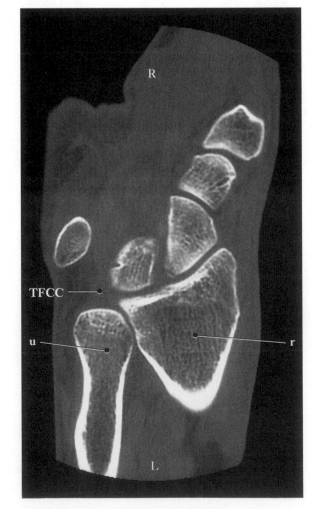

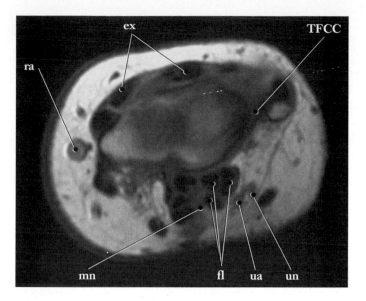

Figure 8.71   Axial MR scan of wrist with triangular fibrocartilage complex.   (R4.D)

Key.   **ex** extensor tendons; **fl** flexor tendons; **mn** median nerve; **ra** radial artery; **TFCC** triangular fibrocartilage complex; **ua** ulnar artery; **un** ulnar nerve.

NEUROVASCULATURE

The main neurovascular structures of the wrist are the **ulnar artery** and **nerve, radial artery,** and **median nerve** (Figures 8.72 and 8.73). The ulnar artery and nerve are located on the palmar medial side of the wrist, whereas the smaller radial artery is situated on the lateral aspect of the radius. The median nerve courses through the carpal tunnel, typically superficial to the flexor tendons (Figures 8.71 and 8.72).

ANSWER TO FIGURE 8.1

There is a flaplike tear of the superior half of the anterior labrum. After the administration of gadolinium and saline solution, the gap between the fragment and the residual blunted margins of the labrum is widened.

Figure 8.73   Coronal view of neurovasculature of wrist.

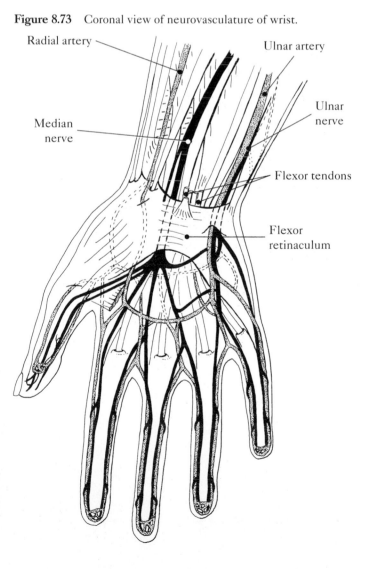

Key.   **c** capitate; **ex** extensor tendons; **fl** flexor tendons; **flr** flexor retinaculum; **h** hamate; **mn** median nerve; **td** trapezoid; **tm** trapezium; **ua** ulnar artery.

Figure 8.72   Axial MR scan with neurovasculature of wrist.   (R4.B)

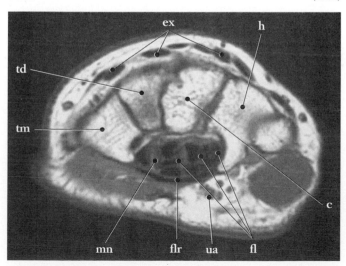

Chapter 9

1

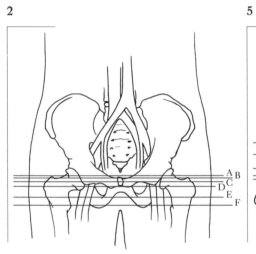

4

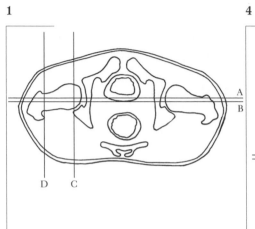

2

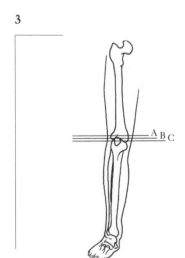

5

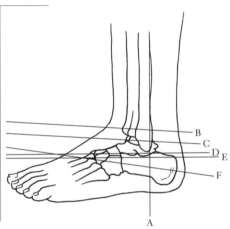

3

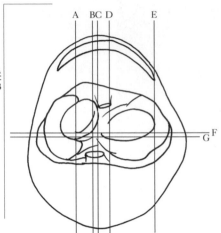

6

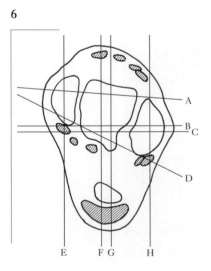

Reference illustrations

Lower Extremity Joints

"And well observe Hippocrates old rule, the only medicine

for the foote is rest."

Thomas Nash (1567-1601)
Summers Last Will and Testament

The complex anatomy of the lower extremity joints is responsible for bearing the entire upper body weight and for accommodating the demands of movement placed on this system.

Hip
bony anatomy
labrum and ligaments
muscle groups
neurovasculature

Knee
bony anatomy
menisci and ligaments
muscles
vasculature

Ankle
bony anatomy
ligaments
tendons

In Figure 9.1, what structure is abnormal? (Answer on p. 287.)

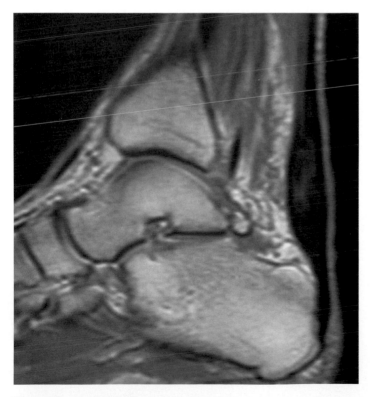

Figure 9.1 Sagittal MR scan of ankle.

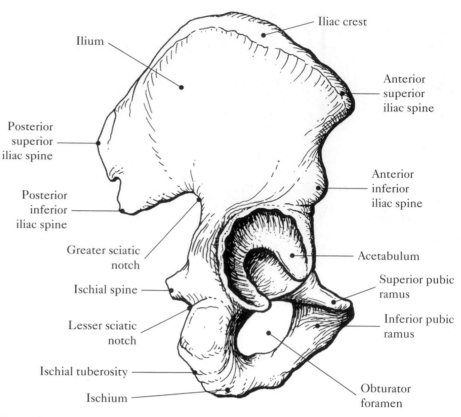

Ilium

Iliac crest

Anterior superior iliac spine

Posterior superior iliac spine

Anterior inferior iliac spine

Posterior inferior iliac spine

Greater sciatic notch

Acetabulum

Ischial spine

Superior pubic ramus

Lesser sciatic notch

Inferior pubic ramus

Ischial tuberosity

Ischium

Obturator foramen

Figure 9.2 Lateral view of acetabulum.

Figure 9.3 Posterior view of proximal femur.

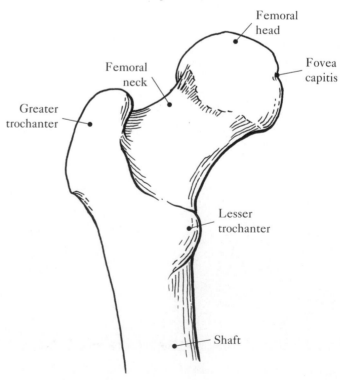

Femoral head

Femoral neck

Fovea capitis

Greater trochanter

Lesser trochanter

Shaft

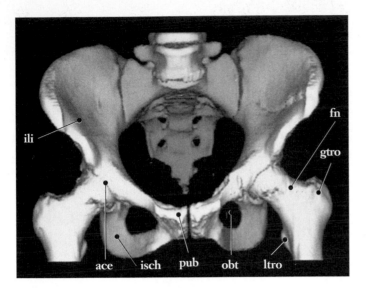

Figure 9.4   3D CT scan of bilateral hips.

Key. **ace** acetabulum; **fn** femoral neck; **gtro** greater trochanter; **ili** ilium; **isch** ischium; **ltro** lesser trochanter; **obt** obturator foramen; **pub** pubic symphysis.

Hip

The hip provides strength to carry the weight of the body in an erect position. This ball-and-socket joint, created by the articulation of the femoral head to the acetabulum, allows for a wide range of motion.

Bony anatomy

A cuplike cavity termed the **acetabulum** is created by the three bones of the pelvis: **ilium, ischium,** and **pubis** (Figures 9.2 through 9.5). In axial cross section, this area can be divided into sections known as the **anterior** and **posterior columns.** Within the acetabulum is a centrally located, nonarticulating depression called the **acetabular fossa,** formed mainly by the ischium, which provides an attachment site for the principal ligaments of the joint. On the proximal portion of the femur is the smooth, rounded femoral head. The femoral head is covered entirely by **articular cartilage,** with the exception of a small centrally located pit termed the **fovea capitis** (Figure 9.5). The fovea capitis is a ligamentous attachment site and a route for transmission of blood vessels to the femoral head. Attaching the head to the femur is the femoral neck. The neck forms an angle with the shaft of the femur, which allows for freedom of the movement. At the distal end of the neck are two large bony prominences termed trochanters (Figures 9.3 and 9.4). The **greater trochanter** is more apparent on the lateral surface of the femoral neck. Inferior to the greater trochanter is the **lesser trochanter,** which is situated on the medial surface of the femoral neck.

Avascular necrosis (AVN) is a major concern following subcapital fractures of the femoral head. Disruption of the arterial supply to the femoral head is the most significant factor leading to AVN.

Key. **ace** acetabulum; **acol** anterior column; **af** acetabular fossa; **fh** femoral head; **fov** fovea capitis; **pcol** posterior column.

Figure 9.5   Axial CT scan of hip joint.   (R2.A)

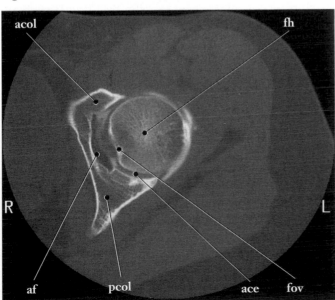

LABRUM AND LIGAMENTS

The femoral head is held to the acetabulum by several major ligaments.
The **acetabular labrum (cotyloid ligament), transverse ligament, iliofemoral ligament, ischiofemoral ligament, pubofemoral ligament,** and
ligamentum teres are addressed in
this section (Figures 9.6 and 9.7). The
acetabular labrum, or cotyloid ligament, creates a fibrocartilaginous rim
attached to the margin of the acetabulum. This labrum closely surrounds
the femoral head, aiding to hold it in
place and deepening the acetabular
fossa, which adds increased stability to
the joint. The inferior margin of the
acetabulum is incomplete and is reinforced by the transverse ligament, a
portion of the cotyloid ligament,
which spans the acetabular notch on
the inferior edge of the acetabulum
(Figure 9.8). The iliofemoral ligament
is among the strongest of the body,
with many stabilizing functions as it
spans from the anterior inferior iliac
spine and rim of the acetabulum to insert on the intertrochanteric line of
the femur (Figure 9.9). A primary
function of this ligament is to provide
a thick reinforcement to the anterior
part of the hip joint.

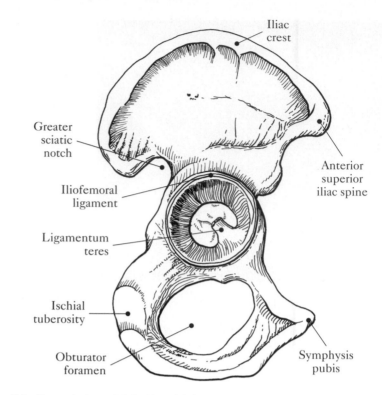

Figure 9.6 Lateral view of right hip with femur removed.

Figure 9.7 Anterior view of hip with iliofemoral ligament.

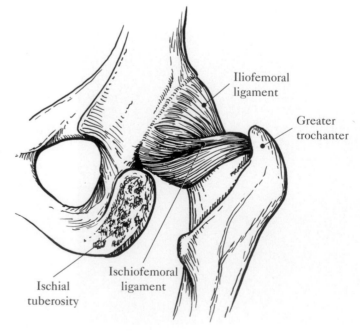

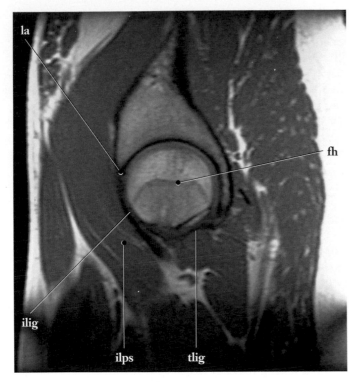

The ischiofemoral and pubofemoral ligaments, though difficult to distinguish, present a spiral configuration of femoral attachment. The ischiofemoral ligament arises from the ischium and courses in a spiral above the femoral neck to insert on the trochanteric fossa, whereas the pubofemoral ligament arises from the superior pubic ramus to radiate and insert into the iliofemoral ligament and intertrochanteric line. The spiral configuration of these two ligaments is unique to humans and ensures the stability and function in controlling the overall position of the lower limb. Extending from the acetabular fossa to the fovea capitis of the femoral head is the ligamentum teres, which can prevent further displacement when the hip is dislocated. This ligament also contains the artery to the head of the femur (Figure 9.10).

Figure 9.8   Sagittal MR scan of hip with iliofemoral ligaments.   (R1.C)

Key.   **fh** femoral head; **ilig** iliofemoral ligament; **ilps** iliopsoas; **la** labrum; **obi** obturator internus; **sar** sartorius; **sGem** superior gemellus; **tere** ligamentum teres; **TFL** tensor fascia latae; **tlig** transverse ligament.

Figure 9.9   Axial MR scan of hip with iliofemoral ligaments.   (R2.B)

Figure 9.10   Coronal MR scan of hip with iliofemoral ligaments.   (R1.A)

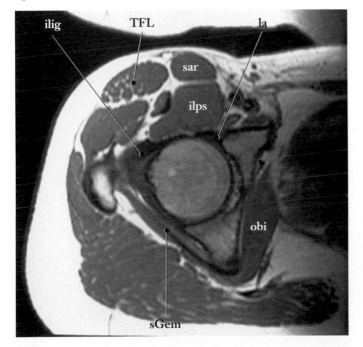

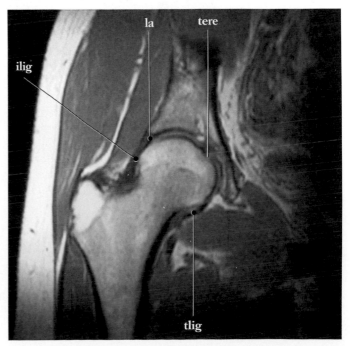

MUSCLE GROUPS

The multiple muscles identified in an examination of the hip can be understood best by dividing them into anterior, posterior, medial, and lateral muscle groups (Figures 9.11 through 9.14).

ANTERIOR MUSCLE GROUP.   Located within the anterior muscle group are the **quadriceps femoris, iliopsoas,** and **sartorius muscles.** The quadriceps femoris muscle originates as four heads (vastus lateralis, vastus medialis, vastus intermedius, rectus femoris) to create a powerful extensor that inserts on the patella. The strongest flexor of the hip is the iliopsoas muscle, which begins in the iliac fossa at the union of the psoas and iliacus muscles to insert on the lesser trochanter. The sartorius muscle is known as the longest muscle in the body; it extends from the anterior superior iliac spine to the medial surface of the tibia near the tuberosity. This muscle acts to flex and rotate the leg (Figures 9.15 through 9.18; see also Figure 9.11).

POSTERIOR MUSCLE GROUP.   The posterior muscle group includes the **obturator internus, obturator externus quadratus femoris,** and **piriformis muscles.** These muscles are known as the lateral rotators of the thigh, and they also act to stabilize the hip joint. Originating from the obturator foramen are the obturator internus muscle, which inserts on the greater trochanter, and the obturator externus muscle, which inserts on the trochanteric fossa. Two gemelli muscles form a portion of the obturator internus muscle, with the **superior gemellus muscle** originating from the ischial spine and the **inferior gemellus muscle** originating from the ischial tuberosity. The quadratus femoris muscle is a cube-shaped muscle originating on the ischial tuberosity and extending to the intertrochanteric crest. Several slips of muscle originate from the anterior sacrum and greater sciatic notch to form the pirifomis muscle, which inserts at the greater trochanter (Figures 9.19 through 9.22; see also Figures 9.13 and 9.15).

Figure 9.11   Anterior view of iliopsoas, pectineus, and sartorius muscles.

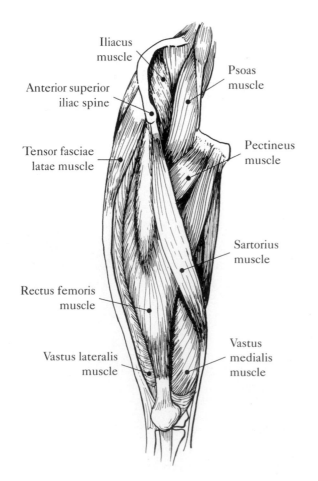

Figure 9.12   Anterior view of adductor, pectineus, and gracilis muscles.

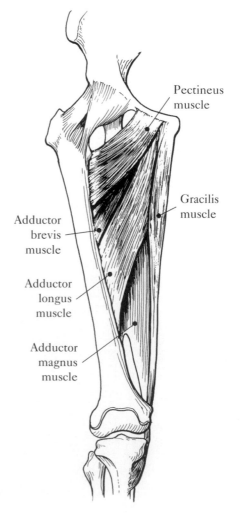

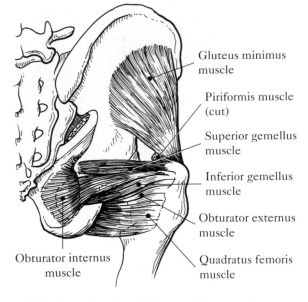

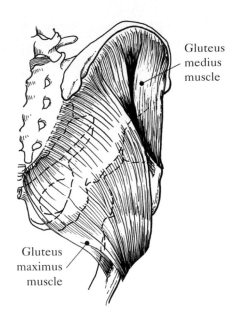

Figure 9.13 Posterior view of obturator internus, obturator externus, and piriformis muscles.

Figure 9.14 Posterior view of gluteus medius and maximus muscles.

Table 9.1 Muscles of the hip

GROUP NAME	ORIGIN	INSERTION	ACTION
ANTERIOR			
Quadriceps femoris			
Rectus femoris	Anterior inferior iliac spine	Patella	Flex hip, extend knee
Vastus intermedius	Anterolateral femur	Patella	Extend knee
Vastus medialis	Medial femur	Patella	Extend knee
Vastus lateralis	Greater trochanter	Patella	Extend knee
Iliopsoas	Iliac fossa	Lesser trochanter	Flex hip
Sartorius	Anterior superior iliac spine	Medial tibia	Flex and rotate leg
POSTERIOR			
Obturator internus	Obturator foramen	Greater trochanter	Rotate thigh laterally, stabilize hip joint
Obturator externus	Obturator foramen	Trochanteric fossa	Rotate thigh laterally, stabilize hip joint
Quadratus femoris	Ischial tuberosity	Intertrochanteric crest	Rotate thigh laterally, stabilize hip joint
Piriformis	Anterior sacrum, greater sciatic notch	Greater trochanter	Rotate thigh laterally, stabilize hip joint
MEDIAL			
Pectineus	Pubic bones	Lesser trochanter	Adduct thigh
Adductors	Pubic bone	Medial aspect of femur	Adduct thigh
Gracilis	Symphysis pubis	Medial surface of tibia	Adduct thigh
LATERAL			
Gluteus			
Maximus	Ilium, sacrum, coccyx	Distal to greater trochanter	Extend thigh
Medius	Iliac crest	Greater trochanter	Abduct and medially rotate thigh
Minimus	Ala of ilium	Greater trochanter	Abduct and medially rotate thigh
Tensor fasciae latae	Anterior superior iliac spine	Distal to greater trochanter	Abduct and medially rotate thigh

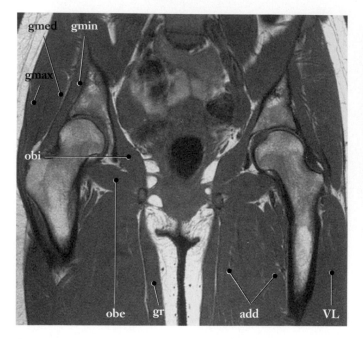

Figure 9.15 Coronal MR scan of hip with hip muscles. (R1.B)

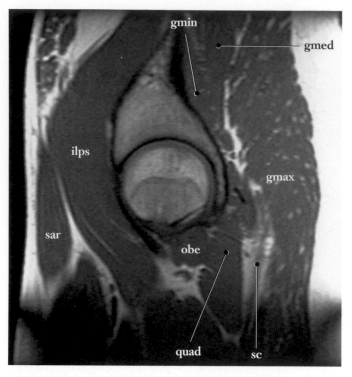

Figure 9.16 Sagittal MR scan of hip with hip muscles. (R1.C)

Key. add adductors; **gmax** gluteus maximus; **gmed** gluteus medius; **gmin** gluteus minimus; **gr** gracilis; **gtro** greater trochanter; **ilps** iliopsoas; **obe** obturator externus; **obi** obturator internus; **quad** quadratus femoris; **RF** rectus femoris; **sar** sartorius; **sc** sciatic nerve; **sGem** superior gemellus; **TFL** tensor fascia latae; **VL** vastus lateralis.

Figure 9.17 Axial MR scan of hip, midjoint with hip muscles. (R2.B)

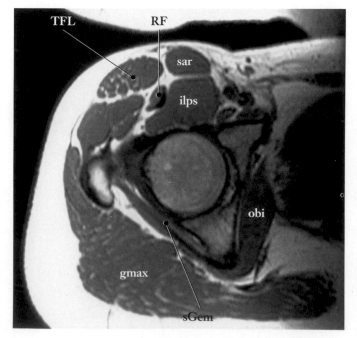

Figure 9.18 Axial CT scan of hip, midjoint with hip muscles. (R2.F)

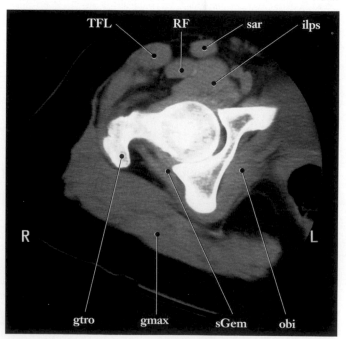

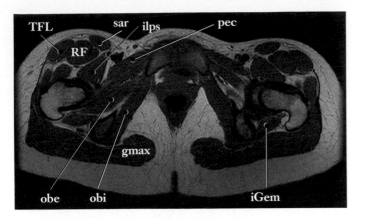

Figure 9.19   Axial MR scan of hip with pectineus muscle.   (R2.D)

MEDIAL MUSCLE GROUP. The medial muscle group consists of the **pectineus, adductor,** and **gracilis muscles** (Figures 9.12 and 9.15). The main action of this group is to adduct the thigh. The triangular-shaped pectineus muscle originates on the pubic bone and courses obliquely to insert just distal to the lesser trochanter. The adductor muscle group is composed of three muscles (adductor brevis, adductor longus, and adductor magnus) that originate at the pubic bone and fan out to insert along the length of the medial aspect of the femur. The most medial of the muscles is the gracilis muscle, which extends from the symphysis pubis to the medial surface of the tibia (see Figures 9.19 through 9.22).

Key. **br** adductor brevis; **gmax** gluteus maximus; **gmed** gluteus medius; **iGem** inferior gemellus; **ilps** iliopsoas; **lo** adductor longus; **ma** adductor magnus; **obe** obturator externus; **obi** obturator internus; **pec** pectineus; **quad** quadratus femoris; **RF** rectus femoris; **sar** sartorius; **TFL** tensor fascia latae; **VL** vastus lateralis.

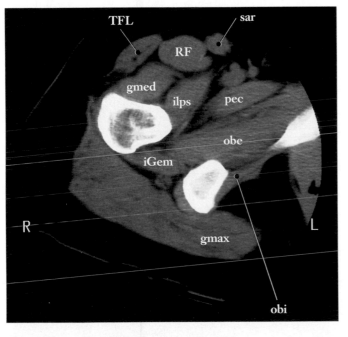

Figure 9.20   Axial CT scan of hip with pectineus muscle.   (R2.E)

Figure 9.21   Axial MR scan with adductor muscles.   (R2.F)

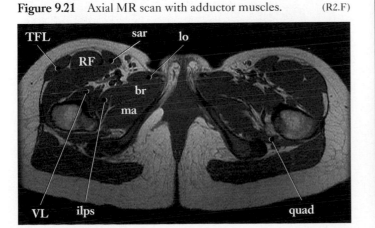

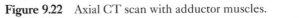

Figure 9.22   Axial CT scan with adductor muscles.   (R2.F)

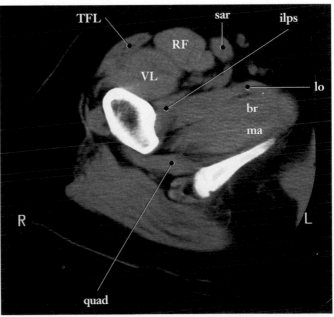

LATERAL MUSCLE GROUP.   The lateral group consists of the three **gluteus muscles (maximus, medius, and minimus muscles)** and the **tensor fasciae latae muscle.** The gluteus maximus muscle is the largest and most superficial of the gluteal muscle group, originating from the ilium, sacrum, and coccyx to insert just distal to the greater trochanter. The gluteus medius muscle originates from the iliac crest, and the gluteus minimus muscle originates from the middle of the ala; both share an insertion site at the greater trochanter. The gluteus maximus muscle acts as an extensor of the thigh, whereas the gluteus medius and minimus muscles abduct and medially rotate the thigh. The tensor fasciae latae muscle is located most lateral within the gluteal region, originating from the anterior superior iliac spine and extending distally to the greater trochanter (see Figures 9.14 through 9.18).

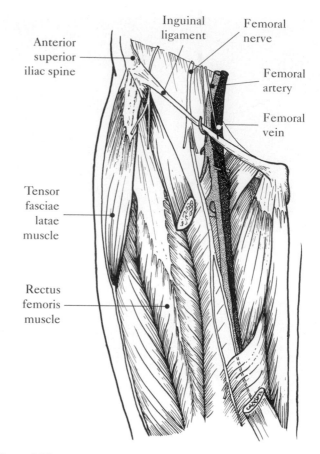

Figure 9.23   Anterior view of femoral artery and vein.   (R3.A)

Key. quad quadratus femoris; **RF** rectus femoris; **sc** sciatic nerve; **VI** vastus intermedius.

Figure 9.24   Sagittal MR scan with sciatic nerve.   (R1.D)

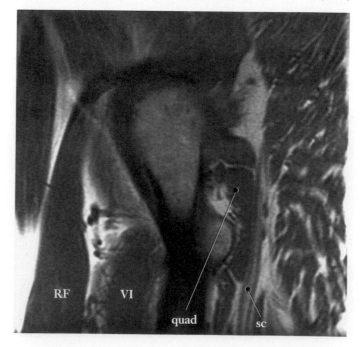

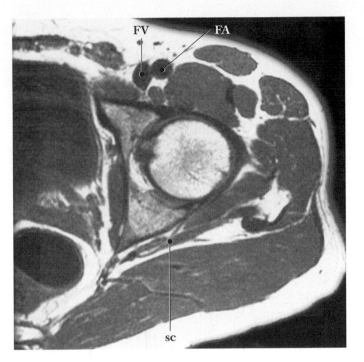

Figure 9.25   Axial MR scan of hip with neurovasculature.   (R2.B)

NEUROVASCULATURE

Several important neurovascular structures can be identified on cross-section images of the hip (Figure 9.23). The primary nerve of interest in this region is the **sciatic nerve,** which is an extension of the sacral plexus. This nerve runs deep to the gluteus maximus muscle and posterior to the obturator internus, quadratus femoris, and adductor muscles (Figure 9.24). It is the largest peripheral nerve in the body, innervating the flexor muscles of the thigh and all the muscles of the distal leg and foot. Traveling vertically along the anteromedian aspect of the hip are the **femoral artery** and **vein.** The femoral artery, an extension of the external iliac artery, is located lateral to the femoral vein. The femoral vein, a continuation of the popliteal vein, ascends to the pelvis to become the external iliac vein (Figures 9.25 and 9.26).

Key.   **FA** femoral artery; **FV** femoral vein; **sc** sciatic nerve.

Figure 9.26   Axial CT scan of hip with neurovasculature.   (R2.A)

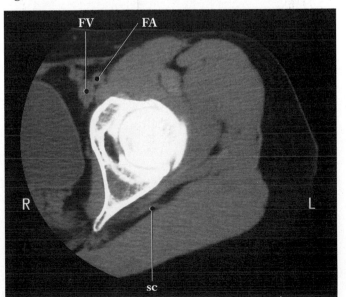

KNEE

The knee is a complex hinge joint that adapts to a variety of stresses. A supporting network of menisci, ligaments, tendons, and muscles operate together to meet the demands made on the knee.

BONY ANATOMY

The bones that contribute to the knee joint are the **femur, tibia,** and **patella** (Figure 9.27). The distal portion of the femur has two projections called the **medial** and **lateral condyles,** which articulate with the tibia at flattened surfaces termed **tibial plateaus.** The tibial plateaus are separated at the midline by the **tibial spine (intercondylar eminence),** which serves as an attachment site for ligaments, increasing the stability of the knee joint (Figure 9.28). On the anterior surface of the tibia is a roughened area called the **tibial tuberosity,** which is the insertion site for the patellar ligament (Figure 9.29). The largest sesamoid bone of the body is the patella, a flat, triangular-shaped bone, located on the anterior surface of the knee joint. It protects the anterior joint surface and functions to increase the leverage of the quadriceps extensor (Figure 9.29 and 9.30).

Cartilage covers the articular surfaces of the femur, tibia, and patella and helps to provide smooth movement within the knee joint (Figure 9.29).

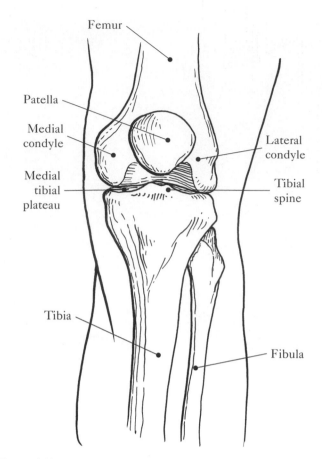

Figure 9.27   Anterior view of knee joint.

Key. fi fibula; **lcon** lateral femoral condyle; **mcon** medial femoral condyle; **tibs** tibial spine.

Figure 9.28   Coronal MR scan of knee joint.   (R4.F)

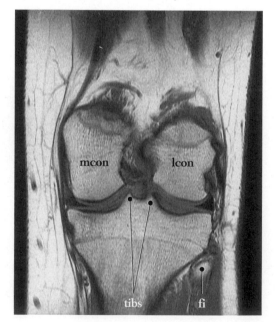

Key.   c cartilage; **f** femur; **p** patella; **tt** tibial tuberosity.

Figure 9.29   Sagittal MR scan of knee joint with tibial tuberosity.   (R4.A)

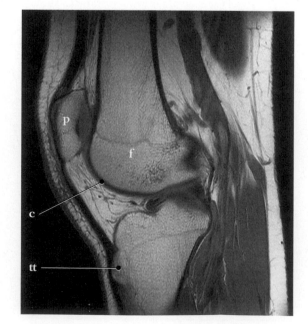

MENISCI AND LIGAMENTS

Located between the femoral condyles and tibial plateaus are the paired **menisci.** These C-shaped menisci, composed of fibrous connective tissue, cushion the articulation of the femoral condyles and the tibial plateaus and are commonly divided into anterior and posterior horns (Figures 9.31 through 9.34).

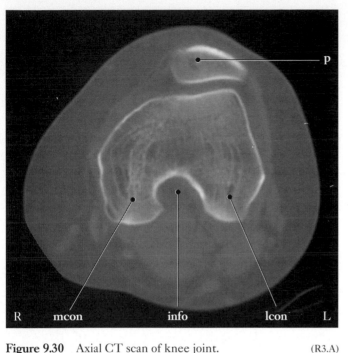

Figure 9.30   Axial CT scan of knee joint.   (R3.A)

Key. **info** intercondylar fossa; **lcon** lateral femoral condyle; **mcon** medial femoral condyle; **p** patella.

Figure 9.31   Anterior view of meniscus and ligaments of knee.

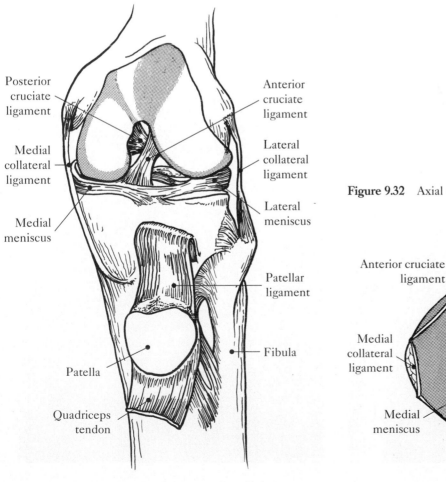

Figure 9.32   Axial view of meniscus and ligaments of knee.

Major ligaments of the knee include the **collateral** and **cruciate ligaments.** Collateral ligaments provide support for the knee by reinforcing the joint capsule on the medial and lateral sides. The **medial (tibial) collateral ligament** is a flattened triangular ligament that originates on the medial femoral condyle and fuses with the medial meniscus. The round **lateral (fibular) collateral ligament** has its proximal attachment on the lateral femoral condyle and distal attachment on the fibular head (Figures 9.31 and 9.33). Cruciate (cross-shaped) ligaments are strong bands of fibers that provide anterior and posterior stability to the knee. They are broken into anterior and posterior ligaments, depending on their site of attachment to the tibia. The **anterior cruciate ligament** extends from the medial aspect of the lateral femoral condyle to the anterior tibial spine. It prevents anterior displacement of the tibia (Figure 9.35). The **posterior cruciate ligament** is the stronger of the two and extends from the medial femoral condyle to the posterior aspect of the tibia (Figure 9.36).

Key. **ACL** anterior cruciate ligament; **gas** gastrocnemius muscle; **lcal** lateral collateral ligament; **lmen** lateral meniscus; **lmena** lateral meniscus, anterior horn; **lmenp** lateral meniscus, posterior horn; **mcol** medial collateral ligament; **mmen** medial meniscus; **PCL** posterior cruciate ligament; **pl** patellar ligament; **pop** popliteus muscle; **qten** quadriceps tendon; **sol** soleus muscle.

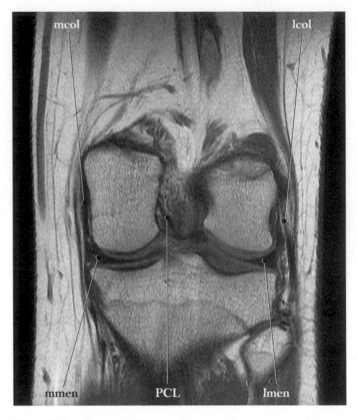

Figure 9.33   Coronal MR scan of knee with meniscus and ligaments of knee.   (R4.G)

Figure 9.34   Sagittal MR scan of knee with meniscus and ligaments of knee.   (R4.E)

Figure 9.35   Sagittal MR scan of knee with anterior cruciate ligament.   (R4.D)

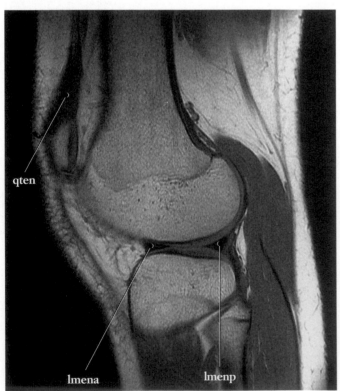

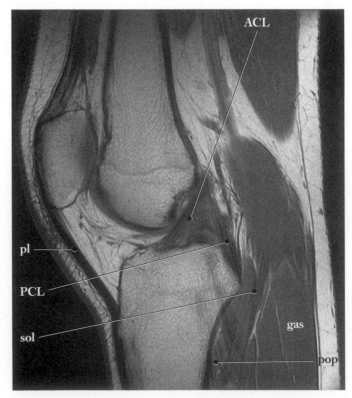

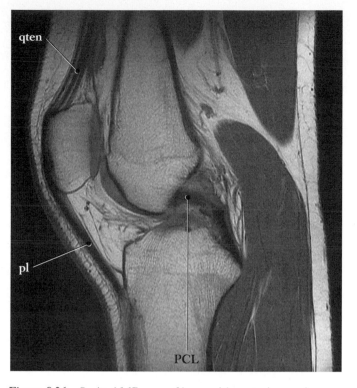

Covering the anterior surface of the patella is the quadriceps tendon, which continues as the **patellar ligament** to insert on the tibial tuberosity. The patellar ligament helps maintain the position of the patella within the knee joint (Figures 9.36 to 9.38).

Figure 9.36   Sagittal MR scan of knee with posterior cruciate ligament.   (R4.C)

Key.   ACL anterior cruciate ligament; **lcol** lateral collateral ligament; **mcol** medial collateral ligament; **pl** patellar ligament; **PCL** posterior cruciate ligament; **qten** quadriceps tendon.

Figure 9.37   Axial MR scan of knee with cruciate and collateral ligaments.   (R3.B)

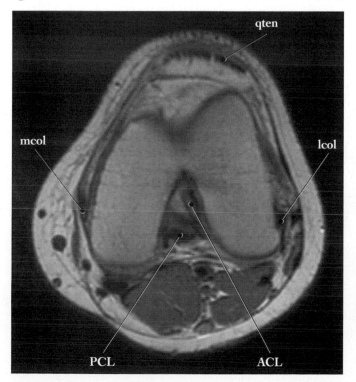

Figure 9.38   Axial CT scan of knee with cruciate and collateral ligaments.   (R3.A)

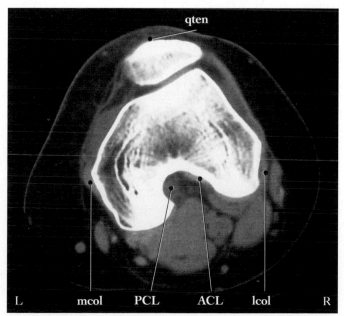

MUSCLES

Prominent muscles of the knee include the **quadriceps femoris group**, the **hamstring group**, the **popliteus muscle**, and the **gastrocnemius muscle** (Figures 9.39 through 9.41). The quadriceps femoris group, the largest muscle group in the body, originates from four heads (rectus femoris, vastus lateralis, vastus medialis, vastus intermedius) about the hip joint and inserts on the patella. This muscle group covers almost all the anterior surface and sides of the femur and functions as a very powerful extensor of the leg. The hamstring muscles span the posterior aspect of the hip and knee joints, hence they are extensors of the thigh and flexors of the leg. This group is composed of three muscles (biceps femoris, semitendinosus, semimembranosus) that originate from the ischial tuberosity and insert on the fibula and medial tibial condyle and shaft. The popliteus muscle flexes the leg and rotates the femur laterally. It extends from the lateral aspect of the lateral femoral condyle and attaches to the posterior surface of the tibia (Figure 9.42). The gastrocnemius muscle is a prominent flexor of the leg. It consists of two heads arising from the medial and lateral femoral condyles and spans the posterior aspect of the knee to insert on the calcaneus via the Achilles tendon (Figures 9.43 and 9.44).

VASCULATURE

Two major vascular structures, the **popliteal artery** and **vein**, are located within the popliteal fossa on the posterior aspect of the knee. Another prominent vessel is the **great saphenous vein,** which ascends the medial aspect of the leg and thigh, to drain into the femoral vein near the hip joint (Figures 9.43 through 9.45).

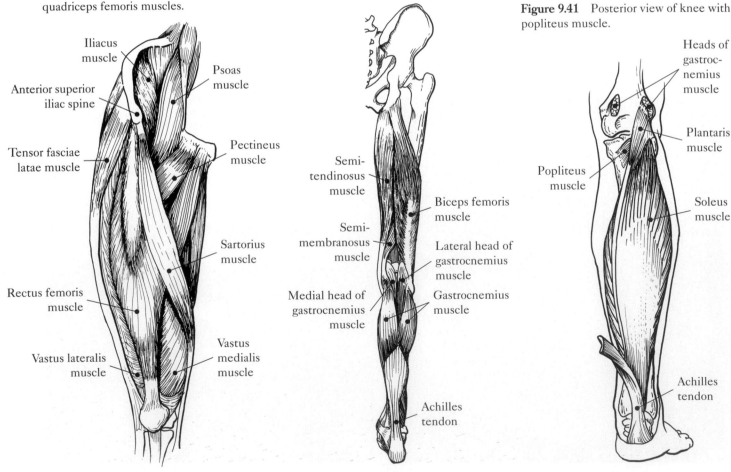

Figure 9.39   Anterior view of thigh with quadriceps femoris muscles.

Figure 9.40   Posterior view of thigh with hamstring and gastrocnemius muscles.

Figure 9.41   Posterior view of knee with popliteus muscle.

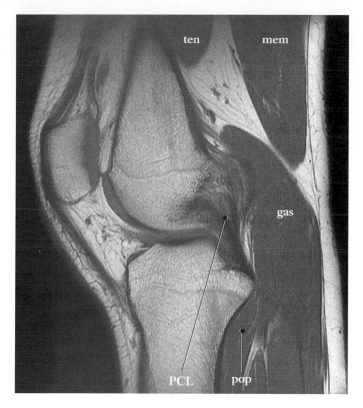

Figure 9.42 Sagittal MR scan of knee with hamstring, gastrocnemius, and popliteus muscles.

(R4.B)

Key. **bft** biceps femoris tendon; **gas** gastrocnemius; **lgas** lateral head of gastrocnemius; **mem** semimembranosus; **memt** semimembranosus tendon; **mgas** medial head of gastrocnemius; **PCL** posterior cruciate ligament; **pop** popliteus; **popA** popliteal artery; **popV** popliteal vein; **sar** sartorius; **SaV** great saphenous vein; **ten** semitendinosus.

Figure 9.44 Axial CT scan of knee with neurovasculature.

(R3.B)

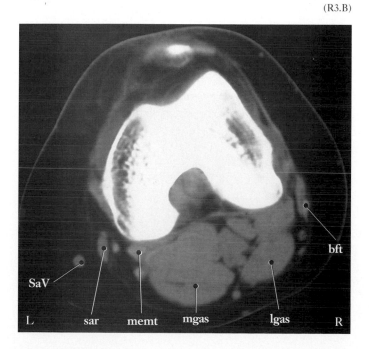

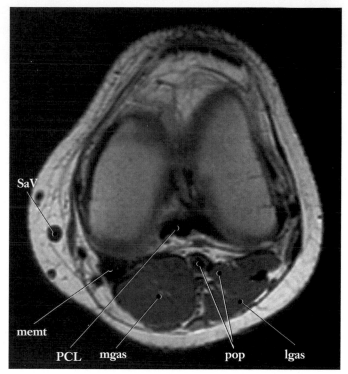

Figure 9.43 Axial MR scan of knee with neurovasculature.

(R3.C)

Figure 9.45 Anterior view of popliteal artery and vein and great saphenous vein.

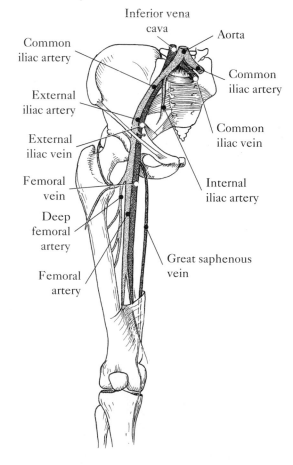

ANKLE

The ankle joint is arranged in a hingelike structure, allowing for plantar flexion and dorsiflexion.

BONY ANATOMY

The ankle joint is created by the articulations between the **tibia, fibula,** and **talus (astragalus);** Figures 9.46 and 9.47). The tibia and fibula rest on the talus to form what is commonly termed the mortise joint. Both the tibia and fibula terminate distally in projections termed **malleoli,** which prevent medial and lateral displacement of the talus. The talus transmits the weight of the entire body to the foot as it rests on the **calcaneus (os calcis),** the largest bone of the foot. The articulation between the talus and calcaneus is termed the **subtalar joint,** which is composed of three articulations formed by the **anterior, middle,** and **posterior facets** (Figures 9.48 and 9.49). The smallest of the three is the anterior facet, which can be independent of or continuous with the middle facet. The middle facet lies on a ledge of bone projecting off the medial surface of the calcaneus called the **sustentaculum tali.** This shelf and the entire middle facet joint provide weight-bearing support to the medial side of the ankle. The posterior facet joint is the largest and provides support for most of the body of the talus. Separating this facet from the middle and anterior facet joints is the tarsal canal. This canal, containing blood vessels, fat, and the interosseous ligament, widens laterally to form the **sinus tarsi** (Figure 9.49).

In addition to the talus and calcaneus, the **cuboid, navicular,** and three **cuneiform bones** comprise the remaining five tarsal bones of the foot (Figures 9.50 and 9.51). Lateral and anterior to the calcaneus is the cuboid bone, which articulates anteriorly with the base of the fourth and fifth metatarsal bones. The navicular bone articulates posteriorly with the talus and anteriorly with the cuneiform bones on the medial side of the foot. The cuneiform bones are numbered from medial to lateral and articulate anteriorly with the first three metatarsal bones.

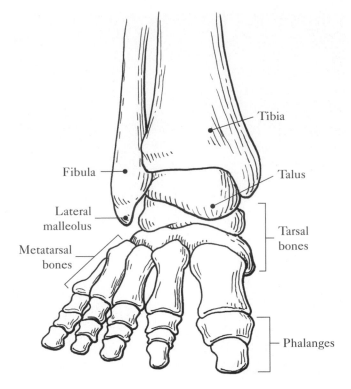

Figure 9.46   Anterior view of ankle joint.

Key.   C calcaneus; **fi** fibula; **ta** talus; **ti** tibia.

Figure 9.47   Coronal CT scan with tibia, fibula, and talus.

(R6.B)

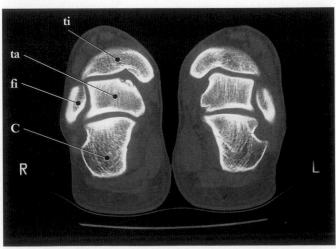

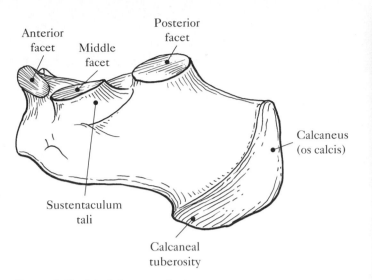

Figure 9.48 Medial aspect of calcaneus.

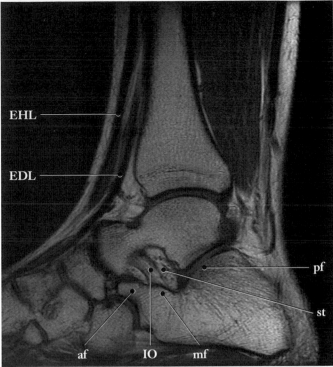

Figure 9.49 Sagittal MR scan of calcaneus.   (R6.G)

Key. **af** anterior facet; **EDL** extensor digitorum longus; **EHL** extensor hallucis longus; **IO** interosseous ligament; **mf** medial facet; **pf** posterior facet; **st** sinus tarsi.

Figure 9.50 Dorsal view of foot.

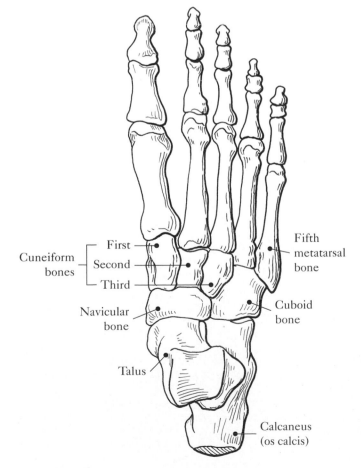

Key. **C** calcaneus; **cu** cuboid; **n** navicular; **tali** sustentaculum tali; **I** medial cuneiform; **III** lateral cuneiform.

Figure 9.51 Axial CT scan of ankle with tarsal bones.   (R5.E)

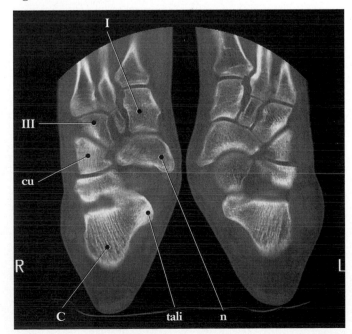

LIGAMENTS

The ankle has a complex architecture of multiple ligaments that provide necessary support. The main support structures of the ankle include the **deltoid ligament, lateral ligaments, spring (plantar) ligament,** and **interosseous ligament** (Figures 9.52 through 9.54). The deltoid ligament provides medial support and is the strongest ligament in the ankle joint (Figure 9.55). It arises from the medial malleolus and fans out into three bands: **tibiotalar ligament, tibiocalcaneal ligament,** and **tibionavicular ligament** to insert on the talus, calcaneus, and navicular bone, respectively (Figures 9.56). The lateral border of the ankle joint is strengthened by several ligaments termed the **anterior talofibular, calcaneofibular, posterior talofibular, anterior tibiofibular,** and **posterior tibiofibular ligaments.** All of these ligaments originate at the fibular malleolus and insert on the adjacent bone structures (Figure 9.57). The spring (plantar) ligament is a triangular-shaped band of fibers that arises from the sustentaculum tali and attaches to the posterior surface of the navicular bone. It is an important ligament in maintaining the longitudinal arch of the foot. A strong band of tissue binding the talus to the calcaneus is the **interosseous (talocalcaneal) ligament,** which is obliquely oriented in the sinus tarsi (see Figure 9.49).

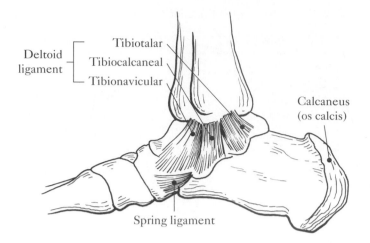

Figure 9.52   Medial view of ankle with deltoid ligament.

Figure 9.54   Posterior view of ankle ligaments.

Figure 9.53   Lateral ligaments of ankle.

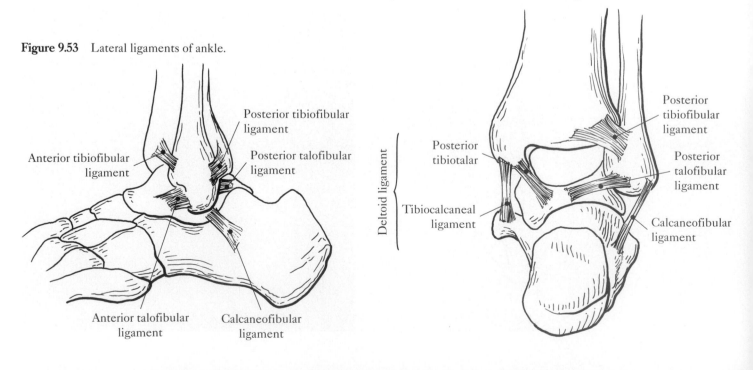

Table 9.2   Ligaments of the ankle

NAME	ORIGIN	INSERTION	ACTION
Deltoid ligament			
Tibiotalar	Medial malleolus	Talus	Provide medial support
Tibiocalcaneal	Medial malleolus	Calcaneus	Provide medial support
Tibionavicular	Medial malleolus	Navicular bone	Provide medial support
Lateral ligaments			
Anterior talofibular	Fibular malleolus	Anterior talus	Provide lateral support
Calcaneofibular	Fibular malleolus	Calcaneus	Provide lateral support
Posterior talofibular	Fibular malleolus	Posterior talus	Provide lateral support
Anterior tibiofibular	Fibular malleolus	Anterior tibia	Provide lateral support
Posterior tibiofibular	Fibular malleolus	Posterior tibia	Provide lateral support
Spring (plantar)	Sustentaculum tali	Posterior surface of navicular bone	Maintain longitudinal arch
Interosseous (talocalcaneal)	Talus	Calcaneus	Bind talus to calcaneus

Key. **C** calcaneus; **del** deltoid ligament; **ta** talus; **ti** tibia.

Key. **AT** Achille's tendon; **ATF** anterior talofibular ligament; **PTF** posterior talofibular ligament; **TBN** tibionavicular ligament; **TBT** tibiotalar ligament.

Key. **CF** calcaniofibular ligament; **PTBF** posterior tibiofibular ligament; **PTF** posterior talofibular ligament.

Figure 9.55   Coronal MR scan of ankle with deltoid ligament.   (R6.A)

Figure 9.56   Axial MR scan of ankle with ligaments.   (R5.C)

Figure 9.57   Coronal MR scan of ankle with lateral ligaments.   (R5.A)

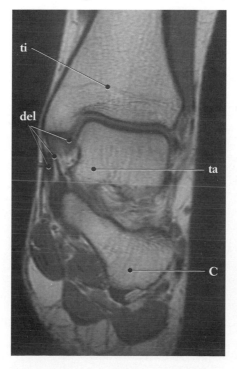

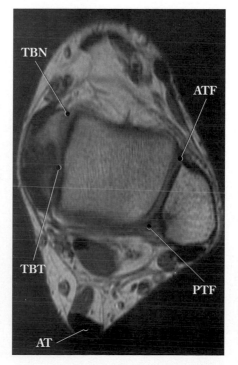

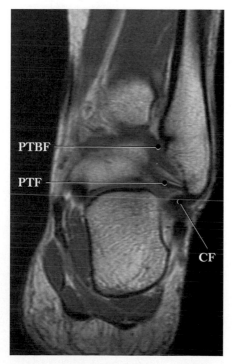

TENDONS

The musculotendinous structures of the ankle can be divided into posterior, anterior, medial, and lateral groups (Figures 9.58 and 9.59).

POSTERIOR GROUP.   The posterior group is composed of the single **Achilles tendon,** the largest and most powerful tendon of the body. The Achilles tendon arises from the **gastrocnemius** and **soleus muscles** and attaches to the calcaneal tuberosity on the posterior aspect of the calcaneus (Figures 9.59 through 9.63).

ANTERIOR GROUP.   The anterior group is made up of the **tibialis anterior, extensor hallucis longus,** and **extensor digitorum longus tendons,** which are named medial to lateral and act to extend and dorsiflex the foot. The tibialis anterior muscle becomes tendinous at the distal tibia and attaches to the plantar and medial aspect of the first cuneiform and metatarsal bones. The tendon of the extensor hallucis longus muscle originates from the anterior fibula and inserts on the great toe. The most lateral of this group is the extensor digitorum longus tendon, which originates at the level of the lateral malleolus and inserts on the second through the fifth digits (Figures 9.59 and 9.60).

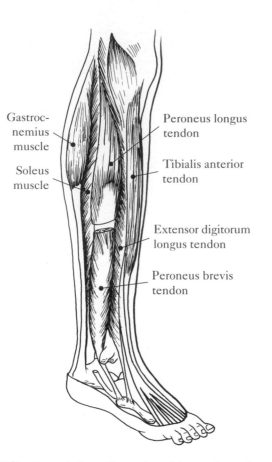

Figure 9.58   Lateral view of lower leg with muscles and tendons.

Key. af anterior facet; **EDL** extensor digitorum longus; **EHL** extensor hallucis longus; **IO** interosseous ligament; **mf** medial facet; **pf** posterior facet; **sol** soleus muscle.

Figure 9.60   Sagittal MR scan of lower leg with anterior group of tendons.   (R6.G)

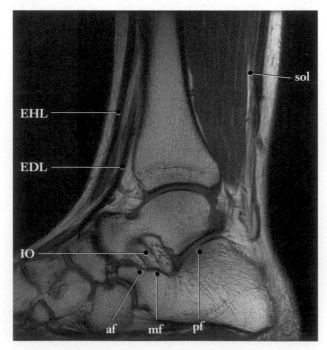

Figure 9.59   Anterior view of lower leg with extensor and tibialis anterior tendons.

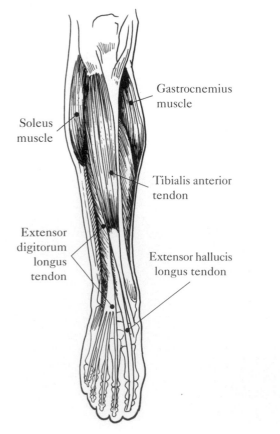

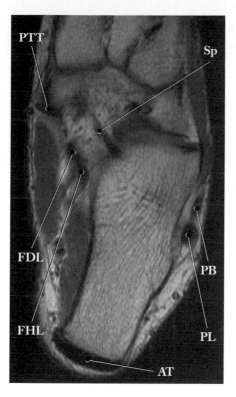

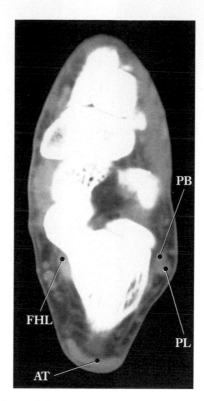

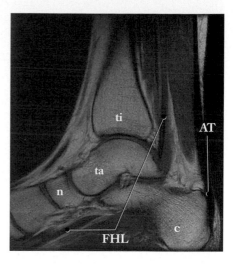

Figure 9.63 Sagittal MR scan of lower leg with posterior group of tendons.

(R6.F)

Figure 9.61 Axial MR scan of lower leg with medial and lateral tendon groups.

(R5.F)

Figure 9.62 Axial CT scan of lower leg with medial and lateral tendon groups.

(R5.D)

Key. **AT** Achille's tendon; **EDL** extensor digitorum longus; **EHL** extensor hallucis longus; **FDL** flexor digitorum longus; **FHL** flexor hallucis longus; **n** navicular; **PB** peroneus brevis; **PL** peroneus longus; **PTT** posterior tibialis tendon; **Sp** spring ligament; **ta** talus; **TAT** tibialis anterior tendon; **ti** tibia.

Figure 9.66 Lateral side of ankle with tendons.

Figure 9.65 Axial MR scan of ankle with tendons.   (R5.B)

Figure 9.64 Medial side of ankle with tendons.

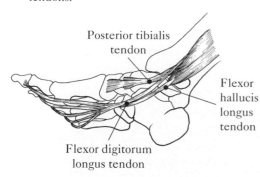

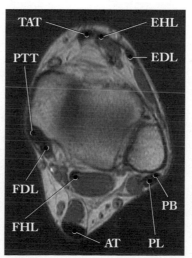

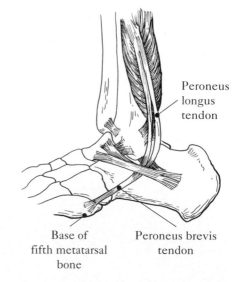

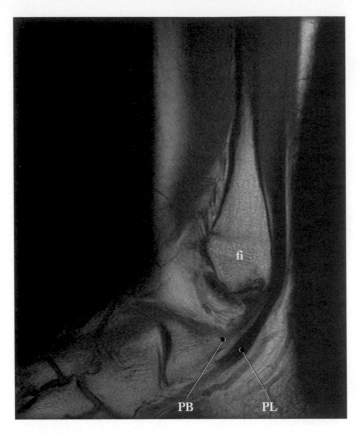

Figure 9.67 Sagittal MR scan of ankle with lateral group of tendons. (R6.H)

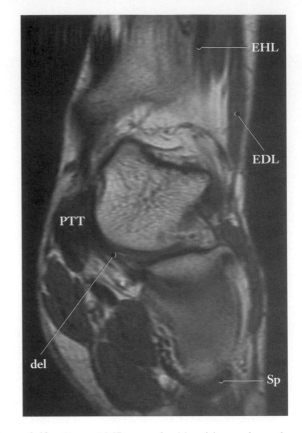

Figure 9.68 Coronal MR scan of ankle with anterior and medial tendon groups. (R6.D)

Key. **ATF** anterior talofibular ligament; **del** deltoid ligament; **EDL** extensor digitorum longus; **EHL** extensor hallucis longus; **fi** fibula; **FDL** flexor digitorum longus; **FHL** flexor hallucis longus; **PB** peroneus brevis; **PL** peroneus longus; **PTT** posterior tibialis tendon; **Sp** spring ligament; **TAT** tibialis anterior tendon.

Figure 9.69 Sagittal MR scan of ankle with medial group of tendons. (R6.E)

Figure 9.70 Coronal MR scan of ankle with medial and lateral tendon groups. (R6.C)

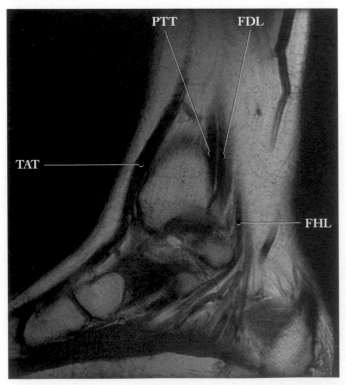

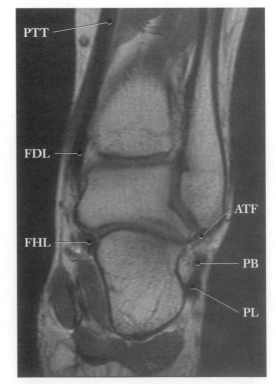

Table 9.3   Tendons of the ankle

GROUP	ORIGIN	INSERTION	ACTION
POSTERIOR GROUP			
Achilles	Gastrocnemius and soleus muscles	Calcaneal tuberosity	Plantar flex foot and flaxes lower leg
ANTERIOR			
Tibialis anterior	Level of distal tibia	1st cuneiform and metatarsal bones	Extend and dorsiflex foot
Extensor hallucis longus	Anterior surface of distal fibula	Great toe	Extend and dorsiflex foot
Extensor digitorum longus	Level of lateral malleolus	2nd-5th phalanges	Extend and dorsiflex foot
MEDIAL			
Posterior tibialis	Posterior tibia	Sustentaculum tali, navicular and 1st cuneiform bones	Invert and plantar flex foot
Flexor digitorum longus	Posterior to posterior tibialis tendon	2nd-4th phalanges	Invert and plantar flex foot
Flexor hallucis longus	Under sustentaculum tali	Great toe	Invert and plantar flex foot
LATERAL			
Peroneus longus	Posterior to lateral malleolus	Base of 1st metatarsal bone	Provide lateral stability; evert and plantar flex foot
Peroneus brevis	Posterior to lateral malleolus	Base of 5th metatarsal bone	Provide lateral stability; evert and plantar flex foot

MEDIAL GROUP. The medial group is composed of the **posterior tibialis tendons, flexor digitorum longus,** and **flexor hallucis longus tendons,** which as a group act to invert and plantar flex the foot. The posterior tibialis tendon fans out in multiple strands that insert on the plantar aspect of the sustentaculum tali, navicular bone, first cuneiform bone, and second through fourth metatarsal bones. Coursing posterior and lateral to the posterior tibialis tendon is the flexor digitorum longus tendon, which at its terminal portion inserts on the second through fourth phalanges. The tendon of the flexor hallucis longus muscle curves under the sustentaculum tali and then courses along the plantar surface of the foot to insert on the great toe (Figures 9.61 to 9.65 and 9.68 to 9.70).

LATERAL GROUP. The two **peroneus tendons, peroneus longus** and **peroneus brevis,** make up the lateral group and act to evert, weakly plantar flex the foot, and stabilize the ankle joint laterally. These two tendons share a common tendinous sheath behind the lateral malleolus. Below the malleolus, they diverge into separate tendon sheaths, with the peroneus brevis tendon inserting on the base of the fifth metatarsal and the peroneus longus tendon curving beneath the calcaneus to insert on the base of the first metatarsal and medial cuneiform bones (Figures 9.61, 9.62, 9.65, 9.66, 9.67, and 9.70).

ANSWER TO FIGURE 9.1

The patient demonstrates round thickening of the Achilles tendon greater than 1 cm. There is a vertical tear of the peripheral portion of the medial aspect of the Achilles tendon just above the insertion site.

Appendix

BODY PLANES

Cross sectional images are acquired and displayed according to one of the four fundamental, anatomic planes that pass through the body (see Figure A-1). The four anatomic planes are defined as:

1. Sagittal plane: a vertical plane that passes through the body, dividing it into right and left portions
2. Coronal plane: a vertical plane that passes through the body, dividing it into anterior (ventral) and posterior (dorsal) portions
3. Axial (horizontal) plane: a transverse plane that passes through the body, dividing it into superior and inferior portions
4. Oblique plane: a plane that passes diagonally between the axes of two of the other planes

BODY CAVITIES

The body can be divided into two large cavities: the thoracic cavity and the abdominal cavity, which can be further subdivided into smaller cavities. The thoracic cavity is subdivided into two lateral pleural cavities and a single, centrally located cavity called the mediastinum. The abdominal cavity can be divided into the abdominal and pelvic cavities (see Figure A-2). The structures located in each cavity are listed in Table A.1.

EXTERNAL LANDMARKS

External landmarks of the body help the health care professional identify the location of many internal structures. The commonly used external landmarks are shown in Figures A-3 and A-4.

Table A-1 Body cavities

CAVITY	CONTENTS
THORACIC	
Mediastinum	Heart, great vessels, trachea, esophagus, and pericardium
Pleural	Lungs, pleural membranes
ABDOMINAL	
Abdominal	Peritoneum, liver, gall bladder, pancreas, spleen, stomach, intestines, kidneys, ureters, and blood vessels
Pelvic	Rectum, urinary bladder, and parts of the male and female reproductive system

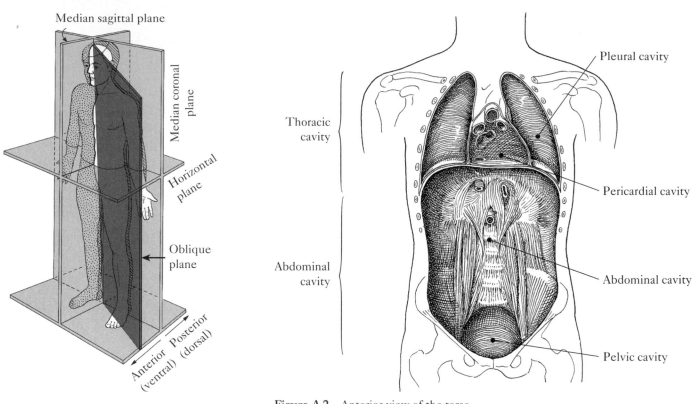

Figure A.1   Planes of the body.

Figure A.2   Anterior view of the torso.

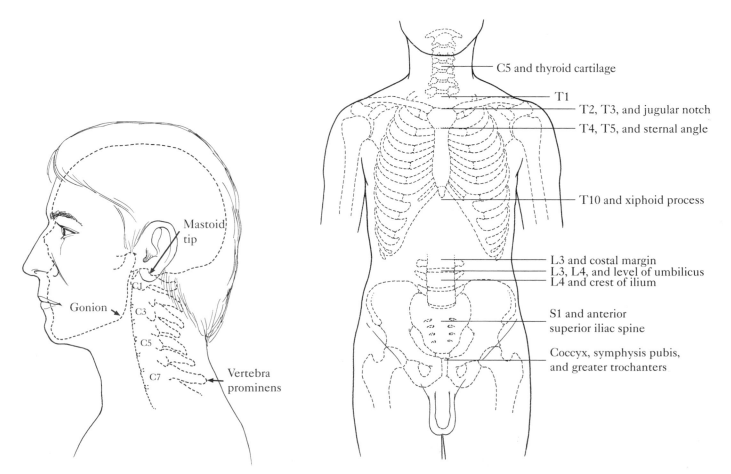

Figure A.3   Surface landmarks of the head and neck.

Figure A.4   Surface landmarks of the torso.

Bibliography

Agur AM: *Grant's atlas of anatomy*, Baltimore, 1996, Williams and Wilkins.

Ballinger PW: *Merrill's atlas of radiographic positions and radiologic procedures*, St. Louis, 1986, Mosby.

Blackwell GC: *MRI: cardiovascular system*, New York, 1992, Raven Press.

Corbett JV: *Laboratory tests and diagnostic procedures with nursing diagnoses*, ed 4, Stamford, Conn, 1996, Appleton and Lange.

Deutsch AL, Mink JH, et al: *MRI of the foot and ankle*, New York, 1992, Raven Press.

England MA, Wakely CN: *Color atlas of the brain and spinal cord*, St. Louis, 1991, Mosby.

Firooznia H, Golimbu CN et al: *MRI and CT of the musculoskeletal system*, St. Louis, 1992, Mosby.

Gutierrez FR, Brown JJ et al: *Cardiovascular magnetic resonance imaging*, St. Louis, 1992, Mosby.

Harnsberger HR: *Handbook of head and neck imaging*, ed 2, St. Louis, 1995, Mosby.

Hayman LA: *Clinical brain imaging: normal structure and functional anatomy*, St. Louis, 1992, Mosby.

Kucharczyk W: *MRI: central nervous system*, Philadelphia, 1990, Gower Medical.

Mancuso AA: *Workbook for MRI and CT of the head and neck*, ed 2, Baltimore, 1989, Williams and Wilkins.

Martin JH: *Neuroanatomy: text and atlas*, Stamford, Conn, 1996, Appleton and Lange.

Martini FH: *Fundamentals of anatomy and physiology*, ed 3, Englewood Cliffs, NJ, 1995, Prentice-Hall.

Miller SW: *Cardiac radiology: the requisites*, St. Louis, 1996, Mosby.

Modic MT, Masaryk TJ et al: *Magnetic resonance imaging of the spine*, St. Louis, 1994, Mosby.

Moore KL, Agur AM: *Essential clinical anatomy*, Baltimore, 1996, Williams and Wilkins.

Osborn AG: *Diagnostic neuroradiology*, St. Louis, 1994, Mosby.

Rhoades RA, Tanner GA: *Medical physiology*, United States of America, 1995, Little, Brown, & Co.

Ros PR, Bidgood WD: *Abdominal magnetic resonance imaging*, St. Louis, 1993, Mosby.

Ryan SP, McNicholas MMJ: *Anatomy for diagnostic imaging*, Philadelphia, 1994, WB Saunders.

Seeley PR, Stephens TD et al: *Anatomy and physiology*, St. Louis, 1989, Mosby.

Spence AP: *Basic human anatomy*, Menlo Park, Ill, 1988, Benjamin/Cummings.

Snopek AM: *Fundamentals of special radiographic procedures*, ed 3, Philadelphia, 1992, WB Saunders.

Stoller DW: *Magnetic resonance imaging in orthopaedic sports medicine*, Philadelphia, 1993, JB Lippincott Company.

Taveras JM: *Neuroradiology*, ed 3, Baltimore, 1996, Williams and Wilkins.

Wegener OH: *Whole body computed tomography*, ed 2, Cambridge, Mass, 1992, Blackwell Scientific Publications.

Weir J, Abrahams PH: *An imaging atlas of human anatomy*, St. Louis, 1992, Mosby.

Weissleder R, Wittenberg J: *Primer of diagnostic imaging*, St. Louis, 1994, Mosby.

Index

A

Abdomen, 165-202
 CT scan of, *165*
 muscles of, 199, *199, 200*
  origin, insertion, and function of, 200t
 organs of, 165
Abdominal aorta, 190, *231*
 anterior view of, *190*
 paired branches of, 194, *194*
 unpaired branches of, 191
Abdominal cavity
 divisions of, 166
 peritoneum of, 166
 sagittal view of, *166*
 structures of, 165
Abdominopelvic muscle(s), *209*
Abducens nerve, 78, *78*
 type, foramen, and function of, 81t
Abscess in neck, *111*
Accessory nerve, 80, *81*
 type, foramen, and function of, 81t
Acetabular fossa, 265
Acetabular labrum, 266
Acetabulum, 204, *204*
 bones of, 265
 CT reformat with, *206*
 lateral view of, *264*
 MR scan of, *206, 207*
Achilles tendon(s)
 origin, insertion, and action of, 287t
 thickening of, 287
Acromioclavicular joint, 238, *240*
Acromion, 238, *238*
Adductor muscle(s), 271, *271*
 origin, insertion, and action of, 269t
Adenohypophysis, 55
Adenoids, 114
Adrenal glands, 182, *182*
 abnormal, *201*
 common configurations of, *182*
 MR scan of, *182, 183*
Ala, 204
Alar ligament(s), 96, *96*
Alveolar process, 12, 17

Ambient cistern, 44
Ampulla of Vater, 178
Amygdala, functions of, 51
Anal canal, 219
Ankle, 280, 282-284, 286
 anterior view of, *280*
 bony anatomy of, 280, *280*
 ligaments of, 282, *282, 283*
  origin, insertion, and action of, 283t
 MR scan of, *263*
 tendons of, 284, *284, 285, 286*
  lateral group, 287
  medial group, 287
  origin, insertion, and action of, 287t
Annular ligament(s), 249, *250*
Annulus fibrosus, 85
Antrum of Highmore, 24
Anus, 219
Aorta
 abdominal, 165, 190, *190, 231, 232*
  paired branches of, 194, *194*
  unpaired branches of, 191
 ascending, 151, *152*
 bifurcation of, *232*
 descending, 151, *152*, 231
Aortic arch, 151, *151, 152, 155*
 branches of, 155, *156, 158*
 MRI of, *155*
Aortic hiatus, 161
Aortic semilunar valve, 148
Apophyseal joints, 85
Appendix, 189
Aqueduct of Sylvius, 40
Aqueous humor, 33
Arachnoid villi, 42
Arnold-Chiari malformation, 60
Arteriovenous malformation, 81
Articular cartilage, 265
Articular disk, 19, *19*
Articular process, 85
Aryepiglottic folds, 117
Arytenoid cartilage, 114, *116*
Ascites, 174
Astragalus, 280
Atlas, 87, *87, 88*
 congenital anomaly of, 109
Atrioventricular valves, 148
Auditory meatus, *18, 19*, 27, *29*

Page numbers in italics indicate illustrations; page numbers followed by a *t* indicate a table.

Auditory meatus—cont'd
    axial CT scan of petrous portion of, *28*
    external, 4
Auditory ossicles, 27
Avascular necrosis of femoral head, 235, 265
Axis, odontoid process of, *88,* 89
Azygos venous system, 159, *159*

B

Basal ganglia, *52, 53*
    structures and functions of, 52-53
Basilar artery(ies), 65, *66*
Biceps brachialis muscle(s), *252,* 253
Biceps brachii muscle(s), *252,* 253
Biceps tendon(s), 241
Bicipital groove, 238
Bicuspid valve, 148
Bile duct, common, 178, *179*
Biliary system, 178, *178*
Bladder, urinary; *see* Urinary bladder
Blood, circulation of, through heart, 153
Blood-brain barrier, function of, 63
Bony nasal septum, 15
Brachial artery(ies), 254, *254*
Brachial plexus, *104,* 105
    innervation of, 106t
    MR scan of, *105*
Brachial veins, 254, *254*
Brachiocephalic artery(ies), 130
Brachiocephalic trunk, 155
Brachiocephalic veins, *158*
Brachioradialis muscle(s), 253, *253*
Brain, 37-81
    abnormal, coronal MR scan of, *38*
    with cranial nerves, *72*
    subarachnoid space of, 42
    vascular supply of; *see* Cerebral vascular system
Brain stem, 55-57
    in Arnold-Chiari malformation, 60
    midsagittal MR scan of, *55*
    MR scan of, *55*
    segments of, 55
    structures of, 37
Breast, layers of, 137, 163, *163*
Bronchi, 137
    divisions of, 143
Bronchial tree, *142*
Buccinator muscle, 123
    location and action of, 129t
Bulbourethral glands, 229, *230*

C

Calcaneofibular ligament(s), of ankle, 282, *282*
    origin, insertion, and action of, 283t
Calcaneus, 280, *281*
    MR scan of, *281*

Capitate bone, 257, *257*
Cardiac notch, 140
Cardiophrenic sulcus, 140
Carditis, 148
Carina, 118, *118,* 143
    MR scan at, *143*
Carotid artery(ies), 130, *130, 131, 132,* 155
    internal, *63,* 63-64, *64*
Carotid canals, 4
Carotid sheath, 135, *135*
Carotid siphon, 63
Carpal bones, CT scan of, *257*
Carpal tunnel, 259
Carpal tunnel syndrome, 259
Cartilage of knee, 274
Cauda equina, *100*
Caudate nucleus, 52, *52*
Caval hiatus, 161, 196
Cavernous sinuses, 69, *76*
Cecum, CT scan of, *189*
Celiac trunk, 191
    anterior view of, *191*
    CT scan of, *192*
    MR scan of, *177, 192*
Cerebellar artery(ies), 65t
    regions supplied by, 65t
Cerebellar peduncles, 61, *61*
    MR scan of, *62*
Cerebellopontine angle cistern, *43,* 44
Cerebellum, 60-61
    in Arnold-Chiari malformation, 60
    dentate nuclei of, 61
    functions of, 60
    hemispheres of, 60, *60*
    tonsils of, 60, *60*
Cerebral aqueduct, 40
Cerebral artery(ies), middle, in stroke, 53
Cerebral cortex, *37*
    axial view of, *46*
    coronal MR scan of, *46*
    lobes of, 47, 47t, *48, 49, 49, 50*
        functions of, 47t
    sagittal view of, *45*
    structures of, 45, 47
Cerebral peduncles, 55, *55, 56, 57*
Cerebral vascular system, 37, 63-71
    arterial supply of, 63
    circle of Willis, 67, *67*
    internal carotid arteries in, *63,* 63-64, 64t
    venous, *68*
    venous drainage of, 69, *70, 71*
        dural sinuses, 68, 69
        superficial cortical and deep veins, 69, *71*
    vertebral arteries in, 65, *65, 66*
Cerebrospinal fluid, 39
Cerebrospinal fluid system, 40-44
    ventricular component of, 40, *40, 41,* 42

Cerebrum
  arterial supply of, *62*
  fissures of, 49, *49*
  gyri of, 49, *49*
  structures and functions of, 45
  structures of, 37
Cervical enlargement, 101
Cervical plexus, *104*, 105
  innervation of, 106t
Cervix, 221
Chest
  CT scan of, *137, 143*
  with pulmonary trunk, *153*
  with pulmonary veins, *154*
Chickenpox, latent herpes zoster virus following, 102
Choroid plexus, 42, *42*
Circle of Willis, 67, *67*
Cisterna magna, 42, *43*
Cisterns, subarachnoidal, 42, *42, 43*, 44
Claustrum, 52, *52*
Clavicle, 238, *238*
Clinoid processes, 7
Clivus, 3, *3*
Coccygeus muscle(s), 214, *215, 217*
  origin, insertion, and function of, 216t
Coccyx, *91*, 92, *92*, 204, *204*
Cochlea, 29
Collateral ligaments of knee, 274, *276, 277*
Colliculi, 55, *55*
  superior and inferior, 56, *56*
Colon
  sigmoid, 189, *189*
  transverse, 189, *189*
Common bile duct, 178, *179*
Common hepatic duct, 178
Common iliac vein, *232*
Condyles
  lateral, 3
  medial and lateral, 248
    of knee, 274
Condyloid process, 17, *19*
Conus medullaris, *100*, 101, *101*
Cooper's ligament(s), 163
Coracoacromial ligament(s), *244*, 245
Coracoclavicular ligament(s), *245, 245*
Coracoid process, 238, *238*
Cornu, 92
Coronary artery(ies), 149, *149*
Coronoid process, 17, 248
Corpora cavernosa, 229
Corpora spongiosum, 229
Corpus callosum
  axial MR scan of, *46*
  axial view of, *46*
  divisions of, 45, *45, 46*
Costal cartilages, 138, *138*

Costal facets, 91
Costophrenic sulcus, 140
Costotransverse joints, 91
Costovertebral joints, 91
Cowper's gland, 229
Cranial fossa
  middle, 4, *4*
  posterior, *3*
  3D CT scan of, *4*
Cranial nerves, 37, 72-81; *see also* individual nerves
  abducens, 78, *78*
  accessory, 80, *81*
  facial, 78, *79*
  glossopharyngeal, 80, *80*
  hypoglossal, 80, *81*
  localization of, 72
  oculomotor, 75, *75, 76*
  olfactory, 73, *73*
  optic, *74*, 75
  trigeminal, 76, *77*
  trochlear, *75, 76*
  type, foramina, and functions of, 81t
  vagus, 80, *80*
  vesticulocochlear, 78, *79*
Craniosynostosis, 11
Cranium, *9, 10*
  bones of, 3-11
  inferior view of, *3, 4, 6, 13*
  structures of, 1
  3D CT scan of lateral surface of, *11*
Cribriform plate, 7, *8*
Cricoid cartilage, 114, *117*
Crista galli, 7, *8*
Cruciate ligament(s), 276, *276, 277*
Crura, 161, *162*
Cubital veins, 254, *254*
Cuboid bone, 280
Cuneiform bones, 280
Cyst, follicular, 224
Cystic artery(ies), 191
Cystic duct, 178

D

Deltoid ligament of ankle, 282, *282*
  origin, insertion, and action of, 283t
Deltoid muscle(s), 241
Dementia, hippocampus in, 51
Dentate nucleus, 61
Denticulate ligament(s), 101
Diaphragm, 140, 161
  inferior view of, *162*
Disks, vertebral, 85
Dopamine, decreased production of, in Parkinson's
    disease, 57
Dorsal root ganglion, *102*, 103
Douglas, pouch of, 224

Duct of Wirsung, 178
Duodenum, 188
  CT scan of, *188*
  MR scan of, *179*
Dura mater, 38
Dural sinuses, 38, *68*, 69

E

Ear
  coronal view of, *27*
  inner, axial MR scan of, *27*
  structures of, 29, 29t
Ejaculatory duct, 227
Elbow, 247-249, 251, 253-254
  anterior view of, *247*
  bones of, 247
  bony anatomy of, 248
  CT scan of, *248*
  lateral view of, *247*
  ligaments of, 249, *249*
  MR scan of, *248*
  muscles of, *250*, 251, *251*, 252, 253, *253*
    anterior group, *252*, 253
    lateral group, 253, *253*
    medial group, 253, *253*
    posterior group, *252*, 253
  neurovasculature of, 254, *254*, *255*
  tendons of, 251
Embolism, pulmonary, 151
Endocardium, 145
Endometrium, 221
Epicardial fat, 145
Epicardium, 145
Epicondyles, 248
Epididymus, *226*
Epidural fat, 100
Epidural hematoma, 39
Epiglottis, 114, 116
  MR scan of, *116*
Epiglottitis, 116
Epinephrine, production of, 182
Erector spinae muscle(s), 97
Esophageal hiatus, 161
Esophagogastric junction, *186*, 187
Esophagus, 118, *118*
  anterior view of, *158*
Ethmoid air cells, 7, *8*
Ethmoid bone, *8*
  anatomy of, 7, *8*
Ethmoid bulla, 26
Ethmoid sinuses, 22, *22*
  axial CT scan of, *14*
  groups of, 22, *23*
Extensor digitorum longus tendon(s), 284, *284*
  origin, insertion, and action of, 287t
Extensor hallucis longus tendon(s), 284, *284*
  origin, insertion, and action of, 287t

Extensor tendons of wrist, *258*, *259*
External oblique muscle, origin, insertion, and function
    of, 200t
Eye
  bony orbit of
    anterior view of, *30*
    axial view of, *32*
    at lacrimal gland, *33*
    sagittal view of, *34*
  globe of, structures of, 33
  muscles of, 35, *35*, 35t

F

Face
  bones of, 1
    anatomy of, 12
    anterior view of, *12*
    axial CT scan of, *14*
    inferior view of, *13*
    lateral view of, *12*
    3D CT scan of oblique aspect of, *13*
  muscles of, *122*, 123
  traumatized, 3D CT scan of, *1*
Facet joints, 85
Facial nerve, 78, *79*
  type, foramen, and function of, 81t
Falciform ligament(s), 168, *168*, 173
Fallopian tubes, *221*, *222*, 225
Falx cerebelli, 39
Falx cerebri
  axial CT scan of, *39*
  sagittal view of, *38*
Femoral artery(ies), 231, *234*, *272*, 273
Femoral head, avascular necrosis of, 265
Femoral vein, *234*, *272*, 273
Femur, 274, *274*
  avascular necrosis of, 235
  proximal, posterior view of, *264*
Fibula, 280
  CT scan of, *280*
Fingers, muscles of, 253, *253*
Flexor digitorum longus tendon(s), origin, insertion, and
    action of, 287t
Flexor hallucis longus tendon(s), origin, insertion, and
    action of, 287t
Flexor muscle(s), 253, *253*
Flexor tendons of wrist, *258*, *259*
Follicular cyst, 224
Foot, dorsal view of, *281*
Foramen(ina)
  cranial, 10t
  intervertebral, 85
  lacerum, 4, *5*
  of Luschka, 42
  of Monro, 40, *41*
  ovale, *6*, 7

Foramen(ina)—cont'd
    rotundum, 7
    spinosum, *6*, 7
Forearm, tendons of, 259
Fornix, functions of, 51
Fovea capitis, 265
Frontal bone, 9, *9*
    axial CT scan of, *9*
    coronal CT scan of, *9*
Frontal sinuses, 22, *22*
    coronal CT scan of, *25*

G

Galen, vein of, *71*
Gallbladder, 178
    with common bile duct, *179*
Gastric artery(ies), 191
    MR scan of, *191*
Gastrocnemius muscle(s), 278, *278*, *279*
Gastroduodenal artery(ies), 191
Gerota's fascia, 170, 185
Glans penis, 229
Glenohumeral ligament(s), 245, *245*
Glenoid, 238
Glenoid fossa, 238
Glenoid labrum, *244*, 245, *245*
Glossopharyngeal nerve, 80, *80*
    type, foramen, and function of, 81t
Glottis, 117
Gluteus muscle(s), 210, *210*, *211*, *269*, *272*
    origin, insertion, and action of, 269t
Gonadal artery(ies), 195
Gonadal veins, 197, *197*
Gonion, 17
Gracilis muscle(s), 268, *268*, 271
    origin, insertion, and action of, 269t
Gray matter, 45
    in cervical and lumbar regions, 103
    periaqueductal, 57
Great saphenous vein, 278, *279*
Great vessels, 150, *151*
    in mediastinum, *157*
Greater trochanter, 265, *265*
Greater tubercle, 238
Gyri, 49, *49*

H

Hamate bone, 257, *257*
Hamstring muscle(s), 278, *278*, *279*
Hand, posterior view of, *256*
Heart
    chambers of, 146, *146*, *147*
    circulation of, 153
    with coronary arteries, 149, *149*
    with epicardial fat, *145*
    and great vessels, *150*

Heart—cont'd
    MR scan of, *146*
    structures of, 145, *145*
    ventricles of, 146, *146*, *147*
Heart valves, 148
Hematoma, epidural, 39
Hemiazygous veins, 159, *159*
Hepatic artery(ies), 176, *176*, 191
    with celiac trunk, *177*
Hepatic duct, common, 178
Hepatic flexure, 189
Hepatic veins, 176, *177*, 198
Hernia, inguinal, 210
Herpes zoster virus in ventral horns of spinal cord, 102
Highmore, antrum of, 24
Hilum, 140, *141*
Hip(s), 265-273
    bony anatomy of, 265
    CT scan of, *265*
    with iliofemoral ligament, *266*
    labrum and ligaments of, 266-267
    lateral view of, *266*
    MR scan of, *267*
    muscles of, 268, *270*, 271-272
        anterior, 268, *268*
        lateral group, 269, *270*, *272*
        medial, 271, *271*
        origin, insertion, and action of, 269t
        posterior, 268
    neurovasculature of, 273, *273*
Hippocampus
    axial view of, *50*
    coronal views of, *51*
    function of, 51
Hormones, female, 224
Humerus, 238, *238*, 247
    MR scan of, *248*
Hyoid bone, 127
Hypertension, portal, 174
Hypoglossal canals, 3
Hypoglossal nerve, 80, *81*
    type, foramen, and function of, 81t
Hypophysis, 55
Hypothalamus
    MR scan of, *54*
    structure and functions of, 55

I

Ileum, 188
    CT scan of, *188*
Iliac artery(ies), 231, *233*
Iliac crest, 204
Iliac fossa, 189, 204
Iliac spines, 204
Iliac veins, *233*
Iliacus muscle(s), 212, *213*
    origin, insertion, and function of, 216t

Iliocostalis muscle(s), 97
  location and action of, 98t
Iliofemoral ligament(s), *266, 267*
Iliopsoas muscle(s), *210,* 212, *214,* 268, *268*
  origin, insertion, and action of, 269t
Ilium, 204, 265
Immune response, 181
Inferior vena cavae, 151
Infracolic compartments, *168*
Infrahyoid muscle(s), *126,* 127
  location and action of, 129t
Infraspinatus muscle(s), 241
  origin, insertion, and function of, 241t
Infundibulum, 26, 55, *73*
Inguinal hernia, 210
Inguinal ligament(s), 210
Innominate trunk, 155
Insula, *48, 49*
  functions of, 47
Intercondylar eminence, 274
Internal oblique muscle, origin, insertion, and function
    of, 200t
Interosseous ligament of ankle, 282, *282*
Interpeduncular cistern, 44
Intervertebral foramina, 85
Intestines, 188-189
  anterior view of, *188*
  large, 189
    regions of, 189
Ischial bone, *208*
Ischial ramus, 205
Ischial tuberosity, 205, *208*
Ischiofemoral ligament(s), 266, 267
Ischiopubic ramus, 205
Ischium, 204, 265

J

Jejunum, 188
  CT scan of, *188*
Joints
  of lower extremity; *see* Lower extremity joints
  of upper extremity; *see* Upper extremity joints
Jugular notch, 138
Jugular veins, 69, *71,* 133, *133, 134, 157*
  external, 157, *157*
  internal, 157, *157*
  thrombosis of, 135

K

Kidney(s), 184, *184*
  CT scan of, *185*
  MR scan of, *171, 185*
Knee, 274-276, 278
  bony anatomy of, 274, *274*
  CT scan of, *275*
  ligaments of, *275,* 275-276

Knee—cont'd
  meniscus of, 275, *275*
  MR scan of, *274*
  muscles of, 278
  neurovasculature of, *279*
  vasculature of, 278
Kyphotic curves, *84,* 85

L

Labrum, 266
Lacrimal bones
  anatomy of, 12
  oblique view of, *13*
Lacrimal canals, 12
Lacrimal gland, 33, *33*
Lambdoidal suture, 11
  axial CT scan of, *11*
Lamina terminalis, 40
Large intestine, 189
Laryngopharynx, 114, *114*
Larynx, 114, *115*
  with cricoid cartilage, *117*
  sagittal section of, *115*
  with vocal cords, *117*
Latissimus dorsi muscle(s), 97
  location and action of, 98t
Lentiform nucleus, 52, *52*
Lesser trochanter, 265, *265*
Lesser tubercle, 238
Levator ani muscle(s), 214, *215, 216*
  origin, insertion, and function of, 216t
Levator scapulae muscle(s), 127, *127*
  location and action of, 129t
Ligamentum flava, *94,* 95
Ligamentum nuchae, 95, *95*
Ligamentum teres, 173, 266
Ligamentum venosum, 173
Limbic system
  sagittal view of, *50*
  structures of, 51
Linea alba, 199
Lingual tonsils, 114
Liver
  anterior and posterior views of, *172*
  CT scan of, *172, 173*
  lobes of, 173
  MR scan of, *172, 173*
  segments of, 173, *173*
  vasculature of, 176
Longissimus muscle(s), 97
  location and action of, 98t
Lordotic curves, *84,* 85
Lower extremity joints, 263-287; *see also* Ankle; Hip(s);
    Knee
Lumbar plexus, 106, *106,* 106t
  innervation of, 107t

Lumbar veins, 197, *197*
Lumbosacral enlargement, 101
Lunate bone, 257, *257*
Lungs
    CT scan of, *141*
    divisions of, 140, *140*
    at hilum, *141*
    MR scan of, *141*
    structures of, 137
Luschka, foramen of, 42
Lymph nodes
    in mediastinum, 158
    of neck, *119*, 122, *122*
    of pelvic region, 234

M

Malleoli, 280
Mamillary bodies, function of, 51
Mammary gland, 163, *163*
Mandible
    anatomy of, 17
    lateral view of, *17*
    sagittal oblique CT reformat of, *17*
Mandibular fossa, 4, 17
Mandibular nerve, type, foramen, and function of, 81t
Mandibular notch, 17
Manubrium, 138
Masseter muscle(s), location and action of, 129t
Mastication, muscles of, 20, *21*, 124, *124*, *125*
Mastoid, 4
Maxilla
    anatomy of, 12
    coronal CT scan of, *14*
Maxillary sinuses, 22, *22*
    axial CT scan of, *24*
    coronal CT scan of, *23*
Meckel's cave, 77
Median nerve
    compression of, 259
    of wrist, 259
Mediastinum, *154*
    great vessels in, *157*
    lymph nodes in, 158
    organs of, 137
    structures of, 144
Medulla oblongata, 55
    structures of, 59, *59*
Medullary velum, 40, *41*
Melatonin, secretion of, 47
Memory, loss of, 51
Meningeal artery(ies), 38
Meninges, 100, *100*
    coronal cross section of, *38*
    structures of, 38
Meniscus, 275, *275*, *276*
Mesencephalon, 55; *see also* Midbrain

Mesenteric artery(ies)
    anterior view of, *192*
    CT scan of, *193*
    inferior, 193, *193*
    MR scan of, *192*
    superior, 193, *193*
Mesenteric veins, 174, *175*, *176*, 178
Mesentery, 166
Midbrain
    MR scan of, *57*
    structures of, 55-56
Mitral valve, 148
Monro, foramen of, 40, *41*
Morison's pouch, 168, *169*
Motor control, dentate nuclei in, 61
Multifidus muscle, location and action of, 98t
Mumps virus, 120
Myocardium, 145
Myometrium, 221

N

Nasal bones
    anatomy of, 12
    coronal CT scan of, *14*
    oblique view of, *13*
Nasal conchae
    coronal CT scan of, *16*
    inferior, 15, *16*
        axial CT scan of, *16*
    superior, 25
Nasal meatus
    sagittal CT reformat of, *15*
    sagittal view of, *15*
Nasal septum, bony, 15
Nasopharynx, 112
Navicular bone, 280
Neck, 111-135
    abscess in, *111*
    midsagittal view of, *112*
    muscles of, 123-124, 127
        anterior, *125*
        within anterior triangle, 124, *125*
        in facial expression, *122*, 123
        infrahyoid, *126*, 127
        location and action of, 129t
        in mastication, 124, *124*, *125*
        within posterior triangle, 127, *128*
        suprahyoid, *126*, 127
    organs of, 112-122
        esophagus and trachea, 118, *118*
        larynx, 114, *115*
        lymph nodes, 122, *122*
        parathyroid glands, 120, *121*
        pharynx, 112, *113*, 114
        salivary glands and thyroid gland, 119, *119*, *120*

Neck—cont'd
  structures of, 111
  vascular structures of, 130, 133, 135
    brachiocephalic artery, 130
    carotid arteries, 130, *130, 131, 132*
    jugular veins, 133, *133, 134*
    retromandibular vein, *134*
    vertebral arteries, *131*, 133
Neonate, sutures of, 11
Nerve plexuses, *104*
Nerve roots
  afferent, 103
  efferent, 103

O

Oblique muscle(s), abdominal, 209, *209*, 210
Obturator externus muscle(s), 268, *269*
  origin, insertion, and function of, 216t
Obturator foramen, 205
Obturator internus muscle(s), 268, *269*
  origin, insertion, and function of, 216t
Obturator muscle(s), 212, *212*
  origin, insertion, and action of, 269t
Occipital bone
  anatomy of, 3
  axial CT scan of
    at level of clivus, *3*
    at level of foramen magnum and lateral condyles, *3*
  inferior surface of, *3*
  sagittal CT reformat of, *4*
  sagittal MR scan of, *4*
Oculomotor nerve, type, foramen, and function of, 81t
Odontoid process, of axis, *88*, 89
Olecranon fossa, 248
Olfactory bulbs, function of, 51
Olfactory nerve, *72*, 73, *73*
  type, foramen, and function of, 81t
Olive, 57, *57*
Omentum, greater and lesser, 166
Ophthalmic artery(ies), 35
Ophthalmic vein, 35
Optic canal, 31, *31*
  oblique 3D CT scan of, *30*
Optic nerves, *74*, 75
  sagittal view of, *34*
  structures of, 35
  type, foramen, and function of, 81t
Optic tract, *74*
Orbital fissures, 31, *31*
Oropharynx
  CT scan of, *113*
  MR scan of, *113*
Os calcis, 280
Os coxae
  bones of, 204
  lateral view of, *205*

Osteomeatal complex
  coronal aspect of, *26*
  structures of, 26
Ovarian artery(ies), 195
Ovarian ligament(s), 224, *224*
Ovaries, *221*, 224, *224*

P

Palate
  hard, 12
    axial CT scan of, *13*
  soft, 112, *113*
Palatine bone, anatomy of, 12
Palatine tonsils, 114
Palmar tendon group, 259
Pancreas, 178
  arteries supplying, 191
  CT scan of, *170*
  MR scan of, *170, 179, 180*
Pancreatic duct, 178, *180*
Pancreatitis, acute, 178
Paracolic gutters, 169, *169*
Paranasal sinuses, 22
  anterior view of, *22*
  drainage locations for, 25t
  lateral view of, *22*
  structures of, 1
Pararenal space, 170
Parathyroid glands, 120, *121*
Parietal bone, *10*
  anatomy of, 11
Parietal pleurae, 143
Parkinson's disease, decreased dopamine production in, 57
Parotid glands, 119, *119, 120*
  mumps virus infection of, 120
Patella, 274, *274*
Patellar ligament(s), *277*
Pectineal line, 204
Pectineus muscle(s), 268, *268*, 271, *271*
  origin, insertion, and action of, 269t
Pectoralis muscle(s), function of, 160
Pelvic brim, 204, *207*
Pelvic diaphragm, 214, *215*
  muscles of, *215*
Pelvic region
  with bifurcation of inferior vena cava, *235*
  lymph nodes of, 234
  muscles of, 203, 209-214
    extrapelvic, *209*, 209-210, *210*
    origin, insertion, and function of, 220t
    of pelvic diaphragm, 214, *215*
    pelvic wall, 212, *212, 213*
  vasculature of, 231, *231, 232, 233*
  viscera of, 203, 217, 219, 221-222, 224-229
Pelvis, 203-235
  anterior view of, *204*

Pelvis—cont'd
　　bony, 203
　　　　structures of, *204*, 204-205, *205*, *206*, *207*, *208*
Penis, 219, 229
　　CT scan of, *230*
Pericardium, 145
Perimetrium, 221
Perirenal space, 171
Peritoneal cavity, inflammation of, 166
Peritoneal spaces, 168
　　location of, 171t
Peritoneum
　　axial view of, *166*
　　CT scan of, *167*
　　MR scan of, *167*
　　structures of, *167*
Peritonitis, 166
Peroneus brevis tendon(s), origin, insertion, and action of, 287t
Peroneus longus tendon(s), origin, insertion, and action of, 287t
Petrosal sinuses, 69
Pharyngeal tonsils, 114
Pharynx, 112, *113*, 114
Phrenic nerve, severed, 105
Pia mater, 39
Pineal gland, *46*, *56*
　　functions of, 47
Piriformis muscle(s), 212, *212*, 268, *268*, *269*
　　origin, insertion
　　　　and action of, 269t
　　　　and function of, 216t
Pisiform bone, 257, *257*
Pituitary gland
　　CT scan of, *54*
　　functions of, 55
　　lobes of, *55*, 55
　　MR scan of, *54*
Plantar ligament of ankle, 282, *282*
　　origin, insertion, and action of, 283t
Platysma muscle, 123
　　location and action of, 129t
Pleural cavity, 137, *142*, 143
Pleural effusion, *142*
Plexuses, 83, 104-106; *see also* specific plexuses
　　nerve, *104*
　　spinal segment and innervation of, 107t
　　venous, of spine, *108*
Pons, *43*, 58, *58*
Pontine cistern, 44
Pontine vessels, 65, 65t
Popliteal artery(ies), 278
Popliteal muscle, *278*, *279*
Popliteal vein, *279*
Portal hepatic system, 174, *174*
Portal vein, 174, *174*

Posterior cranial fossa, *3*
Pouch of Douglas, 224
Pronator teres muscle(s), 253, *253*
Prostate gland, 228, *228*, *229*
　　cancer of, 228
Psoas muscle(s), 185, *185*, 199, *199*, 209, *209*
　　MR scan of, *201*
　　origin, insertion, and function of, 200t
Pterygoid hamulus, 7
Pterygoid muscle(s), *19*, 20, *21*
　　location and action of, 129t
　　medial and lateral, *19*, *124*
Pterygoid process, 7
Pubic bone, 204, *208*, 265
Pubic ramus, 204, 205
　　inferior, *208*
　　superior, *207*
Pubofemoral ligament(s), 266, 267
Pulmonary artery(ies), 151
Pulmonary embolism, 151
Pulmonary semilunar valve, 148
Pulmonary veins, 151, *154*
Pyloric atrum
　　CT scan of, *187*
　　MR scan of, *187*
Pyloric sphincter, 187
Pyramids of medulla oblongata, 59, *59*
Pyriform sinuses, 114

Q

Quadratus lumborum muscle(s), 199, *199*
　　MR scan of, *201*
　　origin, insertion, and function of, 200t
Quadriceps femoris muscle(s), 268, 278, *278*
　　origin, insertion, and action of, 269t
Quadrigeminal cistern, 44, *44*

R

Radial artery(ies), 254, *254*, 261
Radial collateral ligament(s), 249, *249*
Radial notch, 248
Radial styloid process, 257
Radial tuberosity, 248
Radiohumeral articulations, 247
Radius, 247
　　MR scan of, *248*
Ramus, 17
Rectum, 189, 219
Rectus abdominis muscle(s), 199, *199*, 209, *209*
　　origin, insertion, and function of, 200t
Rectus femoris muscle(s), origin, insertion, and action of, 269t
Renal artery(ies), 194, *194*, 195
　　stenosis of, 195
Renal cortex, function of, 184
Renal fascia, 170

Renal pelvis, 184, *184*
Renal pyramids, function of, 184
Renal veins, 198, *198*
Reproductive system
    female, *221*, 221-222, 224-225
        MR scan of, *221*
        pelvic spaces of, *221*, *223*, 224
    male, 225, *225*, 227-229
Retina, 33
Retromandibular vein, *134*
Retroperitoneal spaces
    location of, 171t
    structures of, 170
Retroperitoneum, structures of, 170, *170*
Retropubic space, 224
Rhomboid muscle(s), function of, 160
Ribs, 138
Rima glottidis, 117
Rostrum, 45, *45*
Rotator cuff, 241
    function of, 241
    lesions of, 241
    muscles of, *242*
        origin, insertion, and function of, 241t

S

Sacral hiatus, 92
Sacral plexus, 106, *106*
    innervation of, 106t
Sacral promontory, 204
Sacroiliac joints, *91*, 92, 204, *204*
    CT scan of, *205*
    MR scan of, *206*
Sacrum, *91*, 92, *92*, 204
    CT scan of, *103*
    MR scan of, *103*
    venous plexus of, *109*
Salivary glands, 119, *119*, *120*
    mumps virus infection of, 120
Sartorius muscle(s), 268, *268*
    origin, insertion, and action of, 269t
Scalene muscle(s), 127, *127*, *128*
    function of, 160
    location and action of, 129t
Scaphoid bones, 257, *257*
Scapula, 238, *238*
    lateral view of, *239*
    posterior view of, *239*
Scapular spine, 238
Sciatic nerve, *272*, *273*
    MR scan of, *106*
Sciatic notch, 205
Sella turcica, 25
    sagittal CT reformat of, *6*
Semicircular canals, 29
Semilunar valves, 148

Seminal fluid, 227
Seminal vesicles, 227, *227*
Septal vein, 69, *71*
Septum pellucidum, 40
Serratus muscle(s), function of, 160
Serratus posterior muscle(s), 97
    location and action of, 98t
Shingles, 102
Shoulder
    with acromioclavicular joint, *240*
    bony anatomy of, 238, *238*
    with coracoclavicular ligament, *245*
    with glenoid labrum, *244*
    ligaments of, *244*
    MR scan of, *237*
    muscles of, 241, *241*, *242*, *243*
    sagittal view of, *239*
    with subacromial-subdeltoid bursa, 245, *245*
    tendons of, 241
Shoulder girdle, *238*
Sigmoid colon, 189, *189*
Sigmoid sinuses, 69
Sinus tarsi, 280
Sinuses; *see also* specific sinuses
    cavernous, 69, *70*, *76*
    confluence of, 69
    dural, *68*, 69
    petrosal, 69
    pyriform, 114
    sagittal, 69
    sigmoid, 69
    straight, 69
    transverse, 69
    venous, *68*, *71*
Skull
    anterior view of, *2*
    fracture of, 39
    lateral view of, *2*
Soft palate, 112, *113*
Sperm, storage of, 226
Spermatic cord, 227, *227*
Sphenoid bone
    anatomy of, 7
    axial CT scan of, with foramen ovale and spinosum, *6*
    coronal CT scan of, 7
    inferior surface of, *6*
    lateral view of, 7
    superior surface of, *6*
Sphenoid sinuses, *6*, 7, 22, *22*, 25
    axial CT scan of, *23*
    coronal MR scan of, *24*
Spinal cord, 100-104
    at lumbar level, *102*
    meninges of, 100, *100*
    nerve roots of, *102*, 103, *103*
    segments of, *100*, 101, *101*
    structures of, 83

Spinal fluid, 100
Spinal nerves, 103
Spinalis muscle(s), 97
   location and action of, 98t
Spine, 83-109; *see also* Vertebra(e); Vertebral column
   cervical, *86*
      alar ligaments of, 96, *96*
      with central canal, *102*
      with spinal ligaments, 93, *93*
   functions of, 83
   lateral view of, *84*
   lumbar, *86*
      arterial supply of, *107*
      with neural foramina, *103*
      with spinal ligaments, *94*
      venous drainage of, *109*
   muscles of, 97, 97-98, *98, 99*
      location and action of, 98t
   sagittal section of, with neural foramina, *102*
   thoracic, with spinal ligaments, *94*
   vasculature of, 83, 107-108
      arterial, 107
      venous, 108, *108*
Spinous process, 85
   bifid, *89*
   of thoracic vertebrae, 91
Spleen, 181
   anterior view of, *180*
   CT scan of, *181*
   MR scan of, *181*
Splenic flexure, 189
Splenic vein, 174, *174*
   CT scan of, *175*
   MR scan of, *175*
Splenium, 45, *45*
Splenius capitus muscle, 127
   location and action of, 129t
Splenomegaly, 174
Spring ligament of ankle, origin, insertion, and action
     of, 283t
Squamous suture, 11
Sternal angle, 138
Sternoclavicular joints, 138
Sternocleidomastoid bone, location and action of, 129t
Sternocleidomastoid muscle(s), 124, *125*
Sternum, 138
Steroids, production of, 182
Stomach, 187
   anterior view of, *186*
   MR scan of, *186*
Stroke, middle cerebral artery in, 53
Subacromial-subdeltoid bursa, 245, *245*
Subarachnoid space, 42
   coronal cross section of, *38*
Subclavian artery(ies), 155
Subdural space, 39

Subhepatic spaces, 168, *169*
Sublingual glands, 119, *119, 120*
Submandibular glands, 119, *119, 120*
Subphrenic spaces, 168, *168*
Subscapularis muscle(s), 241
   origin, insertion, and function of, 241t
Substantia nigra, MR scan of, 57, *57*
Subtalar joint, 280
Superior vena cavae, tributaries of, 157
Supinator muscle(s), 253, *253*
Supracolic compartments, 168, *168*
Suprahyoid muscle(s), *126,* 127
   location and action of, 129t
Suprarenal artery(ies), 194, *194*
Suprasellar (chiasmatic) cistern, 44, *44*
Supraspinatus muscle(s), 241, *243*
   origin, insertion, and function of, 241t
Supraspinatus tendon(s), 241, *243*
Supraspinous ligament(s), *94,* 95
Sustentaculum tali, 280
Sutures
   anatomy of, 11
   neonatal, 11
Sylvius, aqueduct of, 40
Symphysis pubis, *207*

T

Talocalcaneal ligament of ankle, 282, *282*
Talofibular ligament of ankle, 282, *282*
   origin, insertion, and action of, 283t
Talus, 280
   CT scan of, *280*
Tarsal bones, *281*
Tectum, structures of, 56, *56*
Tegmentum, 57
Temporal bones
   anatomy of, 4
   axial CT scan of, with foramen lacerum, *5*
   divisions of, 4
   inferior surface of, *4*
   lateral view of, *5*
   petrous portion of, 27
      coronal CT reformat of, *29*
   sagittal CT reformat of, *5*
Temporalis muscle(s), location and action of, 129t
Temporomandibular joint, 17
   anatomy of, bony, 18, *18*
   with articular disk, sagittal MR scan of, *19*
   articular disk and ligaments of, *18,* 19, *20*
   axial CT scan of, *21*
   axial MR scan of, *21*
   coronal view of, *20*
   lateral view of, *18, 20*
   ligaments of, *18,* 19
   muscles of, 20, *21*
   sagittal CT reformat of, *18*
   structure of, 1

Tensor fasciae latae muscle(s), 272
   origin, insertion, and action of, 269t
Tentorium cerebelli, 38
   sagittal view of, *38*
Teres minor muscle(s), 241
   origin, insertion, and function of, 241t
Testes, *226*
Testicular artery(ies), 195
Thalamostriate veins, 69, *71*
Thalamus, 52, *52*
   function of, 53
Thoracic cage, 138, *138*
Thoracic duct, 159
   and azygos venous system, *159*
Thoracic inlet, 139, *139*
Thoracic outlet, 139, *139*
Thorax, 137-163
   apertures of, 139
   bony, 137
      structures of, 138, *138*
   muscles of, 137, 160, *160*, *161*
      intercostal, 161
   structures of, 137
Thymus gland, 144, *144*
   in children, 144, *144*
Thyroid cartilage, 114, *116*
Thyroid gland, 119, *119*, 120, *120*, *121*
Tibia, 274, *274*, 280
   CT scan of, *280*
Tibial plateaus, 274
Tibial spine, 274
Tibial tuberosity, 274, *274*
Tibialis anterior tendon(s), 284, *284*
   origin, insertion, and action of, 287t
Tibialis tendon(s), origin, insertion, and action of, 287t
Tibiocalcaneal ligament of ankle, origin, insertion, and action of, 283t
Tibionavicular ligament of ankle, origin, insertion, and action of, 283t
Tibiotalar ligament of ankle, 282, *282*
   origin, insertion, and action of, 283t
Tonsils
   lingual, 114
   palatine, 114
   pharyngeal, 114
Torcular Herophili, *68*, 69
Trachea, 118, *118*, 143
   anterior view of, *158*
Transverse process, 85
Transversospinal muscle(s), 98
Transversus abdominis muscle(s), origin, insertion, and function of, 200t
Trapezium, 257, *257*
Trapezius muscle(s), 97, 127, *127*, *128*
   function of, 160
   location and action of, 98t, 129t

Trapezoid, 257, *257*
Triangular fibrocartilage complex of wrist, 260, *260*
Triceps anconeus muscle(s), 252, 253
Triceps brachii muscle(s), 252, 253
Tricuspid valve, 148
Trigeminal nerve, 76, 77
   type, foramen, and function of, 81t
Trigone, 217
Triquetral bone, 257, *257*
Trochanter
   greater, 265, *265*
   lesser, 265, *265*
Trochlear nerve, 75, 76
   type, foramen, and function of, 81t
Trochlear notch, 248
Tuberculum sellae, 7
Turbinates, 7

U

Ulna, 247
   MR scan of, *248*
Ulnar artery(ies), 254, *254*, 261
Ulnar collateral ligament(s), 249, *249*
Ulnar nerve, 254, *254*, 261
   CT scan of, *255*
   injuries of, 254
   MR scan of, *255*
Ulnar styloid process, 257
Ulnohumeral articulations, 247
Uncinate process, 26
Upper extremity joints, 237-261; *see also* Elbow; Shoulder; Wrist
Ureters, *185*, 217
Urethra, 217
   male, divisions of, 219
Urinary bladder, 185, 217
   female, *218*, 219
   male, *220*
Urinary system, 184, *184*
   anterior view of, *217*
Uterine tubes, *221*, *222*, 225
Uterus, 221
   anterior view of, *221*
   CT scan of, *222*
   with ligaments, *222*
   MR scan of, *222*
   suspensory ligaments of, 222, *222*, *223*
Uvula, 112, *113*

V

Vagina, *218*, *219*, 221, 225
Vagus nerve, 80, *80*, 135
   type, foramen, and function of, 81t
Valves, cardiac, 148
Vas deferens, 227

Vastus intermedius muscle(s), origin, insertion, and action of, 269t

Vastus lateralis muscle(s), origin, insertion, and action of, 269t

Vastus medialis muscle(s), origin, insertion, and action of, 269t

Vater, ampulla of, 178

Vein of Galen, *71*

Vein of Rosenthal, 69, *71*

Vena cavae
    inferior, 151, 153, 165, *231, 233*
        bifurcation of, *235*
        and tributaries, 196, *196*
    superior, 153
        tributaries of, 157

Venous plexuses, spinal, 108, *108*

Vertebrae
    abnormal, *83*
    cervical, 87, *87, 88*
        with back muscles, *98*
        with spinal ligaments, *95*
    lumbar, 90, *90*, 91
        with back muscles, *99*
        CT scan of, *84*
    superior view of, *84*
    thoracic, *90*, 91, 138, *138*
        with back muscles, *99*

Vertebral arch, 85

Vertebral artery(ies), 65, *65, 66, 131, 132*, 133

Vertebral column, 83
    functions of, 85
    structures of, 85

Vertebral end plates, 85

Vesicouterine pouch, 224

Vestibular folds, 117

Vestibulocochlear nerve, 78, *79*
    type, foramen, and function of, 81t

Visceral pleurae, 143

Vitreous, 33

Vocal cords, *116, 117*
    false, 117
    true, 117

Vomer, 15, *16*

W

White matter, 45

Willis, circle of, 67, *67*

Wirsung, duct of, 178

Wrist
    bony anatomy of, 257, *257*
    CT reformat of, *256*
    extensor tendons of, *258, 259*
    flexor tendons of, *258, 259*
    MR scan of, *256*
    muscles of, 253, *253*
    neurovasculature of, 261
    posterior view of, *256*
    with superficial flexor tendons, *258*
    tendons of, 259
    with triangular fibrocartilage complex and ligaments of, 260, *260*

X

Xiphoid process, 138

Z

Zygoma, *16*
    anatomy of, 12
    coronal CT scan of, *14*

Zygomatic arch, 4

Zygomatic process, 4